Developments in Clinical and Experimental Neuropsychology

Developments in Clinical and Experimental Neuropsychology

Edited by
John R. Crawford and Denis M. Parker

King's College
University of Aberdeen
Aberdeen, Scotland, United Kingdom

PLENUM PRESS • NEW YORK AND LONDON

Library of Congress Cataloging in Publication Data

British Psychological Society Conference on Neuropsychology (1987: Rothesay,
Scotland)
   Developments in clinical and experimental neuropsychology / edited by John R.
Crawford and Denis M. Parker.
     p.   cm.
   "Based on the proceedings of a British Psychological Society Conference on Neurop-
sychology, held September 4–7, 1987, at Rothesay, Isle of Bute, Scotland, United
Kingdom"—T.p. verso.
   Includes bibliographies and index.
   ISBN 0-306-43244-7
   1. Clinical neuropsychology—Congresses. 2. Neuropsychology—Congresses. I.
Crawford, John R., 1957–   . II. Parker, Denis M. III. Title.
   [DNLM: 1. Brain—pathology—congresses. 2. Cognition Disorders—congresses. 3.
Dementia—congresses. 4. Diagnostic Imaging—congresses. 5. Organic Mental
Disorders—congresses. 6. Organic Mental Disorders, Psychotic—congresses. WL 300
B8618d 1987]
RC386.2.B75   1987
616.8—dc20
DNLM/DLC   89-16050
for Library of Congress   CIP

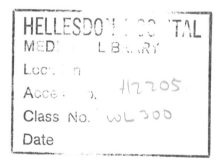
Based on the proceedings of a British Psychological Society
Conference on Neuropsychology,
held September 4–7, 1987,
at Rothesay, Isle of Bute, Scotland, United Kingdom

PREFACE

The chapters published in this volume developed from presentations, and their associated discussions at a conference organised by the Scottish Branch of the British Psychological Society, held at Rothesay, Isle of Bute, Scotland in September 1987. The goal of the conference was to bring together workers across a wide area of neuropsychological research to discuss recent technological advances, developments in assessment and rehabilitation, and to address theoretical issues of current interest. Thus, the chapters in this book include contributions on the use of Magnetic Resonance Imaging and Single Photon Emission Computed Tomography in neuropsychological research, studies of hemispheric specialisation and cooperation, alcoholic and Alzheimer type dementia, prosopagnosia and facial processing, the assessment, management and rehabilitation of memory problems, the assessment of premorbid intellectual status and issues in developmental neuropsychology. Many of those engaged in research and clinical practice in neuropsychology encounter a range of topic at least as wide as this in their professional lives. The opportunity for researchers and clinicians to discuss some of the key issues in the field was invaluable and we hope that readers gain as much from the material presented here as the participants did from the meeting itself.

Our thanks go to those who assisted directly in the preparation and running of the conference, Helen Cable, Hazel Knox, Ken McLeod, Alison Richardson and Nancy Thomson, to Mannell Parker and Jeanette Thorne for their patient help in the preparation of the manuscript for publication and to Elaine Duncan who stepped in at the last minute to help move things to a conclusion.

J.R. Crawford

D.M. Parker

CONTENTS

BRAIN IMAGING TECHNIQUES IN ALZHEIMER'S DISEASE (CT, NMR, SPECT AND PET)

J A O Besson, J R Crawford, D M Parker, P V Best,
H G Gemmell, P F Sharp and F W Smith

INTRODUCTION

The brain imaging techniques described in this chapter allow direct examination of brain structure and function in health and disease states in vivo. The dementias are for the most part age-related conditions and thus the importance of ageing effects on brain structure and function must be taken into account in the interpretation of changes in patients with dementing conditions. In addition to this, the ultimate classification of dementia must rely on postmortem corroboration of macroscopic and microscopic changes in order to be definitive, and ultimately pathological criteria should be used to confirm the clinical and imaging findings.

MORPHOLOGICAL CHANGES IN AGEING AND DEMENTIA

Brain size is reduced with increasing age. Dekaban and Sadowsky (1978) demonstrated a decline with age amounting to 5-10% between the mature adult brain and the brain of those in the 9th decade. The disadvantages of these measures are the marked individual variation in brain weights, the inclusion of CSF trapped within the sulci and the fact that differential rates of atrophy amongst different brain substructures may be measured. However, if one compares brain volume with cranial volume, a more reliable estimate of atrophy can be obtained. Using this technique, it has been demonstrated that significant atrophy does not occur until the 6th decade and thereafter the rate of decline is exponential (Davis & Wright, 1977). More recently, the volume of the cerebral hemispheres and specific structures within these have been measured using image analysing techniques. These studies (Miller et al., 1980) demonstrated that atrophy of the cerebral hemispheres commences after the age of 50 and proceeds at a rate of decline of 2% per decade. This decline was linear rather than exponential and seemed to affect predominantly the cerebral white matter. With regard to the areas of grey matter that show atrophy Tomlinson et al. (1968) have indicated that this was more extensive in the para-saggital frontal and para-sagittal parietal regions than in other areas.

Cortical atrophy is a characteristic feature of presenile cases of dementia Alzheimer type (DAT). The situation in senile cases (SDAT) is less clear-cut with a degree of overlap between age-matched controls and patients. Using morphometric measurements (Hubbard & Anderson, 1981) of individual brain regions and relating these to the cranial capacity as a measure of the original size of the brain, regional variation of atrophy was demonstrated to occur in both grey and white matter. Regional reduction in the grey matter ranged from 13% in the fronto-parietal region to

18% in the temporal region in dements vs. age-matched controls. Reduction in white matter ranged from 8.5% in the occipital region to 26% in the temporal lobe. In the demented group there was a significant reduction of 12.7% in total cerebral tissue, i.e. both grey and white matter, and an increase in ventricular size of 53%. This applies to individuals less than 80 years old. In those over the age of 80 years the ventricles were increased in size by only 9.3% compared to controls, a value that did not reach significance and only in the temporal cortex did significant atrophy occur in the demented group. Using the automated visual analysis technique of assessing atrophy in fixed brain (Miller et al., 1980), a reduction in average hemispheric volume involving both grey and white matter of 18% occurred in demented groups compared with age-matched control groups.

Atrophy, therefore, occurs with ageing. It affects both grey and white matter but in different proportions in different regions. In DAT atrophy occurs predominantly in the pre-senile group.

X-RAY COMPUTERISED AXIAL TOMOGRAPHY

This imaging method utilises the differential penetration by X-rays of the different tissues comprising an organ to create an image of that organ. A number of brain dimensions can be measured using X-ray computed tomography of the brain. These are:

(1) The measurement of the width of the cortical sulci in various brain regions.
(2) Various linear ratios of the sizes of ventricles, e.g. the width between the frontal horns of the lateral ventricles at their maximum point expressed as a ratio of brain width at that level, the width of the 3rd ventricle, etc.
(3) Various area ratios, e.g. the ventricle:brain ratio, the ratio of the area of the lateral ventricles at their maximal dimension to the area of the cerebral hemispheres at that level.
(4) More recently volumetric measures of cerebro-spinal fluid spaces have been obtained.

In addition to this, the state of the cortical tissues themselves can be estimated by measuring the X-ray density of given regions and comparing these in patients and controls.

Linear measures of ventricular dimensions and area measures of ventricle:brain ratios tend to indicate that atrophic changes only reach significance in normal subjects over the age of 60 years (Barron et al., 1976). Sulcal widths and ventricular dilatation have been shown to correlate with each other in control subjects but not in dements. In dements the degree of dementia correlates better with ventricular dilatation, than with sulcal width. This tends to suggest that the atrophic process in ageing and dementia may be different and lends some support to the pathological studies which suggest disproportionate white matter atrophy in DAT. It is now generally accepted that area measures are perhaps more accurate indicators of change than linear measures and more recently the use of volumetric measures of cerebro-spinal fluid space have tended to suggest that brain shrinkage occurs from the 3rd decade, although only achieving significance after the 6th decade (Takeda & Matsuzawa, 1984). Thus CT scans in normal subjects have demonstrated that age-related atrophic changes occur, that these may occur from a surprisingly early age although only reaching significance after the 6th decade and that they involve both ventricular dilatation and sulcal widening, indicating that there is decreased tissue volume. Furthermore, sulcal widening seems to correlate more closely with cognitive decline in normals than it does in dementia.

Studies of patients with senile dementia Alzheimer type (SDAT) have demonstrated that occurrence and severity of ventricular enlargement and sulcal widening is substantially greater than in normals of comparable age and ventricular widening correlated better than sulcal widening with severity of dementia. In one series, for example (Huckman et al., 1975) of 35 demented patients over the age of 60, only 1 had no evidence of atrophy, while two-thirds showed moderate to severe atrophy, the remainder having some evidence of atrophy. In contrast, 8 out of 20 normal subjects over the age of 60 showed no evidence of atrophy, while 3 had moderate to severe atrophy. Brinkman et al. (1981), using age-corrected ventricle:brain ratios of demented patients, showed that by these criteria 50% of patients with DAT showed abnormal values whereas only 1 of the 30 non-demented elderly individuals showed an abnormality. Thus, while atrophy is present in the majority of senile patients with DAT, this is not exclusively so, and similarly while there is a preponderance of normality in non-demented individuals, some show evidence of atrophy.

The usefulness of measures of cerebral atrophy in assisting with the diagnosis of individuals, even when age-related factors have been taken into account, has limitations. This problem may be partly resolved by the use of serial scans taken at approximately 1-2 yearly intervals. Marked increase in ventricular size, particularly the lateral ventricles, occurs in patients with dementia in comparison with normals and separates those changes due to normal ageing and the dementia process (Brinkman & Langen, 1984).

Dementia is associated with histopathological changes in various regions of the brain. These tend to be most marked in the frontal and parieto-temporal areas. Such changes are often not seen on visual examination of CT scans but may be identified by numerical measures of X-ray density of tissues. The X-ray CT numbers, or Hounsfield units, may be obtained for various regions of interest. Patients with SDAT have significantly reduced Hounsfield units in the frontal and medial temporal lobes and the head of the caudate nucleus on both sides (Bondareff et al., 1981). These differences were not related to age nor to the size of the ventricles. Although reductions in CT numbers were also found in patients with pre-senile dementia by Naeser et al. (1980) these findings have not always been replicated (Wilson et al., 1982). Gado (1983) found no differences in density measures of pure grey or white matter samples between SDAT and controls, but there was loss of discriminability between these two tissues. Wilson et al. (1982) did not find any correlations between CT density and presence of dementia nor performance on the Weschler memory scale. Gado et al. (1983) demonstrated no significant differences in density measures of grey or white matter between SDAT and controls nor changes in grey-white discriminability in dementia. They did, however, show that the Digit Symbol subtest of the WAIS and the Reitan Trail-Making Test correlated with grey and white matter density of the right hemisphere, and the Digit Symbol Test showed weaker but significant correlation with grey and white density measures of the left hemisphere. The Benton Visual Retention Test correlated with right hemisphere white matter density. In all cases the greater the impairment on the psychometric test, the higher the density. This technique, however, suffers from problems of instrument variation and patient variation in the X-ray penetration of extra-cerebral tissues and partial volume effects and thus its use in assessing individual cases is limited. These factors may account for some of the variation in results between different studies.

3

The notion of constructing images based on the behaviour of protons in response to magnetic influences (Damadian, 1974; Lauterbur, 1973) has developed (Mallard et al., 1980; Redpath et al., 1987) to the current status of a clinical imaging technique of great value. Protons (hydrogen nuclei) are spinning charged particles. When placed in a static magnetic field generated by large electromagnets, they align themselves in the direction of that field. If the magnetisation is momentarily tilted away from the direction of the original field by application of a radio frequency pulse (RF), the angle at which the protons spin (precess) alters and then gradually recovers (relaxes). A variety of RF pulse sequences have been used. The 'spin echo' technique (Hahn, 1950) involves a one-second sequence of 90° pulses with a 180° pulse at varying time intervals after each 90° pulse. The 'spin warp' technique (Johnson et al., 1981) employs a 2-second sequence of 90° pulses at one-second intervals with a 180° pulse at a varying time before alternate 90° pulses. Signals are detected following the applications of these RF pulses. The decay characteristics of these signals reflect the relaxation behaviour of the protons as they return to their previous position. These signals are detected by the same coils that provide RF pulses. The frequency at which protons precess depends on the magnetic field strength. To achieve spatial discrimination, a magnetic field gradient is employed across the object to be imaged. Small differences in precession frequency generated by this allow position coding of individual voxels imaged.

The pulse sequence employed in 'spin-warp' imaging allows a variety of data to be collected. Proton density (PD) is a measure of the concentration of mobile protons in the imaged tissue. The intensity of the signal resulting from the 90° pulse can be related to the concentration of mobile protons. Relaxation data obtained in the spin warp imaging system are derived from the recovery characteristics of the protons following inversion to 180°. The ratio of signal at the 180° pulse followed by that at 90° allow the spin lattice relaxation characteristics to be calculated. The 90° pulse follows the 180° pulse at a time interval (tau) which can be varied, but in the dementia studies was fixed at 200ms. At this interval the degree of relaxation of the protons would vary from tissue to tissue, and with pathological processes within the tissue. The image constructed, based on data collected at this 90° pulse (following the 180° pulse), is called the inversion recovery (IR) image. The image based on the calculated time taken for the protons to return to their previous resting state is the spin lattice relaxation time (T1). For each pixel the T1 is the average value for that volume of tissue. Images can be constructed based on T1 data (Mallard et al., 1980). From spin echo sequences the faster relaxation properties of the protons following 90°-180° RF pulse sequences give transverse relaxation (T2) data from which images may be constructed.

Relaxation times T1 and T2 reflect the state of water in the tissue imaged. Water is observed in two states - 'free' and 'bound' by virtue of its relationship to larger molecular structures (Mathur-de-Vere, 1979). The contrast in a T1 image of soft tissues depends both on the variation in the proportions of free to bound water and the difference between the T1 values of water in these states. At low magnetic field strengths this difference can be considerable, the T1 of free water being much longer than bound. Thus, a small change in percentage of free water may give a large change in T1. In brain, for instance, T1 of grey matter is longer than white, giving definitions between these two tissues on T1 images. T1 in white matter may be prolonged by a variety of pathological lesions, e.g. demyelination, tumours or infarcts.

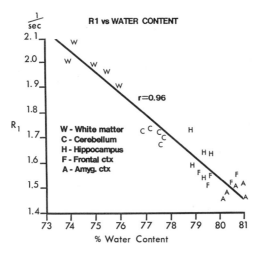

Figure 1. R1 plotted against water content of five brain regions

The relationship between relaxation times and water content for various normal brain tissues may be explored using animal tissue and in vitro proton NMR spectrometry (Besson et al., 1989). Using this, the relationship between the relaxation rate R1 (1/5) and water content can be examined for various brain tissues of the rat (Fig.1). The graph shows a strong correlation (r=0.96) between water content and R1 across rat brain regions.

NMR imaging may be used to measure various brain compartment ratios in the same way as X-ray computed tomography. However, in addition to

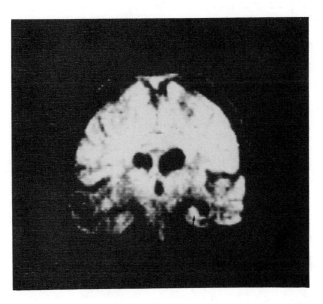

Figure 2. MRI coronal section through brain in Dementia Alzheimer Type showing enlarged lateral ventricles and atrophied hippocampus (arrowed)

5

this, because of the multiplanar nature of the imaging technique, coronal and sagittal displays can be examined. The coronal section is particularly useful for the examination of the temporal lobes. Direct identification of the hippocampus is possible (Fig.2) on a Tl weighted image obtained by subtraction of the SR and IR pulse sequences.

NMR is particularly sensitive in identifying changes that take place in white matter and more so than X-ray CT (Erkinjuntti et al., 1987) in patients with DAT and MID. The inversion recovery and Tl displays give good contrast between grey and white matter and in dementia three kinds of lesion can be seen. These are infarcts at various ages and stages of resolution which can be identified by looking at their characteristics on the different image modalities (Besson, 1987). Periventricular white matter change (PVC), identified as a high intensity periventricular signal is present in some normal elderly individuals in addition to some with dementia. It is also a feature in a number of other neurological conditions, for example, multiple sclerosis. On our imaging system the Tl of these periventricular white matter lesions is over 390ms and often well in excess of that figure. When seen in patients with DAT or in normal controls it is confined to the anterior tips of the frontal horns of the lateral ventricles and it does not invade the white matter. In DAT we also see white matter lesions of lower Tl than periventricular white matter change in a Tl band of 310 to 390ms which have different characteristics, a cotton-wool-like appearance on the Tl display or a speckled appearance on the inversion recovery display. These are noted in a majority of patients with DAT. We have not seen these changes in patients with MID or with normal, elderly control subjects (Ebmeier et al., 1987).

Using clinical criteria with particular reference to the score on the Hachinski (Hachinski et al., 1975) rating scale to differentiate between DAT and MID and excluding those who are of mixed type from their intermediate position on the Hachinski score, we find that there is a significant correlation between the presence of infarcts and high Hachinski score. There is also a significant correlation between the presence of infarcts and periventricular change and a high Hachinski score, but not of periventricular change alone. The Tl changes in white matter are increased in the frontal and parietal regions in DAT compared with controls. MID cases can be divided into two types on the basis of image characteristics: those who have periventricular change with Tl greater than 390ms and those who do not. Thus diagnostic separation on the basis of regional white matter Tl values is possible (Ebmeier, 1987).

Differentiating between DAT, Alcoholic dementia (AlcD) and Korsakoff psychosis is also possible on the basis of regional white matter Tl values. In a study of 28 patients with AlcD (mean age 55.2 years), 16 patients with Korsakoff psychosis (mean age 58.9) and 28 normal control subjects (mean age 66.3) there was an increase in Tl in left parietal white matter in Korsakoff as the only finding compared with control. Comparing controls and Alcoholic dements, the latter had increased Tl in right frontal white matter ($296 \pm 5mS$ vs. $280 \pm 4mS$) (significant on t-test p=0.03) and also increased Tl in left frontal white matter (AlcD $288 \pm 4ms$ vs. $276 \pm 4ms$) (significant by t-test p=0.03).

31P-NMR SPECTROMETRY

Information collected using NMR can be displayed as a spectrum. Metabolic processes can be studied by measuring the spectral activity of nuclei of metabolic relevance, e.g. 31P in tissues. Levels of phosphomonoesters (PME) and phosphodiesters (PDE) are believed to reflect cellular phospholipid synthesis and phospholipid turnover respectively.

These are both elevated in the post-mortem brains of Alzheimer's patients. Elevated PME antedates histopathological evidence of cell damage (Pettegrew et al., 1987). In vivo 31P NMR Spectroscopy does not demonstrate change in phospholipid metabolism in DAT but the PDE/total phosphate ratio in the frontal region correlates with specific focal cognitive deficits in those areas and may therefore reflect a metabolic substrate to behavioural change (Gorell et al., 1987).

SINGLE PHOTON EMISSION COMPUTED TOMOGRAPHY (SPECT)

Images of regional cerebral blood flow (rCBF) can be formed from measurements of the rate at which the brain saturates (or desaturates) when an inert diffusible tracer is presented to cerebral tissue at a constant concentration. 133-Xenon inhalation has been used (Obrist et al., 1967) but since the technique requires the measurement of a temporal variation in activity, a number of technical problems are encountered, particularly in producing tomographic images, and image quality is usually poor. However, this technique has demonstrated reduced grey matter blood flow in DAT patients, which in early cases overlapped that found in normal age-matched individuals. Reductions in flow can be related to severity of the dementia, duration and degree of atrophy as measured by X-ray CT (Meyer, 1983). Imaging during task performance (Ravens Progressive Matrices) demonstrated greater grey matter flow increases in mild DAT compared with controls suggesting greater neuronal activation in mildly cortically impaired individuals during problem solving than in normal subjects (Largen et al., 1981).

The Xenon technique requires specialised instrumentation not available in most nuclear medicine departments. Tomographic imaging is, however, available in most centres using a rotating gamma-camera. It was only recently, though, that a suitable radiopharmaceutical became available. Ideally what is required is a tracer which is trapped on its first pass through the brain. The fraction of cardiac output retained in the brain reflects cerebral blood flow. Technetium microspheres have been used but carry a risk of capillary occlusion (Verhas et al., 1976). N-iso-propyl-123 iodoamphetamine (IMP), which became available in 1980, is completely removed on first pass through the brain (Winchell et al., 1980). It is lipophilic and is localised in cerebral tissue, has a high brain:blood ratio and a slow washout from the brain.

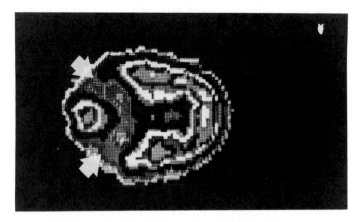

Figure 3. SPECT images of patient with Dementia Alzheimer type showing bilateral reduction of activity in parieto-occipital region (arrowed).

Gemmell et al. (1984) and Sharp et al. (1986) have shown that a specific deficit in rCBF occurs in DAT. This characteristically occurs in the occipito-parieto-temporal region bilaterally and in some cases also frontally (Fig.3). Furthermore, Ebmeier et al. (1987) have shown that the presence of such deficits correlate strongly with a diagnosis of Alzheimer's disease - as defined by clinical criteria and a Hachinski score of <5. Two types of lesion are seen in MID, generalised patchy reductions in uptake of IMP, or focal areas of reduced uptake presumably due to infarcts. In alcoholic dementia there is slight reduction in uptake frontally and fronto-parietally, presumably due to the atrophy identified on NMR imaging of those cases. Similar changes are seen in some patients with Korsakoff psychosis but some are also entirely normal with respect to cerebral blood flow pattern.

More recently a compound, Hexamethylpropylene-amine oxime (HMPAO), which is labelled with the radionuclide 99m Technetium, has been developed. This substance, like IMP, is taken up by cells on first pass through the brain in a manner which reflects cerebral blood flow. It does have the important advantage over IMP of being both cheaper and more readily available. The investigation can be treated as routine and can be performed at short notice. Distribution patterns in DAT and MID occur in a manne similar to IMP (Gemmell et al., 1987). Parker et al. (this volume) have demonstrated that in DAT, there is a good correlation between regional cerebral blood flow deficits and specific tests of regional cognitive deficits.

SPECT can also be used to image the distribution of muscarinic receptors in the brains of patients with DAT. 123-I labelled l quinuclid-inyl-4-iodobenzilate (123I GNB), a muscarinic antagonist, was found to be uniformly taken up but moderately reduced in the cerebral cortex of DAT patients (Holman, 1986).

RELATIONSHIP BETWEEN REGIONAL Tl OF WHITE MATTER AND REGIONAL CEREBRAL BLOOD FLOW DEFICITS, COGNITIVE DEFICITS AND PATHOLOGICAL FINDINGS

Thirteen patients with DAT were studied with NMR and SPECT and were administered a battery of psychometric tests. Tests that reflect parietal lobe deficits are of particular interest in examining brain/behaviour relationships in DAT in view of the persistent findings of deficits in rCBF in the parietal association areas and in the Tl of white matter in the posterior parietal region. Parker et al. (this volume) have demonstrated that performance on the Corsi block tapping test shows a strong negative correlation (r=-0.73, p=0.002) with right occipito-parietal perfusion compared with left (r=-0.45, n.s.). The Corsi block tapping test also shows a significant negative correlation (r=-0.61, p=0.006) with Tl of the white matter in the right occipito-parietal region but not of the left (r=0.4, ns). Thus, impairment of visuo-spatial task activity is related to reduced regional blood flow in the relevant area and to NMR evidence of structural impairment in deep white matter areas lying adjacent to the cortex. Similarly, scores on a facial memory task (Munn test) correlate negatively with the occipito-parietal perfusion score on both sides (on the left r=-0.82, p=0.001 and on the right r=-0.74, p=0.002) but not with frontal perfusion scores. A weak but significant correlation occurs (r=0.44, p=0.05) between Tl in the right posterior parietal white matter and the Munn score. The Munn Test is a measure of facial memory and is presumably more influenced by changes in right than left hemisphere. Brun and Englund (1987) have pointed out that areas of greatest grey matter pathology in DAT correspond to these areas of reduced cortical blood flow and reduced metabolic activity. In the present sample plots of the right and left occipito-parietal grey matter perfusion scores against Tl of the white matter lying deep to those areas show a significant correlation (r=0.46, p=0.03 on the right; and r=0.63, p=0.003 on the left). This suggests that grey matter pathology as reflected by reduced cortical function in the occipito-parietal region is associated with white matter pathology as reflected by increased Tl.

The brains of two patients, both with abnormal scores on Corsi Block Tapping and Munn Test, have been examined pathologically. Both had pre-senile onset of DAT; one died at 66 years of age, the other at 72. In each brain Alzheimer-type disease was the only significant pathological feature and in one it was associated with mild amyloid angiopathy. Al-though the parietal white matter had shown increased Tl in the range 310-390ms (in the individual cases 311ms and 340ms on the left, 362ms and 324ms on the right), there was no evidence of ischaemic damage or macro-phage infiltration in these areas. Mild fibrous sclerosis of some arter-ioles was present, but this did not significantly narrow the vessel lumen and none was thrombosed. Brun and Englund (1985) have suggested that white matter lesions in DAT may arise because of infarcts or incomplete infarcts, particularly as vascular anastomosis in the white matter is poor compared with the grey. While, indeed, this may be the case, it does not seem to be associated with the common kind of white matter changes that we have observed with a Tl between 310 and 390ms. It may be associ-ated, however, with the very high Tl lesions seen in multi-infarct dem-entia, but can occur in other situations. Areas of intermediate Tl change (310-390ms) seem to be associated wih rarefaction in the white matter as revealed in preparations stained for myelin with luxol fast blue (Besson et al., 1988). It seems likely that these atrophic changes in the white matter may be secondary to events occurring in the grey matter and it has been demonstrated that this may be associated with a reduction in the quantities of cerebrosides and sulphatides (Brun & Englund, 1987). It is possible that the atrophic changes in axons are associated with an in-crease in water content of the tissue or, on the other hand, the incresed Tl may be a reflection of the increased free:bound ratio of water conse-quent upon the breakdown of myelin sheaths. The precise explanation for these changes is as yet undetermined. Therefore, it seems that white matter lesions in the dementias cannot be automatically assumed to be generated by vascular disease, but are of two entirely different patho-genetic mechanisms, and that only those of very high Tl may be vascular in origin. This must be taken into consideration in the interpretation of white matter lesions on magnetic resonance images as a diagnostic indic-ator of the dementias and can really only be entirely resolved when a large series of cases has been examined pathologically.

POSITRON EMISSION TOMOGRAPHY

Like SPECT, positron emission tomography (PET) is a method of imag-ing the distribution of a pharmaceutical in the body. It uses positron emitting radionucleides as the label for the pharmaceutical and these produce pairs of gamma-rays which travel in diametrically opposite direc-tions. This makes tomographic imaging a simpler process, in theory, than that employing the conventional single gamma-rays used in SPECT. However, the production of positron emitting radionucleides requires an on-site cyclotron, specialised radiochemical facilities for labelling the pharma-ceutical and an expensive imaging device. It does have the major attrac-tion that many of the biologically interesting elements, such as carbon, oxygen, nitrogen, have positron emitting isotopes but not suitable single gamma-ray emitting ones. Also, the imaging technique, unlike SPECT, allows precise measurement of the amount of radiopharmaceutical in any region of the organ of interest.

Regional cerebral blood flow (rCBF) can be measured by the inhalation of the positron emitting 15-O in the form of C-15 O2. Inhalation of
this gas at a constant rate results in oxygen 15 being transferred to
circulating water H2 15-O. This labelled water diffuses into the brain
and the balance between diffusion into and diffusion out of the brain
(and the rapid radioactive decay of 15-O) allows regional cerebral blood
flow to be estimated. This test can be followed by the inhalation of
15-O. 15-O will label metabolically produced water. By taking the ratio
of the 15-O distribution image to the C-15 O2 image, an image showing the
regional extraction ratio of oxygen, or OER, can be formed.

With increasing age both cerebral blood flow and cerebral metabolic
rate for oxygen (CMRO2) decline, the latter to a lesser extent. There is
increased oxygen extraction compensating for a fall in cerebral blood
flow maintaining the CMRO2 at higher levels than would be possible if
CMRO2 and CBF fell in parallel (Frackowiack et al., 1984). In dementia,
CBF and CMRO2 both decline. This decline is greater in the more severe
cases. OER is, however, maintained at the same level as in normal subjects. In both degenerative and vascular dementias, CBF and CMRO2 fall
but OER is maintained. Presumably, in vascular cases the oxygen requirements of metabolically active tissue are satisfied in the presence of a
declining blood supply by increasing the level of oxygen extraction, and
in the degenerative cases, reduction in metabolic requirements of ailing
neurons means that lower blood flow adequately meets the oxygen demand
(Frackowiak et al., 1981). This supports the view that chronic global
cerebral ischaemia is not a major mechanism of dementia and, therefore,
merely increasing cerebral blood flow will not improve cerebral functioning. The coupling of cerebral blood flow and oxygen utilisation suggests
that techniques for measuring regional cerebral blood flow alone are
probably a reliable way of looking at cerebral function. This tends to be
further confirmed by the correlations between deficits in regional cerebral perfusion (imaged by single photon emission tomography using the
cerebral blood flow markers IMP and HMPAO) and performance on localising
tests of cognitive dysfunction (see Parker et al., this volume). Similar
findings have been reported with respect to measuring regional cerebral
metabolism using 18F labelled deoxyglucose (18FDG). These studies (e.g.
Foster et al., 1984) show that the mean cerebral metabolic rate for
glucose declines in DAT. In DAT the decline in glucose metabolism is
particularly pronounced over the parietal association areas and the
adjoining region of the occipital lobes and extends into the temporal
lobes. Duration of illness but not age correlated with average cortical
metabolism, and in individual cases with DAT, there was a close relationship between principal psychometric deficit and major hypometabolic
focus, for example, those with language difficulties - left parasylvian
region, visuo-spatial difficulties - right posterior parietal, dyscal-
culia - left angular gyrus, personality changes - frontal lobes (Chase et
al., 1984).

In white matter there is a decrease in glucose utilisation but a
preservation of oxygen consumption suggesting alterations in oxidative
phosphorylation of the glial cells in ageing. Most studies have tended to
agree that there is decreased overall metabolic rate of oxygen and of
glucose in DAT. There is preferential location of this metabolic impairment in the parieto-temporo-occipital association cortex with relative
preservation of the primary visual and sensory motor cortex, prefrontal
cortex, anterior cingulum, basal ganglia, thalamus and cerebellum. Using
FDG studies the parieto:cerebellum metabolic ratio has emerged as an
index best related to severity of dementia (Kuhl et al., 1985). The mechanisms underlying these metabolic alterations in cerebral cortex of DAT
patients seems chiefly related to neuronal losses which are known to
display a cortical regional distribution pattern somewhat similar to that

described above for the PET and SPECT evidence of metabolism and blood flow reductions (Brun & Englund, 1981). It, therefore, seems likely that the PET investigation of brain metabolism provides a mapping of neuronal dysfunction and histopathology in vivo. Another approach to metabolic measurements has been the study of brain function following cognitive or sensory activation to assess how in DAT cortical function is integrated by comparison with those of normal subjects. In one study (Foster et al., 1986) the ability to mimic skilled movements or to mime them in response to spoken command was compared with psychometric performance and with regional glucose metabolism using FDG. Praxis scores both on tests to command and to imitation were significantly lower in the Alzheimer patients. Imitation scores correlated best with performance on tests with visuo-spatial ability and with cortical metabolism in the right parietal lobes. Command scores related more closely with results of tests reflecting verbal proficiency and with cortical metabolism in the left cerebral hemisphere, especially frontally; thus response to command and to imitation may reflect neuronal dysfunction in distinct cerebral regions in patients with DAT.

Coupling of cerebral blood flow and cerebral metabolic rate for oxygen has been a consistent finding in patients and normal subjects studied under resting conditions. However, regional uncoupling of cerebral blood flow and cerebral metabolic rate for oxygen was found during neuronal activation induced by somatosensory stimulation (Fox & Raichle, 1986). Stimulus-induced focal augmentation of cerebral blood flow, amounting to some 29%, far exceeded the associated local increase in tissue metabolic rate which increased by 5%. Stimulus duration had no significant effect on the response magnitude or on the degree of uncoupling observed. This suggests that the dynamic physiological regulation of cerebral blood flow is dependent on neuronal firing but independent of the cerebral metabolic rate for oxygen. The precise mechanisms of this, however, are unknown, and these results have not as yet been replicated.

[11]C-labelled methionine has been used in the study of DAT (Bustany & Cumar, 1985). This amino acid acts as a marker for protein synthesis. In early cases of DAT there is a 20% decrease in proton synthesis in the cerebral cortex while in the more advanced cases a decrease of up to 75% has been reported, particularly in the parieto-temporal and frontal cortex. Cortical protein synthesis rate, therefore, appears to be a very sensitive indicator of Alzheimer's Disease and may perhaps be altered long before glucose utilisation is impaired. This is particularly relevant as there has been a suggestion that the primary disturbance of DAT may be related to disturbance of nucleic acid metabolism (Mann, 1982).

CONCLUSION

Morphological imaging using X-ray CT and NMR has confirmed the post-mortem findings in terms of gross atrophic changes of the whole brain in DAT. The ability to pick out differential regional atrophy is not nearly as good. NMR has been shown to be more sensitive than X-ray CT in the identification of white matter lesions which occur in both DAT and MID. The significance of relaxation measurements (T1, T2) in differentiating between pathological processes aetiologically relevant in dementia represents the current status of the application of this technique.

Functional imaging using SPECT and PET is more sensitive and more specific than structural imaging in identifying pathological processes. PET is invasive and expensive but provides more information in the form of more precise quantification of data than SPECT. The latter is inexpensive, more readily available and less uncomfortable for the patient and thus has wider clinical application. NMR Spectroscopy using 31P is new and currently being evaluated. Poor spatial resolution means that as yet it is not as useful as PET, but further refinements of the technique will no doubt improve on this in the future.

REFERENCES

Barron, S.A., Jacobs, L. & Kinkel, W.R. (1976). Changes in size of normal lateral ventricles during ageing determined by computerised tomography. Neurology, 26, 1011-1013.

Besson, J.A.O. (1987). Electrophysiological and brain imaging techniques. in: B. Pitt (ed.). Dementia. Edinburgh: Churchill Livingston.

Besson, J.A.O., Ebmeier, K.P., Best, P.V. & Smith, F.W. (1988). Do white matter changes on MRI and CT differentiate vascular dementia from Alzheimer's Disease? Journal of Neurology, Neurosurgery and Psychiatry, 51, 318-19.

Besson, J.A.O., Greentree, S.G., Foster, M.A. & Rimmington, J.E. (1989). Regional variation in rat brain proton relaxation times and water content. Magnetic Resonance Imaging, in press.

Bondareff, W., Baldry, R. & Levy, R. (1981). Quantitative computed tomography in senile dementia. Archives of General Psychiatry, 38, 1365-1368.

Brinkman, S.D. & Langen, J.W. (1984). Changes in ventricular size with repeated CAT scans in suspected Alzheimer's Disease. American Journal of Psychiatry, 141, 81-83.

Brinkman, S.D., Sarwar, M., Levin, H.S. & Morris, H.H. (1981). Qualitative indices of computed tomography in dementia and normal aging. Radiology, 138, 89-92.

Brun, A. & Englund, E. (1981). Regional pattern of degeneration in Alzheimer's Disease: removal loss and histopathological grading. Histopathology, 5, 549-564.

Brun, A. & Englund, E. (1986). A white matter disorder in dementia of Alzheimer type: a pathoanatomical study. Annals of Neurology, 19, 253-262.

Brun, A. & Englund, E. (1987). Brain changes in dementia of Alzheimer's type relevant to new imaging diagnostic methods. Progress in Neuropsychopharmacology and Biological Psychiatry, 10, 297-308.

Bustany, P. & Cumar, D. (1985). Protein synthesis evaluation in brain and other organs in humans by PET. in: I. Reivich & J. Alan (eds.). Positron Emission Tomography. New York: A.R. Liss.

Chase, T.N., Foster, N.L., Fedio, P., Brooks, R., Mansi, L. & Di Chiro, G. (1984). Regional cortical dysfunction in Alzheimer's Disease as determined by positron emission tomography. Annals of Neurology, 15, Suppl., 170-174.

Damadian, R. (1974). Apparatus and method for detecting cancer in tissue. U.S. Patent 3789823. 1972.

Davis, P.M.J. & Wright, E.A. (1977). A new method of measuring cranial cavity volume and its application to the assessment of atrophy at autopsy. Neuropathology and Applied Neurobiology, 3, 341-358.

Dekaban, A.S. & Sadowsky, D. (1978). Changes in brain weights during the span of human life. relation of brain weights to body heights and body weights. Annals of Neurology, 4, 346-356.

Ebmeier, K.P., Besson, J.A.O., Crawford, J.R., Palin, A.N., Gemmell, H.G., Sharp, P.F., Cherryman, G.R. & Smith, F.W. (1987). Nuclear magnetic resonance imaging and single photon emission tomography with radio iodine labelled compounds in the diagnosis of dementia. Acta Psychiatrica Scandinavica, 75, 549-556.

Erbinjuntti, T., Ketonen, L., Sulkana, R., Sipponen, J., Vuoriallo, M., Iivanainen, M. (1987). Do white matter changes on MRI and CT differentiate vascular dementia from Alzheimer's Disease? Journal of

Neurology, Neurosurgery and Psychiatry, 50, 37-42.

Foster, N.L., Chase, T.N., Mansi, L., Brooks, R., Fedio, P., Patronas, N.J. & Di Chiro, G. (1984). Cortical abnormalities in Alzheimer's Disease. Annals of Neurology, 16, 649-654.

Fox, P.T. & Raichle, M.E. (1986). Focal physiological uncoupling of cerebral blood flow and oxidative metabolism during somatosensory stimulation in human subjects. Proceedings of the National Academy of Sciences, U.S.A., 84, 1140-1144.

Frackowiak, R.S.J., Pozzilli, C., Legg, N.J., Du Boulay, G.H., Marshall, J., Lenzi, G.L. & Jones, T. (1981). Regional cerebral oxygen supply and utilisation in dementia. Brain, 104, 753-778.

Frackowiak, R.S.J., Wise, R.J.S., Gibb, J.M. & Jones, T. (1984). Positron emission tomographic studies in ageing and cerebrovascular disease at Hammersmith Hospital, Annals of Neurology, 15, Suppl., 112-118.

Gado, M., Danziger, W.L., Chi, D., Hughes, C.P. & Coben, L.A. (1983). Brain parenchymal density measurements by CT in demented subjects and normal controls. Radiology, 147, 703-710.

Gemmell, H.G., Sharp, P.F., Besson, J.A.O., Crawford, J.R., Ebmeier, K.P., Davidson, J. & Smith, F.W. (1987). Differential diagnosis in dementia using 99mTc in HMPAO: a new cerebral blood flow agent. Journal of Computed Assisted Tomography, 11, 398-402.

Gemmell, H.G., Sharp, P.F., Evans, N.T.S., Besson, J.A.O. & Lyall, D. (1984). Single photon emission tomography with 123Iodoamphetamine in Alzheimer's Disease and multi infarct dementia. Lancet, ii, 1348.

Gorell, J.M., Brown, G., Bueri, J.A., Levine, S.R., Gordowska, J., Bruce, R., Kensora, T., Welch, K.M.A. & Smith, M.B. (1987). Cerebral 31P NMR Spectroscopy in Alzheimer's and Parkinson's Dementia. Proceedings of the Society for Magnetic Resonance in Medicine, 999.

Hahn, E.L. (1950). Spin Echoes. Physics Review, 80, 580-594.

Holman, B.L., Gibson, R.E., Hill, T.C., Eckelman, W.C., Albert, M. & Reka, M.C. (1985). Muscarinic acetylcholine receptors in Alzheimer's Disease. In vivo imaging with 123I labelled 3 quinuclidinyl 4 iodo benzlate and emission tomography. Journal of the American Medical Association, 254, 3063-3066.

Hachinski, V.C., Linnette, D., Zilhla, E., Du Boulay, G.H., McAllister, V.L., Marshall, J., Ross Russell, R.W. & Symon, L. (1975). Cerebral blood flow in dementia. Archives of Neurology, 32, 632-637.

Hubbard, B.M. & Anderson, J.M. (1981). A quantitative study of cerebral atrophy in old age and senile dementia. Journal of the Neurological Sciences, 50, 135-145.

Huckman, M.S., Fox, J. & Topel, J. (1975). The validity of criteria for the evaluation of cerebral atrophy by computed tomography. Radiology, 116, 85-92.

Kuhl, D.E., Metter, E.J., Benson, F., Wesson-Ashford, J., Riege, W.H., Fujikawa, D.G. & Markham, J. (1985). Similarities of cerebral glucose metabolism in Alzheimer's Disease and Parkinsonian Dementia. Journal of Cerebral Blood Flow and Metabolism, 5 (Suppl.1), 169-170.

Largen, J.W., Shaw, T., Weinman, M. (1981). Order effects and responsiveness of regional cerebral blood flow in early putative Alzheimer's Disease. Journal of Cerebral Blood Flow and Metabolism (Suppl.1), 483-484.

Lauterbur, P.C. (1973). Image formation by induced local interaction: examples employing nuclear magnetic resonance. Nature, 242, 190-196.

Mallard, J.R., Hutchison, J.M.S., Edelstein, W.A., Ling, C.R., Foster, M.A. & Johnson, G. (1980). In vivo NMR imaging in medicine: the Aberdeen approach both physical and biological. Philosophical Transactions of the Royal Society of London, 289B, 519-533.

Mann, D.M.A. (1982). Nerve cell protein metabolism and degenerative disease. Neuropathology and Applied Neurobiology, 8, 161-176.

Mathur-de Vre, R. (1979). NMR studies of water in biological physics, Progress in Biophysics and Molecular Biology, 35, 103-134.

Meyer, J.S. (1983). Cerebral blood flow: use in differential diagnosis of Alzheimer's disease. in: B. Reisberg (ed.). Alzheimner's Disease. New York: Free Press.

Miller, A.K.H., Alston, R.L. & Corsellis, A.N. (1980). Variation with age in the volumes of grey and white matter in the cerebral hemispheres in man: measurements with an image analyser. Neuropathology and Applied Neurobiology, 6, 119–132.

Naeser, M.A., Gebhardt, C. & Levine, H.H. (1980). Decreased computerised tomography numbers in patients with senile dementia. Archives of Neurology, 37, 401–409.

Obrist, W.D., Thompson, H.K., King, C.H. & Wang, H.S. (1967). Determination of regional cerebral blood flow by inhalation of 133Xenon. Circulation Research, 20, 124–135.

Pettegrew, J.W., Kopp, J.J., Minshew, N.J., Glonek, T., Felchsik, J.M., Tow, S.P. & Cohen, M.M. (1987). 31P nuclear magnetic resonance studies of phosphoglyceride metabolism in developing and degenerating brain: preliminary observations. Journal of Neuropathology and Experimental Neurology, 46, 419–430.

Sharp, P.F., Gemmell, H.G., Cherryman, G., Besson, J.A.O., Crawford, J.R. & Smith, F.W. (1986). The application of 123I labelled (IMP) isopropylamphetamine imaging to the study of dementia. Journal of Nuclear Medicine, 27, 761–768.

Takeda, S. & Matsuzawa, T. (1984). Brain atrophy during ageing: a quantitative study using computed tomography. Journal of the American Geriatric Society, 32, 520–524.

Tomlinson, B.E., Blessed, G. & Roth, M. (1968). Observations on the brains of non-demented old people. Journal of the Neurological Sciences, 7, 331–356.

Verhas, M., Schoutens, A., Devol, O., Patte, M., Rokossky, M., Struyven, J. & Cappen, A. (1976). The use of 99mTc-labelled albumen mucospheres in cerebral vascular disease. Journal of Nuclear Medicine, 17, 170–174.

Wilson, R.S., Fox, J.H., Huckman, M.S., Bacon, L.D. & Lobick, J.J. (1982). Computed tomography in dementia. Neurology, 32, 1054–1057.

Winchell, H.S., Horst, W.D. & Braun, L. (1980). N Iso 123I p iodo amphetamine: single pass brain uptake and washout: binding to brain synaptosones and localisation in dog and monkey brain. Journal of Nuclear Medicine, 21, 947–952.

DEMENTIA: CEREBRAL BLOOD FLOW (SPECT) CORRELATES OF COGNITIVE IMPAIRMENT

D M Parker, J R Crawford, J A O Besson,
H G Gemmel and P F Sharp

INTRODUCTION

Since cerebral perfusion is related to cerebral metabolism, measurement of cerebral blood flow (CBF) provides a useful index of cerebral
function (Raichle et al., 1976). There are several techniques currently
available for imaging CBF using radioactive labelled pharmaceuticals. The
available techniques may be conveniently divided into two classes which
use either single-photon-emitting radionuclides or dual-photon-emitting
radionuclides. The former class includes compounds such as 133-xenon,
123-iodine and 99m-technetium which emit a single photon for each nuclear
disintegration and these are used for singlephoton-emission computerised
tomography (SPECT). The latter class, such as 15-oxygen and 18-fluorine,
emit a positron per disintegration and this in turn produces two photons;
these are used in positron emission tomography (PET). The attraction of
PET is that a wide range of biologically relevant compounds can be
labelled enabling studies of selective metabolism to be carried out. It
is expensive, however, because specialised equipment is required for both
radiopharmaceutical production and imaging. Although a much more limited
range of radiopharmaceuticals is available for SPECT, the technique can
be carried out on a routine basis in most nuclear medicine departments
and so is relatively inexpensive. In the present chapter we will briefly
review SPECT and other single-photon techniques with particular reference
to their contribution to the neuropsychology of dementia and then move on
to discuss the results of some of our own recent studies.

Imaging procedures which use single-photon-emitting compounds may
use two dimensional (planar) or three dimensional (tomographic) techniques depending on the detection arrangement available. 133-xenon inhalation and intra-arterial methods have frequently been used with a two
dimensional lateral view of the hemispheres. The non-traumatic inhalation
of a mixture of 133-xenon and air has produced a wealth of data on task
specific brain-behaviour correlations (see Risberg, 1986 for a review).
Studies of dynamic brain-behaviour relationships with compounds other
than 133-xenon have been scanty (Goldenberg et al., 1986). The studies
using 123-iodine and 99m-technetium have been largely employed in the
analysis of regional flow abnormalities with the patient at rest and
sometimes these flow abnormalities have been correlated with the degree
of behavioural deficit. The rapidity with which these latter compounds
become bound in brain tissue makes their use for monitoring task-specific
regional activation of cerebral tissue of very limited value. However
their relative stability allows them to be used satisfactorily for tomographic imaging.

It has been apparent for some time (Freyhan, Woodford & Kety, 1951;

Lassen, Munck & Tottery, 1957) that reductions in total hemisphere blood flow and oxygen uptake occur in organic dementia of diverse aetiologies. Since these early studies it has become clear that, as well as these global reductions in cerebral blood flow, a pattern of regional abnormality is detectable (Simard et al., 1971; Gustafson, Hagberg & Ingvar, 1972). This pattern differs in dementia Alzheimer type (DAT) and multi-infarct dementia (MID). In the former, focal perfusion deficits are particularly apparent in the temporo-parieto-occipital (TPO) area with additional frontal deficits in the more advanced cases (Risberg & Gustafson, 1983; Gemmell et al., 1984; 1987; Sharp et al., 1986). In MID on the other hand the pattern found depends on the imaging medium. If the Xenon (133-Xe) inhalation planar imaging technique is used early cases may show normal flow patterns, because areas surrounding the infarcts, which have relatively normal perfusion, will still influence the detectors - the 'look through effect' (Risberg, 1986). However the expected patchy perfusion pattern has been found with this method (Meyer, 1983) and is also found using SPECT, where the tomographic image allows better resolution of the areas of low perfusion (Gemmell et al., 1987; Neary et al., 1987; Sharp et al., 1986). This finding is important because it represents a step in the direction of diagnosing DAT by the presence of positive signs rather than by the exclusion of other causes. Because the distribution of infarcts is variable in MID it is not uncommon, where these occur in the middle to posterior divisions of the middle cerebral artery, for the perfusion deficit to mimic that of DAT (Gemmell et al., 1987; Sharp et al., 1986) despite a suggestion to the contrary (Jagust et al., 1987). This indicates that cerebral perfusion is currently a less reliable technique for differential diagnosis than one might hope and must be supplemented by other criteria such as those derived from the Hachinski Ischaemic Score (Hachinski et al., 1975). However there is no doubt that the technique is more sensitive than NMR or X-ray CT in identifying functional abnormality although it should be stressed that each technique has its own particular advantages (Besson et al., this volume).

Despite the agreement between a number of studies that hypoperfusion in the TPO area is a characteristic of DAT the proportion of ostensible Alzheimer patients exhibiting this abnormality has been quite variable from one study to another. Derousne et al. (1985) found only 50% of their sample showed the TPO pattern while Neary et al. (1987) found 66%. These proportions are low when contrasted with the 76% of Gemmell et al. (1987) and the 93% of Johnson et al.'s (1987) Alzheimer group which showed TPO perfusion below the lowest level found in a group of age matched controls. Sharp et al. (1986) and Jagust et al. (1987) found 100% of their DAT group showed the TPO pattern, while in Mueller et al.'s (1986) study 100% of the severe group and 80% of the mild to moderate group exhibited the effect. Clearly in a disease process which usually has an insidious onset it would be expected that the kind of pathological change revealed by blood flow imaging would also evolve gradually. Part of the discrepancy between these studies may reflect the severity of illness in the patient groups but it may also reflect varying diagnostic criteria. If clear evidence was available which indicated that the degree of cognitive disintegration was correlated with the degree of perfusion deficit in TPO areas, this would reinforce the view that the degeneration of these regions was of prime importance in the evolution of the disease process. Gustafson and Hagberg (1975) have provided some indication of this association and more recently Jaghust et al. (1987) found a significant correlation of such deficits with impairment on the Mini Mental State Examination (Folstein, Folstein & McHugh, 1975). In the ensuing account of our own research on the relationship between CBF and cognitive function in dementia, particular attention will be paid to the TPO region.

One of the issues that surfaces repeatedly in the literature is the question of differential diagnosis of aetiologically mixed groups of dementing patients. MID may occasionally mimic DAT both in its pattern of cerebral perfusion and in its pattern of cognitive change; in a series of our own patients 68% of those with a diagnosis of DAT showed the very common pattern of severe impairment on visuo-constructional tasks coupled with relatively preserved verbal functions, but so also did 45% of the MID sample. This comparison between relatively preserved verbal skills and impaired visuo-constructional skills is easily indexed by examining the patients' Vocabulary (V) and Block Design (BD) scores on these sub-tests of the Wechsler Adult Intelligence Scale (WAIS). The presence of a profile where V>BD*2 is frequent in dementia (Coolidge et al., 1985) and may show high specificity in DAT although a substantial minority of MID patients also show the profile. Thus the contrast between the two diagnostic groups may aid the discrimination of the truly unique features of DAT.

Clinical subjects were recruited from consecutive referals to the Aberdeen dementia project. Patients eventually diagnosed as suffering from DAT (n=13) and MID (n=9) had a psychiatric interview, neurological examination including EEG and laboratory tests (as recommended by Glen & Christie, 1979) to exclude an endocrine or metabolic cause of the impairment. Initial classification was on the basis of the Diagnostic and Stastical Manual (3rd edition) of the American Psychiatric Association. All cases referred to in this description had the following investigations within normal limits: haemoglobin, ESR, folate, urea and electrolytes, fasting blood glucose, T4, VDRL, serum calcium, phosphorous and alkaline phosphates, chest and skull x-rays. To assist the discrimination of DAT and MID groups the Hachinski scale (Hachinski et al., 1975) was used. This scale records the presence or absence of clinical features associated with cerebrovascular disease and has received partial pathological verification (Rosen et al., 1980). In addition all patients were brain imaged using Nuclear Magnetic Resonance (NMR) and those who had a preliminary diagnosis of DAT but who showed evidence of cerebral infarction were excluded. The SPECT imaging was carried out using one of two radionuclides which previous studies have indicated yield good quality images (Gemmell et al., 1987; Sharp et al., 1986). Patients received either 500 MBq of 99m Tc-hexamethylpropylene-amineoxime (HM-PAO) or 140 MBq of iodine-123 isopropylamphetamine (IMP) intravenously. The SPECT was carried out between 15 and 90 minutes post injection using a Nuclear Enterprises scintillation camera mounted on a rotating gantry and controlled by a DEC PDP 11/34 computer. The camera was fitted with a general purpose, low energy collimator. Sixty views each of 26 seconds duration were collected at 6 degree intervals. The total time taken for each study was 30 minutes allowing for camera movement between views. Reconstruction was by back projection and no correction for attenuation was made. From each set of tomographic data 12 transverse sections at 7mm increments were used for image analysis. A semiquantitative method of image analysis was used. Each of the twelve colour coded transverse sections from each patient was examined by two consultants in nuclear medicine who were ignorant of the diagnostic category of the patient. Each section was divided into 10 regions, 5 per hemisphere (see Fig. 1) and each region was graded as being 0-normal, 1-mild hypoperfusion (<10%), 2-moderate hypoperfusion (10-20%) or 3-severe hypoperfusion (>20%), where the percentages refer to flow reductions relative to surrounding tissue without apparent perfusion abnormality. The scores were then presented as though for a single section; if any abnormality was recorded in a particular region on any section then that was the score assigned to that region even though other sections might have normal uptake in that region. In no

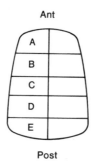

Ant

Post

Figure 1. The location of an abnormality on tomographic sections was indicated by dividing each hemisphere into five approximately equal-size sections labelled A – E.

case did a region have two separate abnormalities present on different tomographic sections. Each patient then had a total of ten perfusion scores representing flow estimates in 5 compartments in each hemisphere. The five compartments thus approximately represented Frontal = A, Fronto-parietal = B, Parietal = C, Occipito-parietal = D and Occipital = F. For the purposes of the present investigation area D most closely approximates the TPO region.

Neuropsychological Tests

The neuropsychological test battery included the following tests: Vocabulary, Digit Span and Block Design subtests of the WAIS (Wechsler, 1955), Orientation, Logical Memory and Visual Reproduction components of the Wechsler Memory Scale – WMS (Wechsler, 1945), Corsi's spatial memory test (Milner, 1971), a test for finger agnosia (Kinsbourne & Warrington,

TABLE 1

Pearson Product Moment correlations between regional cerebral perfusion and performance on four verbal tests, DF = digits forward, DB = digits backward, VOC = WAIS Vocabulary Scale, LM = Logical Memory of WMS, LMD = delayed test of LM. Statistically significant correlations (P<.05) are underlined.

| | LEFT H | | | | | | RIGHT H | | | | |
	F	FP	P	OP	O		F	FP	P	OP	O
DF	.06	.32	.00	.12	.00		.06	.06	.02	.58	.12
DB	.48	.07	.26	.21	.00		.50	.44	.45	.57	.06
VOC	.37	.22	.29	.15	.00		.43	.38	.31	.45	.13
LM	.12	.26	.13	.22	.00		.00	.05	.03	.05	.04
LMD	.40	.09	.34	.30	.11		.36	.40	.33	.22	.28

1962), Raven's Coloured Progressive Matrices - RCPM (Raven, 1965), a test
of facial learning - NFAC (Munn, 1961), a test of remote memory which
involved naming or otherwise identifying photographs of 20 famous individuals widely publicised in the media during the previous 30 years -
RFAC, an assessment of the patients ability to copy designs and Rey's
Auditory-Verbal Learning Test - AVLT (Lezak, 1983). In addition, the
Logical Memory and Visual Reproduction components of the WMS were tested
after a 30 minute interval as well as immediately after presentation.

RCBF - Cognitive Correlations

The rating of regional perfusion indicated that of the thirteen DAT
patients, twelve exhibited bilateral perfusion deficits in the TPO region
(area D). Four of the nine MID patients showed bilateral perfusion deficits in the same region but in only one case was this bilateral abnormality rated as severe. For ease of comprehension all correlations between
cerebral perfusion and performance on behavioural tests are shown as
positive where poor behaviour performance was associated with hypoperfusion. Table 1 shows the relationship between cerebral perfusion and
performance on selected verbally mediated items from the test battery.
It is noteworthy that only three correlations in this table are significant and this is typical of the verbally related items in the test
battery. The measures from the AVLT also fail to show a significant
correlation with ratings of regional perfusion.

In the case of Digits Forward, where the patient simply repeats the
digit list in the same order in which it is heard, only one significant
relation with rCBF is obtained and that is in the right occipito-parietal
region. In the case of Digits Backwards however, where the subject must
reproduce the sequence in the reverse of the presentation order, three
significant correlations are found, with left and right frontal regions

TABLE 2

Pearson Product Moment correlations between regional cerebral
blood flow and DAT patients performance on a range of visuo-
spatial tests. COR = Corsi Block Tapping Test, BD = Block
Design subtest of the WAIS, RCPM, RFAC and NFAC see text, VR =
Visual Recall component of WMS. Statistically significant
correlations are underlined, P<.05 and for P<.01 in bold type.

	LEFT H					RIGHT H				
	F	FP	P	OP	O	F	FP	P	OP	O
COR	.04	.15	.29	.29	.00	.03	.04	.05	**.61**	.01
BD	.12	.32	.21	.53	.14	.06	.06	.10	**.66**	.40
RCPM	.08	.16	.24	.51	.00	.21	.12	.27	**.75**	.32
RFAC	.46	.14	.23	.02	.00	.49	.37	.58	.21	.14
NFAC	.51	.21	.24	.01	.01	.58	.49	**.60**	.32	.02
VR	.31	.25	.48	.31	.00	.42	.46	.38	.48	.17

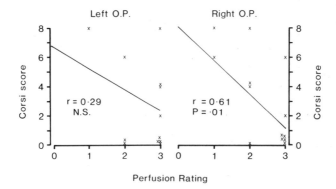

Figure 2.   Score on the Corsi block tapping test
(ordinate) and perfusion rating (abscissa) for left
and right occipito-parietal region in a group of
DAT patients.   The straight lines have been fitted
using the least squares method.

and with the right occipito-parietal region. The appearance of a posterior right hemisphere relationship in these tests is probably due to
the importance of attentional factors in their performance (Lezak 1983).
The frontal involvement in the Digits Backwards task clearly reflects the
importance of these structures in the active reorganisation of the stimulus material which is required in this task.   In the case of the Vocabulary test and the auditory verbal memory tests no significant relationships are found with rCBF.

Turning to the visuo-spatial tests a much more consistent picture
emerges.   Rather more significant correlations are obtained than with the
verbally linked tests (Table 2).   Performance on the Corsi block tapping
tests is correlated with rCBF only for the right occipito-parietal region
and the effect is highly significant.   This association is plotted for
occipito-parietal regions in the left and right hemisphere in Figure 2.
Thus, these results only partly confirm the findings of De Renzi, Faglioni and Previdi (1977) that failure on this task is strongly associated
with damage to posterior zones of either hemisphere. However, they do
demonstrate that an association between the right occipito-parietal region and performance on this test is found in degenerative conditions
like DAT as well as in cases of total brain injury. Data on the test of
finger agnosia was available only for a subset of the DAT group (n=7) but
this test also correlated significantly with occipito-parietal perfusion
in both left (r=0.88, P=.005) and right (r=0.94, P=.001) hemispheres. The
Block Design subtest of the WAIS shows a significant relationship with
both the left (r=0.53) and the right (r=0.66) occipito-parietal region,
reflecting the well established link between damage in these regions and
impairment on constructional tasks (Black & Strub, 1976). The Raven's
Coloured Progressive Matrices task was also significantly linked to perfusion abnormalities in both parieto-occipital regions.   On the Visual
Reproduction component of the WMS, only the left occipito-parietal region
shows a significant relationship. This is in many ways suprising unless
the ability to successfully complete this test is influenced more by the
praxic aspect of the patients performance than by the visuo-spatial aspect. Some indication that this might be the case is indicated by examining the ability of a subset of this group of patients at copying the designs of the WMS. The correlation of this praxic capability with rCBF is
significant only for the right occipito-parietal region (r=.075, P=.026,
n=7) but it approaches significance in the corresponding region of the
left hemisphere (r=0.60, P=.078, n=7).

Of the group of tests which comprised this battery, the facial memory tests showed the largest number of significant correlations with rCBF. The test of remote memory (RFAC) and the test of ability to learn new faces (NFAC) between them show six significant correlations. Both of these tests show relationships (r=0.58 and 0.60 for RFAC and NFAC respectively) with perfusion in the right parietal region and the NFAC also shows a relationship with rCBF in the right front-parietal region. Both tests also show relationships with perfusion in left and right frontal regions although in the case of the RFAC test this effect does not reach significance in the left hemisphere. It is not obvious why such a relationship should emerge for these, but not for other visuo-spatial or memory tests. One possibility that can be considered is that in these tests the patients may have been less constrained by the experimenter to emit a real response to each item than was the case in most of the other tests. In the case of the famous faces test (RFAC) the patient had simply to indicate that they could not recall anything about an individual for the experimenter to pass on to the next item i.e. the patient is not constrained to make any effortful reponse - searching for the name or other identifying detail concerning the face before them. In the case of the facial learning task (NFAC), having been presented with a set of twelve faces to memorise the patient is then presented with these faces mixed up with thirteen distractors. They then indicate by pointing to which faces they remember. The experimenter does not go through each one getting the patient to say yes or no. Both these tasks may then be liable to the failure of self-initiated cognitive activity (Weingartner, 1984) that is characteristic of dementia and is also a feature of frontal lobe pathology (Lezak, 1983). This failure of responsiveness rather than accuracy and its relationship with frontal lobe pathology can be indexed by examining the association between perfusion and total number of responses, regardless of accuracy, given on the NFAC task. When this is done (Table 3) it can be seen that the strongest associations are found between frontal lobe abnormality and the responsiveness of the patient.

In summary then, the DAT group showed little association between perfusion deficit and impaired performance on a number of verbally related tasks but showed several significant relationships between rCBF and visuo-spatial tasks. The failure to find an association between rCBF and the Vocabulary subtest of the WAIS is perhaps worth remarking on. This test has been shown to be highly correlated with general intelligence (Lezak, 1983) and the mean scaled score on this subtest for the DAT group shows it to be significantly below population norms. The mean age-graded scaled score for the Vocabulary subtest was 7.14 (SD=4.15) and it should be bourne in mind that this score should be compared to a population mean of 10.0. Thus despite showing a range of impairment, a relationship with rCBF did not emerge. However, as has already been indicated, verbal processes as assessed by the WAIS Vocabulary test are usually among the best preserved skills in the DAT patients' repertoire. It is possible that a quantitative measure of average reduction in cerebral perfusion would have shown a relationship with this measure whereas the regional rating was sensitive to tasks, such as some of the visuo-spatial tests in the battery, which show greater localising power.

When one examines the association between rCBF and cognitive impairment in the MID group there is a paucity of significant relationships. This could be attributed to two causes. The MID group was smaller than the DAT group and thus any correlation would have to be higher in order to achieve significance. The second possible cause could be the much more erratic distribution of abnormalities in this group with unilateral and subcortical perfusion deficits being present. This latter explanation is probably the more likely of the two. Among the battery of tests only two significant correlations of cognitive deficit with rCBF are found, with

TABLE 3

The relationship between rCBF and total number of responses emitted by a group of DAT patients on the NFAC task. Probabilities are given beneath significant correlations.

	LEFT H					RIGHT H				
	F	FP	P	OP	O	F	FP	P	OP	O
NFAC	.62	.27	.10	.14	.25	.64	.55	.13	.49	.24
P =	(.02)					(.01)	(.03)		(.05)	

Digit Span in the left fronto-parietal area (r=0.58, P=0.05) and with new face learning (NFAC) in the right occipito-parietal region (r=0.71, P=0.02). If one ignores statistical significance and simply looks for correlations of reasonable magnitude then the only additional associations of interest are two correlations of 0.48 with remote face recall (RFAC) and of 0.57 with copying the WMS designs and rCBF in the left occipito-parietal region. The age and educational characteristics of the two groups were very similar although the overall performance of the MID group on tests of intellectual function was higher than the DAT group. Mean age-graded scaled scores on the Vocabulary and Block Design scales were 8.1 and 3.6 respectively. However the range of performance on most of the items in the test battery was as wide in the MID group as in the DAT group, so it was not a restricted performance band that prevented the emergence of relationships. Thus the inconsistent pattern of pathology in this group, which included highly asymmetric patterns of damage and sometimes severe subcortical lesions, probably prevented the emergence of consistent brain-behaviour correlations.

CONCLUSION

It is evident from the data presented above that significant relationships between rCBF and cognitive impairment are readily detected in DAT. It may appear that such effects are more liable to be found with visuo-spatial tasks than with verbal tasks but closer examination of the nature of the tasks and the method of scaling cerebral perfusion advises caution. The visuo-spatial tasks which are associated with regional perfusion deficits are those which can be regarded as useful localising tests e.g. Corsi's block tapping task or facial memory tasks. The Block Design task which is visuo-spatial in nature, but which demands high level intellectual resources for its satisfactory performance, shows much weaker regional associations than these. The verbal tasks which were used cannot be regarded as narrowly localising although one would expect a greater association of abnormality in the left hemisphere with impairments on these tests than in the right. However the perfusion rating was based on the detection of local abnormalities rather than hemisphere-wide deficits. One would expect to find such associations with a measure of cerebral flow which was sensitive to widespread as well as local abnormalities. Thus the method reported by Johnson et al. (1987) which allows objective measurements of whole hemisphere and intrahemisphere flow, by using cerebellar perfusion as a reference, would be expected to show sensitivity to a broader range of perfusion-behaviour relationships.

However, it is worth stressing that a few of the significant correlations indicated that in regions other than TPO perfusion-impairment relationships are obtained with tasks other than those which are visuo-spatial in nature. The relationships between rCBF and lowered responsivenes in frontal regions is one such example.

Despite the caveats mentioned above, it is apparent from the results we have described that the TPO region of the patient suffering from DAT frequently shows perfusion abnormalities and that the magnitude of these abnormalities is associated with cognitive change. In fact in the present study the majority, twelve of thirteen cases, showed such bilateral perfusion deficits and their severity was correlated with impairment on a number of visuo-spatial tasks. This regional abnormality is similar to the metabolic deficit reported by Chase et al. (1985) and Friedland et al. (1987) in their studies of cerebral glucose utilisation using Positron Emission Tomography. The failure of Derousne et al. (1985) and Celsis et al. (1987) to find such effects in the majority of their DAT group is then suprising. It was not the case that all of the patients in the present study were very deteriorated cases. All of them showed severe impairments in retaining new information over time, almost a hallmark of DAT, but the verbal and visuo-spatial skills found in the group spanned a wide range. On the basis of the evidence which we and others have gathered it seems reasonable to conclude that DAT is associated with perfusion abnormalities in the TPO region and the severity of these abnormalities is correlated with severity of symptoms.

REFERENCES

Black, F.W. & Strub, R.L. (1976). Constructional apraxia in patients with discrete missile wounds of the brain. Cortex, 12, 212-220.

Celsis, P., Agniel, A., Puel, M., Rascol, A. & Marc-Vergas, J.P. (1987). Focal cerebral hypoperfusion and selective cognitive deficits in dementia of the Alzheimer type. Journal of Neurology, Neurosurgery and Psychiatry, 50, 1602-1612.

Chase, T.N., Brooks, R.A., Di Chiro, G., Fedio, P., Foster, N.L., Kessler, R.A., Mansi, L., Manning, R.G. & Patronas. N.J. (1982). Focal cortical abnormalities in Alzheimer's disease. in: I. Greitz (ed.), The Metabolism of the Human Brain studied by Positron Emission Tomography. New York: Raven Press.

Coolidge, F.L., Peters, B.M., Brown, R.E., Harsch, T.L. & Crookes, T.G. (1985). Validation of a WAIS algorithm for the early onset of dementia. Psychological Reports, 57, 1299-1302.

De Renzi, E., Faglioni, P. & Previdi, P. (1977). Spatial memory and hemispheric locus of lesion. Cortex, 13, 424-433.

Derousne, C., Rancurel, G., Le Poucin Lafitte, M., Rapin, J.R. & Lassen, N.A. (1985). Variability of cerebral blood flow deficits in Alzheimer's disease on 123-iodoisopropyl-amphetamine and single photon emission tomography. Lancet, i, 1282.

Folstein, M.F., Folstein, S.E. & McHugh, P.R. (1975). Mini Mental State: a practical method for grading the cognitive state of patients for the clinician. Journal of Psychiatric Research, 12, 189-198.

Freyhan, F.A., Woodford, R.B. & Kety, S.S. (1951). Cerebral blood flow and metabolism in the psychosis of senility. Journal of Nervous and Mental Disease, 113, 449- 459.

Friedland, R.P., Jagust, W.J., Budinger, T.F., Berkeley, C.A., Koss, E., Davis, C.A., Ober, B.A. & Martinez, C.A. (1987). Consistency of tempero-parietal cortex hypometabolism in probable Alzheimer's disease (AD): relationship to cognitive decline. Neurology, 37, Suppl.1, 224.

Gemmell, H.G., Sharp, P.F., Evans, N.T.S., Besson, J.A.O., Lyall, D. &

Smith, F.W. (1984). Single photon emission tomography with I-123 isopropylamphetamine in Alzheimers disease and multi-infarct dementia. Lancet, ii, 1348.

Gemmell, H.G., Sharp, P.F., Besson, J.A.O., Crawford, J.R., Ebmeier, K.P., Davidson, J. & Smith, F.W. (1987). Differential diagnosis of dementia using the cerebral blood flow agent 99m Tc HM-PAO: a SPECT study. Journal of Computer Assisted Tomography, 11, 398-402.

Glen, A.I.M. & Christie, J.E. (1979). Early diagnosis of Alzheimer's disease: working definitions for clinical and laboratory criteria. in: A.I.M. Glen & L.J. Whalley (eds), Alzheimer's Disease: Early Recognition and Potentially Reversible Deficits. Edinburgh: Churchill Livingstone.

Goldenberg, G., Podreka, I., Hoell, K. & Steiner, M. (1986). Changes of cerebral blood flow patterns caused by visual imagery. in: D.G. Russell, D.F. Marks & J.T.E. Richardson (eds.), Imagery 2. Dunedin: New Zealand, Human Performance Associates.

Gustafson, L. & Hagberg, B. (1975). Emotional behaviour, personality changes and cognitive reduction in presenile dememtia: related to regional cerebral blood flow. Acta Psychiatrica Scandinavica, Suppl. 257, 39-67.

Gustafson, L., Hagberg, B. & Ingvar, D.H. (1972). Psychiatric symptoms and psychological test results related to regional cerebral blood flow in dementia with early onset. in: J.S. Meyer, et al. (eds.), Research on Cerebral Circulation, Springfield Illinois: Charles C. Thomas.

Hachinski, V.C., Linnette, D., Zilhka, E., Du Boulay, G.H., McAllister, V.L., Marshall, J., Ross Russell, R.W. & Symon, L. (1975). Cerebral blood flow in dementia. Archives of Neurology, 32, 632-637.

Jagust, W.J., Budinger, T.F. & Reed, B.R. (1987). The diagnosis of dementia with single photon emission tomography. Archives of Neurology, 44, 258-262.

Kinsbourne, M. & Warrington, E.K. (1962). A study of finger agnosia. Brain, 85, 47-66.

Johnson, K.A., Mueller, S.T., Walshe, T.M., English, R.J. & Holman, B.L. (1987). Cerebral perfusion imaging in Alzheimer's disease: use of single photon emission computed tomography and Iofetamine Hydrochloride I-123. Archives of Neurology, 44, 165-168.

Lassen, N.A. (1985). Measurement of reginal cerebral blood flow in humans with single photon emission radioisotopes. in: L. Sokoloff (ed.), Brain Imaging and Brain Function. New York: Raven Press.

Lassen, N.A., Munck, O. & Tottery, E.R. (1957). Mental function and oxygen consumption in organic dementia. Archives of Neurology and Psychiatry, 77, 126-133.

Lezak, M.D. (1983). Neuropsychological Assessment. Oxford: Oxford University Press.

Meyer, J.S. (1983). Cerebral blood flow: use in differential diagnosis of Alzheimer's disease. in: B. Reisberg (ed.), Alzheimer's Disease: The Standard Reference. New York: The Free Press.

Milner, B. (1971). Interhemispheric differences in the localisation of psychological processes in man. British Medical Bulletin, 27, 272-277.

Mueller, S.P., Johnson, K.A., Hamil, D., English, R.J., Nagel, S.J., Ichish, M. & Holman, B.L. (1986). Assessment of I-123 IMP SPECT in mild/moderate and severe Alzheimer's. Journal of Nuclear Medicine, 27, 889.

Munn, N.L. (1961). Psychology: The Fundamentals of Human adjustment (4th Edit.). London: Harrap.

Neary, D., Snowden, J.S., Sheilds, R.A., Burjan, A.W.I., Northen, B., MacDermott, N., Prescott, M.C. & Testa, H.J. (1987). Single photon emission tomography using 99m Tc HM-PAO in the investigation of dementia. Journal of Neurology Neurosurgery and Psychiatry, 50, 1101-1109.

Raichle, M.E., Grubb, R.L., Gado, M.H., Eichling, J.O. & Ter-Pogossian, M.M. (1976). Correlation between regional cerebral blood flow and oxidative metabolism. Archives of Neurology, 33, 523-526.

Raven, J.C. (1965). Guide to the Coloured Progressive Matrices. London: H.K.Lewis.

Risberg, J. (1986). Regional cerebral blood flow. in: H.J. Hannay (ed.), Experimental Techniques in Human Neuropsychology. Oxord: Oxford University Press.

Risberg, J. & Gustafson, L. (1983). 133-xenon cerebral blood flow in dementia and in neuropsychiatry research. in: P. Magistretti (ed.), Functional Radionuclide Imaging of the Brain. New York: Raven Press.

Rosen, W.A., Terry, R.D., Fuld, P.A., Katzman, R. & Peck, A. (1980). Pathological verification of ischaemic score in differentiation of dementias. Annals of Neurology, 7, 486-488.

Sharp, P., Gemmell, G., Cherryman, G., Besson, J., Crawford, J. & Smith, F.W. (1986). Application of iodine-123-labelled isopropylamphetamine imaging to the study of dementia. Journal of Nuclear Medicine, 27, 761-768.

Simard, D., Olesen, J., Paulson, O.B., Lassen, N.A. & Skinhoj, E. (1971). Regional cerebral blood flow and its regulation in dementia. Brain, 94, 273-288.

Wechsler, D. (1945). A standardised memory scale for clinical use. Journal of Psychology, 19, 87-95.

Wechsler, D. (1955). Manual for the Wechsler Adult Intelligence Scale. New York: Psychological Corporation.

Weingartner, H. (1984). Psychobiological determinants of memory failures. in: C.R. Squire & N. Butters (eds.), The Neuropsychology of Memory, New York: Guilford Press.

NEUROPSYCHOLOGY AND NEUROIMAGING AFTER TRAUMATIC BRAIN DAMAGE

Klaus D Wiedmann and J T Lindsay Wilson

Studies linking neuropsychology and neuroimaging in head injury research must still be regarded as being in their infancy. In many cases brain damage is diffuse and it is therefore questionable to what extent the issue of structure-function relationships can be elucidated by this approach. However, the understanding of diffuse brain damage forms a challenge in itself and is of considerable theoretical and practical relevance.

We will confine ourselves in this chapter to structural neuroimaging techniques such as Computed Tomography (CT) and Magnetic Resonance Imaging (MRI). Functional neuroimaging techniques (PET and SPECT) are addressed elsewhere in this volume.

BACKGROUND

The relationship between structure and function remains one of the key issues in neuropsychology and the neurosciences at large. However, attempts to correlate brain structure and psychological function have often rested on the implausible assumption that the aim is to demonstrate an underlying one-to-one mapping between structure and performance. This idea was given credence by the discovery of particular language areas in the brain during the last century by Broca (1861) and Wernicke (1874). Experiments using cortical stimulation, at first in the motor cortex but later extending to areas like the temporal lobes (Penfield & Jasper, 1954), seem to have furthered the belief that complete mapping of function could eventually be achieved. However, even as far back as 1917 Leyton and Sherrington noted that repeated stimulation of a particular area does not invariably produce the same response. Lashley's findings in his ablation studies also appeared to contradict early attempts at brain mapping (Lashley, 1950). Still, the paradigm of assigning one particular function to a particular structure seems to prevail in some areas of the behavioural neurosciences. We should therefore at the onset distinguish between two questions:

(1) What is the functional significance of particular structural changes?
(2) What types of brain abnormalities are associated with particular functional deficits?

Head injury research is an area in which these two questions are of importance. Self-evidently the relationship between structure and function is of particular interest here but the two questions are almost as frequently confused as they arise. Examination of the literature reveals that they are either not asked at all or people fail to distinguish them when they are asked: thus assuming that the aim is to establish one-to-one relationships between performance and structure, the effects of traumatic brain damage have been studied systematically within various disciplines over the past two decades. However, the majority of studies have been carried out in isolation and failed to take a more comprehensive approach. Studies aiming at an integration of psychological and neuroimaging findings are the exception. Large scale systematic controlled follow-up studies which could facilitate our understanding of the dynamic processes involved in head injury and recovery of function are lacking entirely at present.

PATHOLOGY OF HEAD INJURY

The effects of traumatic head injury in the brain are variable but are increasingly well characterised. A variety of different kinds of damage may be sustained, and these give rise to a number of areas in which the relationship between structural brain damage and functional deficits can be investigated. Much of our knowledge of the processes involved in severe traumatic brain damage has been derived from neuropathological studies (Adams et al., 1977; 1980; 1982; 1986). However, there is some doubt as to whether these findings are generalisable to survivors of head injury and in addition pathological studies reveal little about the processes involved during the recovery period.

Blunt head injury results primarily in contusions and diffuse axonal injury (Adams et al., 1982), and secondarily in hypoxic-aeschemic damage (Graham, Adams & Doyle, 1978). With conventional methods only large contusions are detected, and the clinical importance of such contusions is often played down, despite the fact that they may relate quite closely to psychological deficits. The most common sites are the temporal lobes, particularly the lateral and inferior surface, and the orbito-frontal cortex (cf. Adams et al., 1980). Diffuse axonal injury is well recognised at post mortem, and is by far the most significant type of direct impact damage (Adams et al., 1977). Yet it has been difficult to answer the question of why patients with this type of injury frequently present with generalized slowing of information processing representing, or probably being responsible for, significant cognitive deficits. It is still unclear why patients with apparently identical lesions differ greatly in their outcome in spite of receiving almost identical management.

NEUROPSYCHOLOGY OF HEAD INJURY

Studies which have attempted to relate psychological function and the results of neuroimaging have often used measures of psychological outcome. Assessment of outcome after head injury is sometimes restricted to physical or neurological indices and the most frequently used categorisation, the Glasgow Outcome Scale, is based on criteria put forward by Jennet and Bond (1975). This scale is limited to four categories: Dead or permanently vegetative, severe disability, moderate disability and good recovery. However, even in its extended format (Jennett et al., 1981) this scale provides insufficient information about the quality of life after head injury and residual cognitive and behavioural deficits. Often patients within the first two categories are excluded from psychological assessment and rehabilitation is limited to control of inappropriate behaviours. The third and fourth category comprise the range in which assessment and rehabilitation may be possible and a greater degree of independence can be achieved by providing appropriate intervention. Moreover, patients categorised as 'good recovery' have been found to suffer from mild to severe cognitive, behavioural and social sequelae

(Brooks, 1984). It is obviously patients in the third and fourth category who demand most of our concern and where a more differentiated approach to categorisation and intervention remains to be achieved.

In some studies localization of function seems to be the primary aim. One of the underlying problems, however, when this is attempted is that there are no psychological test procedures which allow for precise inferences about the localization of specific functions. McFie (1975) suggested that various subtests of the WAIS may indicate the involvement of individual lobes and proposed a scheme to aid localisation of particular deficits. However, most studies concentrating on the cognitive effects of head injury have reported generalized overall impairment in performance and slowing of information processing (Mandleberg & Brooks, 1975; Brooks & Aughton, 1979; Brooks et al., 1980). In many cases head injury patients are found to perform worse on timed tasks whereas performance on untimed and verbal tasks are more frequently preserved. Severity of injury in many studies is correlated with severity of coma as measured by the Glasgow Coma Scale (Teasdale & Jennett, 1974), duration of coma and post-traumatic amnesia (PTA).

Studies of Neuropsychological Outcome

Van Zomeren & Deelman (1978) reported a study of 57 young male head injury patients who were followed up over a period of two years. They found that choice reaction times discriminated better than simple reaction times between subgroups and revealed a highly significant improvement during follow-up. This was shown to be independent of a mere training effect. Levin et al. (1979) assessed 27 long-term survivors of head injury neuropsychologically and found that all severely, and some moderately, disabled patients exhibited unequivocal cognitive and emotional sequelae even three years post injury. McKinlay et al. (1981) interviewed close relatives of 55 head injury patients at 3, 6 and 12 months post injury and found that the most frequently reported residual disorders were emotional disturbances, poor memory and subjective symptoms. Dikmen, Reitan and Temkin (1983) studied 27 patients over a 18 month period during which they were assessed three times. They found that higher level cognitive functions like reasoning, concept attainment and flexibility of thought processes were more vulnerable than lower level functions like finger tapping and grip strength and proved to be more resistant to recovery. Encouraging findings were that improvement appeared to continue in complex as well as simple tasks over a much longer period than previously anticipated. In a similar study Tabaddor, Mattis and Zazula (1984) examined the course of recovery in 68 patients with severe or moderate head injury and observed improvement for all cognitive functions assessed over a one-year period. The authors concluded that all patients sustained significant mental sequelae after severe to moderate head injury but observed that in spite of significant improvement patients continued to show marked impairment in cognitive functions. Williams et al. (1984) used multiple regression statistics to identify the most powerful predictors of outcome in their sample of 96 patients. Best predictors for post-injury IQ were coma grade and premorbid IQ and coma grade, mass lesion, and skull fracture for the Halstead Impairment Index.

Summarizing, it can be said that focal or unilateral deficits after traumatic brain injury are far less common than generalized cognitive and emotional deficits. Attempts to localize functions may therefore be misguided and methods developed to study focal brain lesions may prove inappropriate. Newcombe (1982) advocates 'a different theoretical approach and new techniques' (p.112) for the study of traumatic brain damage.

The progress in neuroimaging over the last two decades with Computed Tomography and Magnetic Resonance Imaging providing dramatically enhanced resolution, has revolutionised our ability to study the brain in vivo. In addition to locating abnormalities in the brain, neuroimaging can supply us with information about the nature of the damage (haematoma, contusion, oedema, brain swelling etc.), about the extent or size of lesions and the number of abnormalities. These categories can be subdivided further for example into extracerebral and intracerebral haematoma, haemorrhagic vs. non-haemorrhagic contusions etc. Furthermore, neuroimaging provides information about ventricular enlargement and cortical atrophy which are common late complications after head injury (Meyers et al., 1983). Studies of ventricular enlargement based on CT have been criticised for suffering from too large an error rate, even when ventricular-brain ratios (VBRs) are determined by digitized computer-aided analysis. Wyper, Pickard and Matheson (1979) state that assessing ventricular enlargement with conventional methods gives an error rate as high as 20% to 30%. However, more recently Condon et al. (1986) have devised a technique based on MRI to determine cerebrospinal fluid (CSF) volume which allows assessment of ventricular size to a much higher degree of accuracy. This technique has been successfully employed in a study by Grant et al. (in press) in determining fluctuations in CSF during the menstrual cycle in females. The potential importance to head injury research is obvious since interactions between CSF and intracranial pressure (ICP) may play a role in the management of acute head injuries and are often responsible for secondary lesions. Precise assessment of ventricular enlargement as a late sequela is also of particular interest because it has been found to correlate with impaired psychological performance (e.g. Levin et al., 1981).

Studies Based on Computed Tomography

Computed Tomography came into use in the early seventies (cf. Ambrose, 1973; New et al., 1974) and within a few years it has become the standard method of investigation in the diagnosis and prognosis of acute head injury. However, even in the well known study by French and Dublin (1977) only 316 out of 1000 consecutive admissions for head injury had undergone CT investigations. Fifty-one per cent of the 316 patients showed abnormalities, and some relationship with neurological findings was demonstrated. 103 patients had further CT investigations and in 52% of those, new lesions, or deterioration in known lesions, were observed. Zimmerman et al. (1978) examined 286 head injury patients on CT and found abnormalities in 58%. They concluded that CT could lead to prompt and more efficient treatment and resulted in a significant improvement in mortality rate and in a decrease in the use of arteriography, skull radiography and surgical intervention. Sweet et al. (1978) studied 140 severe head injury cases of whom 26 had normal scans. The aim of the study was to investigate whether CT information concerning the presence of lesions in the entire brain rather than in only the most affected part could be correlated with neurological status and whether this would be of value in predicting outcome. The authors observed that patients with bi-lateral lesions also had increased ICP and poorer outcome than those who only showed a slight, homogeneous decrease in density of the brain. Cooper et al. (1979) reported findings of serial CT scans in 58 patients with severe head injury. Over half of their patients developed new lesions within seven days of the initial scan. There was a high correlation between absence of new lesions and good outcome. The authors stress the value of serial CT scans in increasing the confidence and accuracy of prognosis in severely head injured patients. Robertson et al. (1979) presented a more moderate view and stated that serial scanning is only necessary under specific circumstances. However, they suggested an obligatory follow-up scan at three months and acknowledged the value of serial scans for research purposes in post-traumatic hydrocephalus, delayed intracerebral haematomas and intraventricular haemorrhage. Van Dongen and Braakman (1980) reported CT results for 97 survivors of a sample of 225 cases of severe head injury. Findings which included infratentorial and focal and diffuse supratentorial atrophy were correlated with overall social outcome, persistent neurological deficit, and prognostic features. The authors suggested a comprehensive model for the classification of cortical atrophy/ventricular enlargement following head injury. Holliday, Kelly and Ball (1982) reviewed the effects of increased ICP in relation to CT scans in 160 patients. They concluded that normal CT in patients with closed head injury and pulmonary injury does not preclude the occurrence of increased ICP and that patients with a normal initial CT in the absence of associated extracranial injuries should make a good recovery. In a multicentre study based on a large number of patients (N=1107) with severe head injuries Gennarelli et al. (1982) argued that predicting outcome reliably requires information about type of lesion in addition to GCS scores indicating depth of coma. They demonstrated that information about severity of coma alone was not sufficient to make sound predictions about mortality and overall outcome, and devised a system of seven lesion categories. The authors state that this would have been impossible without the aid of CT scanning but acknowledge contributory factors such as age, pre-injury medical status and other neurological variables for a valid prognosis. They conclude that their system allows the ranking of head injury lesions according to their importance and that it could help to improve individual management.

CT and neuropsychological outcome. The above studies show that CT findings can be correlated with general measures of functional status such as coma score or broadly defined outcome. However, none of these studies attempted a correlation between CT findings and specific cognitive sequelae. The following studies are examples where such correlations have been sought. Bigler (1981) gives an account of five patients in whom psychological evaluations were obtained together with CT scans for the purpose of assessing their rehabilitation potential. CT and psychological investigations demonstrated concommittant abnormalities in three cases but disagreed in two cases. Dolinskas et al. (1978) followed 153 patients by CT and neurological examinations. Twenty-seven patients underwent psychological evaluation. Cerebral parenchymal disruption was the abnormality most likely to result in a fixed neurological or psychological deficit. The sites of residual parenchymal damage were associated more frequently with deficits found on psychological testing than with neurologically detected deficits. An approach to localization/lateralization of function was taken by Uzzell et al. (1979) who examined 26 patients on CT and the WAIS. Only five of their subjects presented with diffuse bilateral damage whereas the rest were diagnosed as suffering from either left or right hemisphere damage. Using McFie's (1975) scoring method the authors found a significant overall difference between left and right sided lesions and WAIS performance. However, lateralized lesions yielded significant differences for only three individual subtests. The authors concluded that the traditional distinction between Verbal and Performance subtests on the WAIS was valid for CT documented lesions. Tsushima and Wedding (1979) compared the diagnostic conclusions of the Halstead-Reitan battery with a diagnosis based on CT in 45 patients. They claimed that their results indicated no false positive errors from CT with a clinical interpretation of the Halstead-Reitan tests as opposed to a statistical approach. However, only 24 of their patients had a diagnosis of head injury, and CT findings agreed with clinical neuropsychological conclusions in only 56%. Since patients of different oetiology had been pooled it is not clear to what extent their findings apply with respect to head injury. Timming, Orrison & Mikula (1982) studied 30 patients with severe head trauma after they had undergone an extensive in-hospital multidisciplinary rehabilitation program. Patients were assigned to one of four categories based on their CT results. Psychological assessment was carried out if the patient's condition permitted but no correlations were attempted between psychometric and neuroimaging findings due to the small numbers in each category. However, CT findings were related to outcome and achievement of independence. The study also demonstrated clearly that patients with normal CT's although achieving greater independence, can show significant psychological impairment. Rao et al. (1984) studied 30 patients who had undergone CT investigations and found a significant relationship with rehabilitation functional outcome, demographic characteristics and predicted goal achievement.

Ventricular enlargement and neuropsychological outcome. The following studies demonstrate the relevance of ventricular enlargement and cortical atrophy, frequently found after head injury, to neuropsychological test performance. Levin et al. (1981) studied 32 young adults with traumatic brain injury and a control group of similar age. They found enlargement of the lateral ventricles in 72% of the head injured subjects. Enlargement was related to duration of coma and to psychological performance on psychometric assessment. Meyers et al. (1983) studied 39 closed head injury patients and a control group of 51 subjects to assess possible differences in cognitive outcome for early vs. late ventricular enlargement. They found a significant relationship only for the late group on the Verbal and Performance scales of the WAIS. Cullum and Bigler (1985) investigated the effects of haematoma on ventricular size, cortical atrophy and memory in 16 patients and compared them with a group without haematoma matched for age, sex and education but not on measures of severity of injury. The haematoma group showed significantly greater cortical atrophy than controls and was inferior in their performance on memory tests, but results only reached significance when considering the entire battery and only one subtest (Associate Learning) was significant on its own. Finally Cullum and Bigler (1986) assessed ventricular size, cortical atrophy and the relationship to neuropsychological status after closed head injury in 48 patients. They found highly significant correlations between psychological performance and ventricular enlargement. Performance measures showed a stronger relationship than verbal measures and a certain degree of lateralization was observed: performance measures rendered higher correlations for right ventricular enlargement and verbal measures for left ventricular enlargement.

These studies demonstrate the importance of ventricular enlargement and its relationship with neuropsychological performance. Since it is found in a significant proportion of survivors of moderate to severe head injury it is obvious that the precursors and the time course of ventricular enlargement and cortical atrophy deserve further attention and should be studied with methods allowing for a higher degree of accuracy (cf. Condon et al., 1986).

Studies Based on Magnetic Resonance Imaging

Although MRI (NMR) had been in use in physics for decades clinical applications only started in the early seventies. Even by 1981 less than 40 cases had been published on cerebral MR imaging. This changed with the publication of the account by Bydder et al. (1982) reporting brain imaging results for 140 patients of various etiology. General advantages of MRI over CT identified by this study were: the high level of gray-white matter contrast, lack of bone artefact, an abundance of imaging sequences, the possibility of obtaining transverse, saggital and coronal sections, increased sensitivity to pathological change, and the absence of known health risks. Disadvantages like limited spatial resolution, and lack of contrast agents have now been largely overcome. High cost remains a drawback and is primarily a function of lengthy imaging sequences resulting in low 'throughput'. The use of stronger magnetic fields and, most importantly, more efficient software has already cut down on imaging time.

Gandy et al. (1984) described three single cases in whom standard skull radiography and CT had been unremarkable whereas MRI revealed focal intracranial lesions. Sipponen, Sepponen & Sivula (1984) studied five patients with chronic subdural haematoma and found MRI particularly useful in the detection of isodense collections and collections in locations where access is difficult for CT such as the lower aspects of the temporal lobes. The first report with a considerable sample (N=25) applying MRI after head trauma was published by Han et al. (1984). They described various abnormalities visualized by MRI in their patients and also stressed the advantages of multiplanar imaging and increased sensitivity compared to CT but were unable to determine the age of blood collections visualized. Jenkins et al. (1986) studied 50 patients who had MRI within one week of injury. They found abnormalities in 46 patients which was almost twice as many as found with CT. Snow et al. (1986) compared the results of MRI and CT from 35 patients after mild to severe head trauma. MRI was reported to be superior in some aspects but failed to diagnose acute subarachnoid or acute parenchymal haemorrhage within the first three days after injury. They advocated continued use of CT as the procedure of choice in diagnosing head injury less than 72 hours old. Subsequently it has been shown that acute haemorrhage can easily be demonstrated on high field (1.5 Tesla) (Gomari, 1985) and medium field (0.5 T) MR systems (Edelman, 1986) but most recently also on low field (0.15 T) systems (Hadley & Teasdale, in press). A further limitation is described by Barnes et al. (1987) who reported difficulties in discriminating between two types of experimentally induced oedema.

MRI and neuropsychological outcome. All of the above studies confined themselves to descriptions of neuroradiological and clinical aspects and none of them attempted a follow-up or neuropsychological outcome assessment. Levin et al. (1985) gave a detailed description of a patient who had undergone serial neurobehavioural assessment for clinical correlation with abnormalities detected by MRI. The authors attempted to assign deficient psychological performance to structural abnormalities identified by MRI. However, it is possible that their interpretation is somewhat confounded with overall generalized impairment since the patient showed abnormalities in almost every lobe. Levin et al. (1985) described four patients who had MRI and CT investigations and neuropsychological assessment with a wide spread of post injury intervals (3 months to 5 years). All patients showed more abnormalities on MRI than on CT and were impaired on most neuropsychological tests but none displayed signs of hemispheric disconnection. No explicit conclusions concerning localization of function were drawn from this study. However, the authors inferred from their findings that MRI data supported the hypothesis of diffuse nonmissile head injury being in many cases a multifocal insult. Wilson et al. (1988) have recently investigated the ability of CT and MRI to predict psychological outcome. Twenty-five adult head injury patients were studied who had undergone CT and MRI investigations in the acute phase. They were followed up between five and eighteen months (median 11 months) after injury when they underwent further MRI investigation and were given a battery of standard neuropsychological tests. The number of abnormalities detected by MRI outnumbered those detected by CT by a ratio of 2:1 indicating an increased sensitivity of MRI over CT. The majority of patients showed multiple abnormalities which precluded analysis of the data on the basis of traditional models of lateralization or localization. Patients were therefore categorized according to depth of lesion i.e. whether a lesion was discovered in the cortex, in the white matter or whether it was found in the deep white matter or basal ganglia. Patients who presented with ventricular enlargement at follow-up were placed in the last category. Findings in this study showed no correlation between CT results obtained in the acute phase and late neuropsychological outcome. A weak relationship was established between acute MRI findings and late neuropsychological outcome but for MRI performed at the time of neuropsychological assessment the correlation was relatively high (pooled results: $r=0.75$ $p<.001$). A possible explanation for the difference in predictive power of acute and follow-up MRI findings lies in the difficulty of confidently predicting the evolution of lesions during recovery. Thus in some patients abnormalities had completely disappeared whereas others had developed further complications or cortical atrophy/ ventricular enlargement. The predictive power of MRI for outcome based on acute findings therefore seems to depend upon a more profound understanding of the evolution of abnormalities visualized in the acute phase. The findings of Wilson et al. (1988) are consistent with the views of Ommaya and Gennarelli (1974) who proposed that rotational components of accelerative trauma to the head produced a graded centripetal progression of diffuse cortical - subcortical disconnection, which is described as being maximal at the periphery and enhanced at sites of structural inhomogeneity.

A study by Groswasser et al. (1987) underlines the problems of classifying patients with multiple lesions. CT performed during the rehabilitation period were normal for all of their 11 patients but MRI detected abnormalities in all of them. The temporal lobe was invariably involved and in seven patients, in addition, the frontal lobe. However, no attempts were made to relate findings to outcome or cognitive performance in this report.

The studies described illustrate that the combination of MRI and neuropsychological techniques may be of theoretical and practical value. However, too few studies have been reported to date to evaluate the full potential of this approach to head injury research.

FUTURE RESEARCH

One of the primary aims of future research should be the provision of a coherent classification system of underlying brain damage in head injury. The studies reported above suggest that there is little correspondence between lesions in particular areas and specific neuropsychological deficits. Much more convincing relationships have been demonstrated for measures reflecting overall severity of brain damage. This could be an indication that brain damage after head injury is primarily diffuse. Alternatively, this could be due to the fact that the neuropsychological measures employed did not allow for a strong degree of localization. However, it may be possible to identify particular subgroups within the head injury population, groups which are primarily focal, primarily diffuse, or a combination of both. Future investigation of this issue must therefore concentrate on well chosen neuropsychological procedures.

Most studies enumerated above had been conducted at variable times post injury, but few have specifically compared acute and late abnormalities. When follow-up studies have been conducted they have shown that late abnormalities are of greater significance than early abnormalities for psychological outcome and adjustment (Meyers et al., 1983; Wilson et al., 1988). There is thus a pressing need for follow-up studies of head injured patients combining neuroimaging and neuropsychology. Such studies would elucidate the nature of the long-term damage caused by head injury, and allow the evolution of lesions to be investigated. An important question concerns the precursors of atrophy and ventricular enlargement. Such research would address one of the central puzzles of head injury, namely the variability in recovery from apparently similar injuries.

ACKNOWLEDGEMENT: KDW was supported by an MRC grant.

REFERENCES

Adams, J.H., Doyle, D., Graham, D.I., Lawrence, A. & McLellan, D.R., (1986). Deep intracerebral (basal ganglia) haematomas in fatal non-missile head injury in man. Journal of Neurology, Neurosurgery and Psychiatry, 49, 1039-1043.

Adams, J.H., Graham, D.I., Murray, L.S. & Scott, G. (1982). Diffuse axonal injury due to nonmissile head injury in humans: an analysis of 45 cases. Annals of Neurology, 12, 557-563.

Adams, J.H., Scott, G., Parker, L.S., Graham, D.I. & Doyle, D. (1980). The contusion index: a quantitative approach to cerebral contusion in head injury. Neuropathology and Applied Neurobiology, 6, 319-324.

Adams, J.H., Mitchell, D.E., Graham, D.I. & Doyle, D. (1977). Diffuse brain damage of the immediate impact type. Brain, 100, 489-502.

Ambrose, D. (1973). Computerized transverse axial scanning (tomography). British Journal of Radiology, 46, 1023-1046.

Barnes, D., McDonald, M.W., Johnson, G., Tofts, P.S. & Landon, D.N. (1987). Quantitative nuclear magnetic resonance imaging: characterisation of experimental oedema. Journal of Neurology, Neurosurgery and Psychiatry, 50, 125-133.

Bigler, E.D. (1981). Neuropsychological assessment and brain scan results: a case study approach. Clinical Neuropsychology, 2, 13-24.

Broca, P. (1861). Perte de la parole. Ramollissement chronique et destruction partielle du lobe anterieur gauche du cerveau. Bulletin de la Societe Anthropologique, 2, 235-238.

Brooks, D.N. (1984). Closed Head Injury. Psychological, Social and Family Consequences. Oxford: Oxford University Press.

Brooks, D.N., Aughton, M.E., Bond, M.R., Jones, P. & Rizvi, S. (1980). Cognitive sequelae in relationship to early indices of severity of brain damage after severe blunt head injury. Journal of Neurology, Neurosurgery and Psychiatry, 43, 529-534.

Brooks, D.N. & Aughton, M.E. (1979). Psychological consequences of blunt head injury. International Rehabilitation Medicine, 1, 160-165.

Bydder, G.M., Steiner, R.E., Young, I.R., Hall, A.S., Thomas, D.J., Marshall, J., Pallis, C.A. & Legg, N.J. (1982). Clinical NMR imaging of the brain: 140 cases. American Journal of Radiology, 139, 215-236.

Condon, B., Patterson, J., Wyper, D., Hadley, D., Grant, R., Teasdale, G. & Rowan, J. (1986). Use of magnetic resonance imaging to measure intracranial cerebrospinal fluid volume. The Lancet, i, 1355-1356.

Cooper, P.R., Maravilla, K., Moody, S. & Clark, W.K. (1979). Serial computerized tomographic scanning and the prognosis of severe head injury. Neurosurgery, 5, 566-569.

Cullum, C.M. & Bigler, E.D. (1986). Ventricle size, cortical atrophy and the relationship with neuropsychological status in closed head injury: a quantitative analysis. Journal of Clinical and Experimental Neuropsychology, 8, 437-452.

Cullum, C.M. & Bigler, E.D. (1985). Late effects of haematoma on brain morphology and memory in closed head injury. International Journal of Neuroscience, 28, 279-283.

Dikmen, S., Reitan, R.M. & Temkin, N.R. (1983). Neuropsychological recovery in head injury. Archives of Neurology, 40, 333–338.

Dolinskas, C.A., Zimmerman, L.T., Bilaniuk, L.T. & Uzzell, B.P. (1978). Correlations of long-term follow-up neurologic, psychologic and cranial computed tomographic evaluations of head trauma patients. Neuroradiology, 16, 318–319.

Edelman, R.R., Johnson, K., Buxton, R., Shoukimas, G., Rosen, B.R., Davis, K.R. & Brady, T.J. (1986). MR of hemorrhage: a new approach. American Journal of Neuroradiology, 7, 751–756.

French, B.N. & Dublin, A.B. (1977). The value of computerized tomography in the management of 1000 consecutive head injuries. Surgical Neurology, 7, 171–183.

Gandy, S.E., Snow, R.B., Zimmerman, R.D. & Deck, D.F. (1984). Cranial nuclear magnetic resonance imaging in head trauma. Annals of Neurology, 16, 254–257.

Gennarelli, T.A., Spielman, G.M., Langfitt, T.W., Gildenberg, P.L., Harrington, T., Jane, J.A., Marshall, L.F., Miller, J.D. & Pitts, L.H. (1982). Influence of the type of intracranial lesion on outcome from severe head injury. Journal of Neurosurgery, 56, 26–32.

Gomari, J.M., Grossman, R.I., Goldberg, H.I., Zimmerman, R.A. & Bilaniuk, L.T. (1985). Intracranial haematomas: imaging by high field MR. Radiology, 157, 87–93.

Graham, D.I., Adams, J.H. & Doyle, D. (1978). Ischaemic brain damage in fatal non-missile head injuries. Journal of the Neurological Sciences, 39, 213–234.

Grant, R., Condon, B., Lawrence, A., Hadley, D.M., Patterson, J., Bone, I. & Teasdale, G.M. (1989). Hormonal changes in cranial CSF volume. Journal of Computed Axial Tomography, in press.

Groswasser, Z., Reider-Groswasser, I., Soroker, N. & Machtey, Y. (1987). Magnetic resonance imaging in head injured patients with normal late computed tomography scans. Surgical Neurology, 27, 331–337.

Hadley, D.M. & Teasdale, G.M. Magnetic Resonance Imaging of the brain and spine. Journal of Neurology, in press.

Hadley, D.M., Teasdale, G.M., Jenkins, A., Condon, B., McPerson, P., Patterson, J. & Rowan, J.O. (1988). Magnetic Resonance Imaging in acute head injury. Clinical Radiology, 39, 131–139.

Han, J.S., Kaufman, B., Alfindi, R.J., Yeung, H.N., Benson, J.E., Haaga, J.R., El Yousef, S.J., Clampitt, M.E., Bonstelle, C.T. & Huss, R. (1984). Head trauma evaluated by magnetic resonance and computed tomography: a comparison. Radiology, 150, 71–77.

Holliday, P.O., Kelly, D.L. & Ball, M. (1982). Normal computed tomograms in acute head injury: correlation of intracranial pressure, ventricular size and outcome. Neurosurgery, 10, 25–28.

Jenkins, A., Hadley, D.M., Teasdale, G., MacPherson, P. & Rowan, J.O. (1986). Brain lesions detected by magnetic resonance imaging in mild and severe head injury. Lancet, ii, 445–446.

Jennett, B., Snoek, J., Bond, M.R. & Brooks, D.N. (1981). Disability after severe head injury: observations on the use of the Glasgow Outcome Scale. Journal of Neurology, Neurosurgery and Psychiatry, 44, 285–293.

Jennett, B. & Bond, M.R. (1975). Assessment of outcome after severe brain damage. The Lancet, i, 480–484.

Lashley, K.S. (1950). In search of the engram. Symposia of the Society for Experimental Biology, 4, 454–482.

Levin, H.S., Grossman, R.G., Rose, J.E. & Teasdale, G. (1979). Long-term neuropsychological outcome of closed head injury. Journal of Neurosurgery, 50, 412–422.

Levin, H.S., Kalisky, Z., Handel, S.F., Goldman, A.M., Eisenberg, H.M., Morrison, D. & Von Laufen, A. (1985). Magnetic resonance imaging in relation to the sequelae and rehabilitation of diffuse closed head injury: preliminary findings. Seminars in Neurology, 5, 221–232.

Levin, H.S., Handel, S.F., Goldman, A.M., Eisenberg, H.M. & Guinto, F.C.

(1985). Magnetic resonance imaging after 'diffuse' nonmissile head injury. Archives of Neurology, 42, 963-968.

Levin, H.S., Meyers, C.A., Grossman, R.G. & Sarwar, M. (1981). Ventricular enlargement after closed head injury. Archives of Neurology, 38, 623-629.

Leyton, A.S.F. & Sherrington, C.S. (1917). Observations on the excitable cortex of the chimpanze, orang-utan and gorilla. Quarterly Journal of Experimental Physiology, 11, 135-222.

Mandleberg, I.A. & Brooks, D.N. (1975). Cognitive recovery after severe head injury: I Serial testing on the Wechsler Adult Intelligence Scale. Journal of Neurology, Neurosurgery and Psychiatry, 38, 1121-1126.

McFie, J. (1975). Assessment of Organic Intellectual Impairment. London: Academic Press.

McKinlay, W.W., Brooks, D.N., Bond, M.R., Martinage, D.P. & Marsall, M.M. (1981). The short-term outcome of severe blunt head injury as reported by relatives of the injured persons. Journal of Neurology, Neurosurgery and Psychiatry, 44, 527-533.

Meyers, C.A., Levin, H.S., Eisenberg, H.M. & Guinto, F.C. (1983). Early vs. late lateral ventricular enlargement following closed head injury. Journal of Neurology, Neurosurgery and Psychiatry, 46, 1092-1097.

New, P.F.J., Scott, W.R. & Schnur, J.A. (1974). Computerized axial tomography with the EMI scanner. Radiology, 110, 109-123.

Newcombe, F. (1982). The psychological consequences of closed head injury: assessment and rehabilitation. Injury, 14, 111-136.

Ommaya, A.K. & Gennarelli, T.A. (1974). Cerebral concussion and traumatic unconsciousness. Correlation of experimental and clinical observations on blunt head injuries. Brain, 97, 633-654.

Penfield, W. & Jasper, H.H. (1954). Epilepsy and the functional anatomy of the human brain. Boston: Little & Brown.

Rao, N., Jellinek, H.M., Harvey, R.F. & Flynn, M.M. (1984). Computerized tomography head scans as predictors of rehabilitation outcome. Archives of Physical Medicine and Rehabilitation, 65, 18-20.

Robertson, F.C., Kishore, P.R.S., Miller, J.D., Lipper, M.H. & Becker, D.P. (1979). The role of serial computerized tomography in the management of severe head injury. Surgical Neurology, 12, 161-167.

Sipponen, J.T., Sepponen, R.E. & Sivula, A. (1984). Chronic subdural haematoma: demonstration by magnetic resonance. Radiology, 150, 79-85.

Snow, R.B., Zimmerman, R.D., Gandy, S.E. & Deck, M.D.F. (1986). Comparison of magnetic resonance imaging and computed tomography in the evaluation of head injury. Neurosurgery, 18, 45-52.

Sweet, R.C., Miller, J.D., Lipper, M., Kishore, P.R.S. & Becker, D.P. (1978). Significance of bilateral abnormalities on the CT scan in patients with severe head injury. Neurosurgery, 3, 16-21.

Tabaddor, K., Mattis, S. & Zazula, T. (1984). Cognitive sequelae and recovery course after moderate and severe head injury. Neurosurgery, 14, 701-708.

Teasdale, G. & Jennett, B. (1974). Assessment of coma and impaired consciousness. The Lancet, ii, 81-83.

Timming, R., Orrison, W.W. & Mikula, J.A. (1982). Computerized tomography and rehabilitation outcome after severe head trauma. Archives of Physical Medicine and Rehabilition, 63, 154-159.

Tsushima, W.T. & Wedding, D. (1979). A comparison of the Halstead-Reitan neuropsychological battery and computerized tomography in the identification of brain disorder. Journal of Nervous and Mental Disease, 167, 704-707.

Uzzell, B.P., Zimmerman, R.A., Dolinskas, C.A. & Obrist, W.D. (1979). Lateralized psychological impairment associated with CT in head injured patients. Cortex, 15, 391-401.

Van Dongen, K.J. & Braakman R. (1980). Late computed tomography in survivors of severe head injury. Neurosurgery, 7, 14–22.

Van Zomeren, A.H. & Deelman, B.G. (1978). Long-term recovery of visual reaction time after closed head injury. Journal of Neurology, Neurosurgery and Psychiatry, 41, 452–457.

Wernicke, C. (1874). Der Aphasische Symptomencomplex: Eine Psychologische Studie auf Anatomischer Basis. Breslau: Cohn & Weigert.

Williams, J.M., Gomes, F., Drudge, O.W. & Kessler, M. (1984). Predicting outcome from closed head injury by early assessment of trauma severity. Journal of Neurosurgery, 61, 581–585.

Wilson, J.T.L., Wiedmann, K.D., Hadley, D.M., Condon, B., Teasdale, G.M. & Brooks, D.N. (1988). Early and late magnetic resonance imaging and neuropsychological outcome after head injury. Journal of Neurology, Neurosurgery and Psychiatry, 51, 391–396.

Wyper, D.J., Pickard, J.D. & Matheson, M. (1979). Accuracy of ventricular volume estimation. Journal of Neurology, Neurosurgery and Psychiatry, 42, 345–350.

Zimmerman, R.A., Bilaniuk, L.T., Gennarelli, T., Bruce, D., Dolinskas, C. & Uzzell, B. (1978). Cranial computed tomography in diagnosis and management of acute head trauma. American Journal of Roentgenology, 131, 27–34.

COGNITIVE DYSFUNCTION IN LATENT PORTASYSTEMIC ENCEPHALOPATHY

Arthur A Dunk and John W Moore

INTRODUCTION

Portasystemic encephalopathy (PSE) is a neuropsychiatric disorder which occurs as a complication of both acute and chronic liver diseases. This syndrome has traditionally been divided into several crude but easily recognisable clinical grades (Parsons-Smith et al., 1957), ranging from grade I (impairment of concentration, trivial mood changes, impaired ability to draw a five-pointed star) at one extreme through to grade IV (coma) at the other. More recently, the use of psychometric testing has revealed that many cirrhotic patients, who have no evidence of PSE on clinical examination, suffer from significant neuropsychological deficits. These patients are termed to have 'latent' or 'sub-clinical' PSE (Schomerus & Hamster, 1976; Rikkers et al., 1978; Schomerus et al., 1981; Gitlin et al., 1986). This increasingly recognised category of PSE is of importance as the neuropsychological deficits involved are often those of performance skills, and may therefore lead to impairment of a patient's abilities to safely perform important activities of daily living (Rehnström et al., 1977; Rikkers et al., 1978; Schomerus et al., 1981; Gitlin et al., 1986).

FREQUENCY OF LATENT PSE IN PATIENTS WITH CIRRHOSIS

There is no universally agreed definition of what number and what type of psychometric test abnormalities constitute a diagnosis of latent PSE, and it is therefore impossible to give accurate figures of the frequency of this condition in the ambulant non-clinically encephalo-pathic cirrhotic population. Two recent controlled studies do however suggest that latent PSE is present in the majority of the 'healthy' cirrhotic population (Gitlin et al., 1986; Moore et al., submitted for publication). In these studies, in excess of 70% of cirrhotic patients failed two or more of the psychometric tests employed, compared with 10% or less of those in the control groups. However, agreed definitions and much larger studies are needed to more accurately determine the frequency of latent PSE in patients with cirrhosis, and similar studies should also be performed in patients with pre-cirrhotic chronic liver diseases in order to determine whether they too are at risk of latent PSE.

MECHANISMS OF PSE

A detailed review of current opinions on the pathogenesis of hepatic encephalopathy is outside the scope of this chapter. At a simplistic level, the patient with cirrhosis and PSE is characterised by the ability of portal venous blood to enter the systemic and hence the cerebral circulation, without first being metabolised in the liver. This may result either because of the presence of vascular 'shunts' between the portal and systemic venous systems or because of advanced hepatocellular failure. Thus it is likely that PSE is due to impaired hepatic metabolism of gut-derived neurotoxins or neurochemicals. The exact substance(s) involved and their mechanism(s) of action remain incompletely defined and the interested reader is referred to detailed articles on the subject (Zieve, 1981; Borg et al., 1982; Zeneroli, 1985; Jones & Schafer, 1986; Rossi-Fanelli et al., 1987).

NEUROPSYCHOLOGICAL DEFICITS IN LATENT PSE

A study by Zeegen et al. (1970) applied neuropsychological tests to the assessment of cerebral dysfunction in 64 patients following porta-caval anastomosis. This study was important not only because it was the first occasion on which neuropsychological tests were employed in this patient group, but also because over half the patients showed no evidence of clinical encephalopathy. Approximately two-thirds of the patients however had abnormal test scores when compared to controls, and test scores tended to reflect the clinical severity of the encephalopathy. More recent studies dealing specifically with latent PSE are difficult to interpret due to variability in patient selection and to the great diversity of psychometric tests employed. There is however general agreement that performance-based psychometric tests and tests of memory are frequently abnormal in cirrhotics who have no clinical evidence of encephalopathy. Schomerus et al. (1981) and Gitlin et al. (1986) both found significant impairment in Digit Symbol and Block Design WAIS performance subtests relative to controls. They found no significant differences on

TABLE 1

WAIS Subtest Scores in 19 Patients with Cirrhosis
(mean $\pm$ SD)s

WAIS SUBTEST	RESULT
Verbal	
Information	10.4 ± 3.0
Comprehension	10.9 ± 4.1
Arithmetic	10.3 ± 4.1
Similarities	11.2 ± 2.5
Digit Span	10.9 ± 2.6
Vocabulary	11.4 ± 2.8
Performance	
Digit Symbol	10.8 ± 3.4
Picture Completion	10.1 ± 2.7
Block Design	9.6 ± 2.3
Picture Arrangement	9.0 ± 3.6
Object Assembly	9.0 ± 2.7

Total Verbal IQ   = 105.5 ± 16.0
Total Performance IQ = 98.5 ± 13.2

individual verbal subtests scores. A study by Dunk et al. (1988) examined the WAIS subtests scores of a group of 19 patients with cirrhosis and no clinical evidence of encephalopathy (Table 1). Rather than examine each subtest score individually, the data was subjected to the criteria of Field (1960), in order to examine subtest scaled scores scatter. At the 1% significance level, 17 and 12 patients respectively had abnormally scattered subtest scores in the Verbal and Performance scales. This study, which was primarily designed to examine the effect of beta adren-ergic blockade on cognitive functioning, suggests subtle widespread cog-nitive impairment in these patients.

In a controlled study (Moore et al., submitted for publication), a group of non-encephalopathic cirrhotics with oesophageal varices (n=19) and an age, sex and educationally matched control group with normal liver function, underwent a battery of tests of memory and performance. These included the Benton Visual Retention Test, Reitan Trail Tests A and B, and measurement of reaction times to light, sound and choice stimuli. The results are summarised in Tables 2 and 3. Short term visual memory and speed and accuracy of reaction to light, sound and choice stimuli were all significantly impaired in cirrhotic patients. The majority (84%) of patients failed two or more of the seven test parameters examined, though none of the controls did so. These findings are in broad agreement with those of other workers (Rehnstrom et al., 1977; Rikkers et al., 1978; Schomerus et al., 1981; Gitlin et al., 1986). It is of interest that Reitan Trail Test performance, which is frequently used in the assessment of clinically apparent encephalopathy (Conn, 1977), was not impaired in our study, and cannot therefore be recommended as a simple means of screening for latent PSE. Though some authors have suggested that number connection tests are of benefit in diagnosis (Rehnstrom et al., 1977; Rikkers et al., 1978; Schomerus et al., 1981; Sarin et al., 1985; Gitlin

TABLE 2

Memory and Performance-based Psychometric Test Results in Patients with Cirrhosis and in Matched Controls (mean $\pm$ SD) (from Moore et al., submitted for publication)

TEST	CIRRHOTICS	CONTROLS
Benton Visual Retention Test		
No. correct	4.8 $\pm$ 2.1[*]	7.7 $\pm$ 1.7
No. of errors	8.5 $\pm$ 4.8[*]	3.3 $\pm$ 2.3
Reitan Trail Tests (secs)		
A	43.9 $\pm$ 19.0	35.0 $\pm$ 13.0
B	105.0 $\pm$ 66.0	93.0 $\pm$ 36.0
Reaction Times (msecs)		
Light	316.0 $\pm$ 132.0[*]	225.0 $\pm$ 36.0
Sound	361.0 $\pm$ 152.0[*]	236.0 $\pm$ 52.0
Choice	651.0 $\pm$ 190.0[*]	406.0 $\pm$ 101.0

[*] p < 0.05 vs. controls

TABLE 3

Memory and Performance-based Psychometric Test Results in Patients with Cirrhosis: Results for Individual Patients (data from Moore et al., submitted for publication)

SUBJECT	BVRT Correct	BVRT Errors	REITAN A	REITAN B	REACTION TIMES L	S	C	No. TESTS ABNORMAL
1	A	A			A	A	A	5
2					A	A	A	3
3					A	A	A	3
4	A	A				A	A	4
5					A	A	A	3
6		A			A	A	A	4
7						A	A	2
8		A					A	2
9								0
10						A	A	2
11	A	A	A	A	A	A	A	7
12			A			A	A	3
13	A	A						2
14								0
15		A					A	2
16	A	A	A	A		A	A	6
17							A	1
18	A	A				A	A	4
19						A	A	2
No. Subjects Abnormal	6	9	3	2	6	13	16	

Abbreviations: A = abnormal; BVRT = Benton Visual Retention Test; L = light; S = sound; C = choice

et al., 1986), when age is controlled for, as in our studies, it is apparent that these tests are frequently normal (Gilberstadt et al., 1980; Levy et al., 1987). A host of other psychometric tests have been employed in the neuropsychological assessment of patients with cirrhosis. As previously stated, tests of memory and performance skills are frequently impaired, and the interested reader is referred to the individual studies referenced above and to the recent review by Tarter et al. (1986a).

RELATED NEUROPHYSIOLOGICAL AND MORPHOLOGICAL ABNORMALITIES

The electroencephalogram (EEG) is normal in 66%-94% of patients with latent PSE (Rikkers et al., 1978; Schomerus et al., 1981; Gitlin et al., 1986; Dunk et al., 1988). The patients with EEG abnormalities have, as would be expected, more severe abnormalities on psychometric testing than those who do not (Rikkers et al., 1978; Schomerus et al., 1981). More recently, visual evoked potentials (VEPs) have been measured in cirrhotics without clinical evidence of encephalopathy. Prolonged peak latencies have been observed in the presence of normal EEG findings (Zeneroli et al., 1984; Levy et al., 1987), though detailed studies comparing VEP measurement and psychometric testing in the diagnosis of latent PSE are lacking. Brain-stem auditory evoked potentials are occasionally abnormal but less frequently so than VEPs (Pierelli et al., 1985). Somatosensory evoked potentials may also be abnormal in patients without evidence of hepatic encephalopathy (Yang et al., 1985), though this work requires confirmation.

CT scanning (Tarter et al., 1986b; Bernthal et al., 1987) and NMR imaging (Moore et al., submitted for publication) have both demonstrated macroscopic abnormalities of cerebral morphology in cirrhotic patients without clinical evidence of encephalopathy. Bernthal et al. (1987) noted a variety of abnormalities in their detailed studies of a large group of non-alcoholic cirrhotics, some of whom had very mild clinically-apparent PSE. The maximum width of frontal sulci were increased, indicating atrophy of the frontal cortex, and bicaudate diameter, maximum diameter of the third ventricle, and cella media distance were each reduced, possibly indicating focal cerebral oedema. These changes could be significantly associated with a variety of abnormalities in tests of psychomotor efficiency, learning and memory, and perceptual-motor coordination. Our own studies (Moore et al., submitted for publication) were performed on a different patient population (alcoholic and non-alcoholic cirrhotics, none with clinical encephalopathy), used a different imaging technique (NMR), and measured a variety of parameters, some of which were not studied by Bernthal et al. (1987). It is therefore unwise to compare and contrast the two studies closely. We also found numerous morphological changes in cirrhotics. Sulcal width was significantly increased in both parietal lobes and just failed to reach significance in the frontal and occipital areas (both p=0.056). Interhemispheric fissure width was significantly increased in cirrhotics, as was bicaudate diameter. Thus we found evidence of diffuse cortical atrophy in our patient population but could not demonstrate cerebral oedema. We, like Bernthal et al. (1987), could demonstrate numerous significant correlations between the NMR variables and neuropsychological test performance. The precise neuropathology underlying the gross changes found on CT or NMR imaging of patients with latent PSE remains to be determined. As most cirrhotics dying of hepatic disease do so with clinical evidence of encephalopathy, such studies would have to be performed on patients dying of unrelated non-hepatic disorders such as myocardial infarction.

RELATIONSHIP TO ALCOHOL ABUSE

Patients with alcoholic cirrhosis have made up the majority of patients examined in many of the studies already described. It is therefore reasonable to speculate that the neuropsychiatric deficits noted in these studies are the result of alcohol-induced neurotoxicity rather than latent PSE. This subject has recently been addressed by Tarter et al. (1986a). It would appear from the available data that the neuropsychiatric abnormalities are almost certainly attributable to latent PSE occurring as a consequence of liver damage. This is evidenced by the fact

that the neuropsychiatric deficits in alcoholic and non-alcoholic cirrhotics are similar (Rehnström et al., 1977; Gitlin et al., 1986; Moore et
al., submitted for publication) and that these changes improve significantly upon instituting treatment for PSE (Rikkers et al., 1978; McClain
et al., 1984; Egberts et al., 1985).

NATURAL HISTORY OF LATENT PSE

The frequency and rate with which patients with latent PSE pass into
the clinical stages of the disorder remain undetermined. Prospective
follow-up studies are needed in this area.

SIGNIFICANCE OF LATENT PSE

Patients with impaired performance skills put themselves and the
general public at risk when their occupation involves the use of mechan-
ised equipment and when they drive a car (Schomerus et al., 1981; Gitlin
et al., 1986). The question of driving fitness has been specifically
addressed by Schomerus et al. (1981). On the basis of psychometric test
performance 60% of their patients were considered totally unfit to drive
and a further 25% were of dubious driving ability. Thus it would seem
appropriate to treat these patients, even though their encephalopathy is
by definition asymptomatic.

TREATMENT

The psychometric deficits in latent PSE may improve upon protein
restriction (Rikkers et al., 1978), branched chain amino acid supplementation, (Egberts et al., 1985) and lactulose treatment (McClain et al.,
1984). Each of these studies has been short-term, and their long-term
acceptability and efficacy remain to be determined. It is doubtful
whether anything other than specific therapy designed to halt continuing
hepatic damage will be able to prevent patients from eventual progression
into the clinically obvious stages of the disease.

CONCLUSIONS

The majority of 'healthy' ambulant cirrhotic patients have demonstrable neuropsychological deficits which particularly affect memory and
performance skills. They are frequently associated with neurophysiological abnormalities and macroscopic changes in cerebral morphology, and
are not a consequence of alcohol-induced neurotoxicity. Patients with
latent PSE who drive or operate heavy machinery put themselves and others
at risk, and should therefore be offered some form of treatment for PSE.
A variety of treatments have shown efficacy in the short-term but their
long-term effects require evaluation. The natural history of this disorder remains to be determined.

REFERENCES

Bernthal, P., Hays, A., Tarter, R.E., Van Thiel, D., Lecky, J. & Hegedus,
    A. (1987). Cerebral CT scan abnormalities in cholestatic and hepato-
    cellular disease and their relationship to neuropsychologic test
    performance. Hepatology, 7, 107-111.
Borg, J., Warter, J.M., Schlienger, J.L., Imler, M., Marescaux, C. &
    Mack, G. (1982). Neurotransmitter modifications in human cerebro-

spinal fluid and serum during hepatic encephalopathy. Journal of Neurological Science, 57, 343-356.

Conn, H.O. (1977). Trailmaking and Reitan connection tests in the assessment of mental state in portal systemic encephalopathy. American Journal of Digestive Diseases, 22, 541-550.

Dunk, A.A., Moore, J., Symon, A., Dickie, A., Sinclair, T.S., Mowat, N.A.G. & Brunt, P.W. (1988). The effects of propranolol on hepatic encephalopathy in patients with cirrhosis and portal hypertension. Alimentary Pharmacology and Therapeutics, 2, 143-152.

Egberts, E-H., Schomerus, H., Hamster, W. & Jurgens, P. (1985). Branched chain amino acids in the treatment of latent portasystemic encephalopathy: a double-blind placebo-controlled crossover study. Gastroenterology, 88, 887-895.

Field, J.G. (1960). Two types of tables for use with Wechsler's intelligence scales. Journal of Clinical Psychology, 16, 3-7.

Gilberstadt, S.J., Gilberstadt, H., Zieve, L., Buegel, B., Collier, R.O. & McClain, C.J. (1980). Psychomotor performance defects in cirrhotic patients without overt encephalopathy. Archives of Internal Medicine, 140, 519-521.

Gitlin, N., Lewis, D.C. & Hinkley, L. (1986). The diagnosis and prevalence of subclinical hepatic encephalopathy in apparently healthy, ambulant, non-shunted patients with cirrhosis. Journal of Hepatology, 3, 75-82.

Jones, E.A. & Schafer, D.F. (1986). Hepatic encephalopathy: a neurochemical disorder. Seminars in Liver Disease, VIII, 525-540.

Levy, L.J., Bolton, R.P. & Losowsky, M.S. (1987). The use of visual evoked potentials (VEP) in delineating a state of subclinical encephalopathy: a comparison with the number connection test (NCT). Journal of Hepatology, 5, 211-217.

McClain, C.J., Potter, T.J., Kromhout, J.P. & Zieve, L. (1984). The effect of lactulose on psychomotor performance tests in alcoholic cirrhotics without overt hepatic encephalopathy. Journal of Clinical Gastroenterology, 6, 325-329.

Messori, E., Zani, G. & Ventura, E. (1984). Visual evoked potential: a diagnostic tool for the assessment of hepatic encephalopathy. Gut, 25, 291-299.

Moore, J.W., Dunk, A.A., Crawford, J.R., Deans, H., De Lacey, G., Besson, J., Sinclair, T.S. Mowat, N.A.G. & Brunt, P.W. Psychometric deficits and morphological NMR brain scan abnormalities in apparently 'healthy' non-encephalpathic patients with cirrhosis: a controlled study. Submitted for publication.

Parsons-Smith, B.G., Summerskill, W.H.J., Dawson, A.M. & Sherlock, S. (1957). The electroencephalograph in liver disease. Lancet, ii, 867-871.

Pierelli, F., Pozzessere, G., Sanarelli, L., Valle, E., Rizzo, P.A. & Morocutti, G. (1985). Electrophysiological study in patients with chronic hepatic insufficiency. Acta Neurologica Belgica, 85, 284-291.

Rehnstrom, S., Simert, S., Hansson, J.A., Johnson, G. & Vang, J. (1977). Chronic hepatic encephalopathy. A psychometrical study. Scandinavian Journal of Gastroenterology, 12, 305-311.

Rikkers, L., Jenko., P., Rudman, D. & Freides, D. (1978). Subclinical hepatic encephalopathy detection, prevalence and relationship to nitrogen metabolism. Gastroenterology, 75, 462-469.

Rossi-Fanelli, F., Strom, C.R., Cardelli-Gangiano, P., Ceci, F., Muscaritoli, M. & Cangiano, C. (1987). Amino acids and hepatic encephalopathy. Progress in Neurobiology, 28, 277-301.

Sarin, S.K. & Nundy, S. (1985). Subclinical encephalopathy after portasystemic shunts in patients with non-cirrhotic portal fibrosis. Liver, 5, 142-146.

Schomerus, H. & Hamster, W. (1976). Latent portasystemic encephalopathy. Digestion, 14, 5-6.

Schomerus, H., Hamster, W., Blunck, H., Reinhard, U., Mayer, K. & Dolle, W. (1981). Latent portasystemic encephalopathy. 1. nature of cerebral functional defects and their effect on fitness to drive. Digestive Diseases and Sciences, 26, 622-630.

Tarter, R.E., Edwards, K.L. & Van Thiel, D.H. (1986a). Hepatic encephalopathy. in: G. Goldstein & R.E. Tarter (eds.). Advances in Clinical Neuropsychology, Vol.3. New York: Plenum Press.

Tarter, R.E., Hays, A.L., Sandford, S.S. & Van Thiel, D. (1986b). Cerebral morphological abnormalities associated with non-alcoholic cirrhosis. Lancet, ii, 893-895.

Yang, S-S., Chu, N-S. & Liaw, Y-F. (1985). Somatosensory evoked potentials in hepatic encephalopathy. Gastroenterology, 89, 625-630.

Zeegen, R., Drinkwater, J.E. & Dawson, A.M. (1970). Method for measuring cerebral dysfunction in patients with liver disease. British Medical Journal, 2, 633-636.

Zeneroli, M.L. (1985). Hepatic encephalopathy: experimental studies on a rat model of fulminant hepatic failure. Journal of Hepatology, 1, 301-312.

Zieve, L. (1981). The mechanism of hepatic coma. Hepatology, 1, 360-365.

EFFECTS OF ESSENTIAL FATTY ACID SUPPLEMENTATION ON NEUROPSYCHOLOGICAL FUNCTION IN ABSTINENT ALCOHOLICS

L E F MacDonell, F K Skinner, E M T Glen and A I M Glen

INTRODUCTION

Alcohol is known to block the conversion of the essential fatty acid known as linoleic acid (LA) into gamma-linolenic acid (GLA) and thus deprive the body of some of the vital components involved in the structure of cell membranes (Lieber & Spritz, 1966; Reitz, 1979; Alling et al., 1984). Nervi et al. (1980) showed that alcohol inhibits the enzymes involved in the conversion of LA to arachidonic acid. Alcohol is also known to affect liver function adversely and, as well as being the cause of Wernicke-Korsakoff's psychosis, can cause minimal impairments in brain function (Miller & Saucedo, 1983; Shaw & Spence, 1985).

In the past few years there has been an increasing amount of evidence for the role of essential fatty acids (EFAs) in biological systems in man and in animals (Horrobin, 1981). Clinically most work has been undertaken using evening primrose oil (Oenothera biennis), which is 72 per cent LA, 9 per cent GLA and 2 per cent dihomogammalinolenic acid. GLA is not usually found in a normal diet and its uptake is not blocked by alcohol (Horrobin, 1987). Thus, by bypassing the blocked link, the chain might be reactivated.

In 1983, the Highland Psychiatric Research Group in Inverness set up a double-blind trial using EFA supplementation over a 6-month period with recovering male alcoholics aged between 20 and 59. The purpose was to establish whether or not giving EFAs of the n-6 series would have the effect of improving liver function tests, and tests of neuropsychological function in recovering alcoholics more than if they were merely abstinent. Blood samples were taken regularly throughout the trial and analyses of phospholipid levels were carried out in Nova Scotia. Automated neuropsychological testing was carried out at 3, 12 and 24 weeks after admission to hospital. Social-drinking control data (ages 20-59) were obtained from male volunteers in Inverness, as well as being made available by Ronald Draper from St. Patrick's Hospital, Dublin, and Clare Acker from the Institute of Psychiatry in London.

In an earlier trial, we (Glen et al., 1985; 1987) found significant improvements (p<0.02) in gamma-glutamyltransferase (GGT) for the EFA-supplemented group, when compared with the placebo group, when blood samples were taken 48 hours after admission to hospital and then at 3 weeks. This result was later replicated by us (Besson et al., 1987) at the p<0.01 level. It was also found that fatty acid estimation showed that alcoholics, on admission, had significantly less unsaturated n-6 and n-3 fatty acids and significantly more saturated than age- and sex-matched controls.

NEUROPSYCHOLOGICAL IMPAIRMENT IN ALCOHOLICS

This report is concerned with neuropsychological aspects. When selecting neuropsychological tests to measure changes in minimal brain impairments in recovering alcoholics, we first looked at which functions have been found by previous researchers (for example, Ron, 1977; Parsons & Leber, 1981; Goldman, 1983) to be impaired by excessive use of alcohol and at which tests had already been used.

The general level of intelligence in alcoholics has rarely been found to be impaired using either the Wechsler Adult Intelligence Scale (WAIS) or the National Adult Reading Test (NART) (Acker et al., 1987). Thus NART, which is quick and easy to administer, is commonly used to estimate pre-morbid intelligence (see Crawford, this volume). The fact that WAIS Performance score tends to be inferior to the Verbal score in alcoholics could perhaps be said to reflect the fact that their verbal abilities are not generally found to be impaired, whereas their non-verbal are. However Kleinknecht and Goldstein (1972) warn against the use of VIQ-PIQ differences as a diagnostic sign of cerebral impairment in alcoholism because of failure to control for possible peripheral neuropathy. Brandt et al. (1983) found deficits on verbal paired associate learning and verbal short-term memory tasks, and for verbal memory Ryan and Butters (1980) report that the more difficult a task becomes the more the alcoholic's performance deteriorates. It seems overall that it is only when conceptual processing, possibly with new learning, is also involved that verbal abilities are impaired. Most of the evidence cites only non-verbal abilities as being impaired in alcohlics.

The non-verbal abilities which may be affected by abuse of alcohol involve what Brandt et al. (1983) describe as 'the integrity of visuo-perceptual, associative, and psychomotor functions'. Parsons and Farr (1981) report specific cognitive deficits in problem solving involving abstracting, in complex perceptual motor skills and in memory and learning tasks. It seems that alcoholics are able to grasp concepts, but have inefficient strategies for solution (Shaw & Spence, 1985) and an inabiity to process new and complex information or use error responses. Motor speed is only impaired where a perceptual component is also involved. Visual search and spatial orientation, as well as sustained concentration on repetitive tasks, may also be involved. The tests most frequently used to assess these non-verbal impairments have been the performance subtests of the WAIS, most notably the Digit Symbol substitution test, the Halstead Reitan battery and the Trail Making Test (for example, Sanchez-Craig, 1980).

EFA SUPPLEMENTATION AND NEUROPSYCHOLOGICAL FUNCTION

Since it is now possible to measure responses to visual stimuli to a very high degree of accuracy, in milliseconds where appropriate, by using automated tests on a microcomputer, and since this also has the advantage of results printed out at the push of a button, it was decided to use automated tests. An Apple II microcomputer was used with hardware modifications, a Mountain Hardware Clock, two disc drives and two additional special keyboards.

A maximum of 14 GLA-supplemented and 14 placebo patients completed testing on all three occasions and remained abstinent. For data analysis t-tests were performed between patient groups and controls and for the patient groups an analysis of variance and co-variance, with age and IQ as co-variates, was carried out for the 21-week period. There was no age difference between the two groups.

In an endeavour to separate motor time and perceptual processing when analyzing other results from more complex tasks, we selected a series of reaction time tests from Elithorn's neuropsychological battery (Elithorn et al., 1980). Reaction times measured were:

(i)   simple auditory – responding to an intermittently presented tone by pressing a button;
(ii) simple visual – responding to an intermittently presented block by pressing a button;
(iii) visual discrimination – pressing a right or left button appropriately according to the position of the presented block;
(iv) visual discrimination with auditory inhibition – responding with a right or left button only when no tone is present.

The actively treated group and the placebo group of patients did not differ from each other or from control subjects at either 3 or 24 weeks after admission, except in one instance where the placebo group at 24 weeks performed less well than the controls ($p < 0.02$). This seemingly negative set of results leads us to the conclusion that abstinent alcoholics who are past the withdrawal phase do not have slowing of reaction times. Thus, as was confirmed by Shaw and Spence (1985), the motor component on any test should not be impaired and, if there is slowness on other tasks, then some impairment in perceptual processing would be indicated.

The visual memory tests (Wilson et al., 1982), in which subjects have to replace a block which has been removed from a pattern of blocks previously displayed on the screen, also failed to show any difference between our alcoholic sample and controls on either short, 'working', or long, 'stored', visual memory. This may also be a useful finding when attempting to explain any results which do show deficits in alcoholics, since the visual memory component is unlikely to be impaired.

The two problem-solving tests, the Perceptual Maze Test (Elithorn et al., 1982) and Cogfun II (Draper et al., 1983), have already been fully described by us (MacDonell et al., 1987) and reported as being sensitive to known minimal brain impairments in alcoholics. The Perceptual Maze Test is a problem-solving task which evaluates perceptual-motor performance and is thought to detect frontal lobe damage. The subject is required to trace a path through a specified number of dots in each of a series of triangular grids or 'mazes'. The pencil-and-paper rectangular version of this test was found by us (Glen et al., 1985) in a previous trial to be the most sensitive to neuropsychological deficits in recovering alcoholics.

Cogfun, in which the subject has to complete a series of patterns drawn partway through an array of blocks on the screen, is designed to tap conceptual ability and, at the same time, involve tracking and sequencing of data embedded in a maze, test the subjects' spatial orientation, their ability to form and shift cognitive sets and utilize error responses.

Results from these two tests are shown in Table 1, from which it can be seen that at the 3-week testing only 'percentage incorrect' differed significantly from controls in both tests for both patient groups, but that the scores for mean times were significantly different from controls only for Cogfun at 3 weeks. At 24 weeks all patient scores were similar to those for controls. Thus it appears that on both these tests alcoholics are impaired relative to controls in the early weeks of abstinence, but that there is repair after six months of abstinence. This recovery is not affected by EFA supplementation or, if it is, we have not

TABLE 1

Peceptual Maze Test and Cogfun Results for Abstinent
Alcoholics at 3 and 24 weeks after Admission to Hospital
and for Social Drinking Controls

MAZES	EFA-suppl. (n=14)		Placebo (n=13)		Controls (n=34)	
	mean	SD	mean	SD	mean	SD
% incorrect						
at 3 wks	55.8***	18.42	56.25***	20.89	39.71	16.85
at 24 wks	40.18	15.64	36.54	20.23		
Mean time						
at 3 wks	30.79	8.66	29.31	6.51	27.71	7.06
at 24 wks	30.00	5.64	30.69	6.25		

COGFUN	EFA-suppl. (n=13)		Placebo (n=14)		Controls (n=28)	
	mean	SD	mean	SD	mean	SD
% incorrect						
at 3 wks	49.61*	18.25	57.7***	20.57	35.46	21.64
at 24 wks	43.84	24.90	44.53	22.84		
speed						
at 3 wks	3.81*	1.51	5.22****	2.52	2.58	1.7
at 24 wks	3.18	1.63	3.56	1.92		

KEY: Compared with control values: *p = < 0.05; **p = < 0.02;
***p = < 0.01; ****p = < 0.001

identified it at the testing times selected.

The battery also included two subtests from the Bexley-Maudsley
Automated Psychological Screening battery (Acker & Acker, 1982), 'Little
Men' and Symbol-Digit coding. 'Little Men', in which the subject is
required to indicate in which hand the 'little man', who may be standing
on his feet or his head and looking away from or towards the subject, is
holding an object, is a test of spatial orientation. Symbol Digit, in
which the subject has to find numbers which are paired with particular
objects, taps perceptual-motor speed as well as the ability to sustain
attention on a repetitive task. Results from these two tests are shown in
Table 2 and Table 3, from which it can be seen that, whereas at 3 weeks
both patient groups differ consistently from controls on Symbol Digit,
Little Men does not consistently differentiate alcoholics from controls. In
fact, at 24 weeks mean times for the actively treated group are actually superior to control mean times. The analysis of variance favours the
GLA-supplement over the placebo for Head Up Mean Time (p=0.034) and for
Feet Up Mean Time (p=0.033). In Symbol-Digit two of the three mean time
measures for the EFA-supplemented group at 24 weeks show no differences
from controls, whereas levels of significance for the placebo group

TABLE 2

BMAPS 'Little Men' Results for Abstinent Alcoholics
at 3 and 24 weeks after Admission to Hospital and
for Social Drinking Controls

MAZES	EFA-suppl. (n=14)		Placebo (n=14)		Controls (n=44)	
	mean	SD	mean	SD	mean	SD
Head Up % incorrect						
at 3 wks	10.27*	10.57	3.57	4.04	4.26	7.95
at 24 wks	4.91	5.58	4.46	5.71		
Feet Up % incorrect						
at 3 wks	21.88	16.94	29.02**	18.44	15.32	18.40
at 24 wks	20.09	24.04	25.89	27.61		
Head Up Mean time						
at 3 wks	2.42	0.82	2.77	0.88	2.64	0.98
at 24 wks	1.88***	0.64	2.60	0.93		
Feet Up Mean time						
at 3 wks	3.50	1.35	4.53	2.21	3.94	2.00
at 24 wks	2.74*	1.21	4.09	2.06		

Analysis of variance and co-variance results favoring EFA supplement over placebo.

Head Up Mean Time $p = 0.034$
Feet Up Mean Time $p = 0.033$

KEY: Compared with control values: *$p < 0.05$; **$p < 0.02$;
***$p < 0.01$; ****$p < 0.001$

remain unchanged from 3 weeks. The analysis of variance favors the EFA-supplemented group on all three measures: 1st 20 MT, $p=0.05$; 2nd 20 MT, $p=0.032$; 3rd 20 MT, $p=0.037$.

The facts that there were virtually no significant differences in the reaction time tests and that detoxified alcoholics perform similarly to controls enable us to discount the simple motor factor in other tests. However, it is the measures of speed and not of accuracy whch have shown differences between EFA-supplemented patients and placebos. It is likely therefore that it is the speed of perceptual processing which is being improved differentially and not the motor speed itself. So far as we know this is the first time that such differential improvements as the result of therapeutic intervention have been identified. In the case of Symbol-Digit, impairments on similar tests have previously been shown to endure for periods in excess of one year (Parsons, 1983; Brandt et al., 1983).

TABLE 3

BMAPS Symbol-Digit Results for Abstinent Alcoholics at
3 and 24 Weeks after Admission to Hospital and for
Social Drinking Controls

	EFA-supp. (n=14)		Placebo (n=14)		Controls (n=44)	
	mean	SD	mean	SD	mean	SD
1st mean time						
at 3 wks	2.42***	0.44	2.49****	0.39	2.04	0.34
at 24 wks	2.23	0.37	2.47****	0.41		
2nd 20 mean time						
at 3 wks	2.18****	0.51	2.32****	0.39	1.79	0.28
at 24 wks	2.07***	0.33	2.29****	0.40		
3rd 20 mean time						
at 3 wks	2.1**	0.70	2.25****	0.4	1.80	0.26
at 24 wks	1.92	0.29	2.18****	0.38		

Analysis of variance and co-variance results favoring EFA supplement
over placebo.

1st 20 Mean Time   p=0.05
2nd 20 Mean Time   p=0.032
3rd 20 Mean Time   p=0.037

KEY: Compared with control values: *p < 0.05; **p < 0.02;
        ***p < 0.01; ****p < 0.001

If EFA-supplemented subjects return to normal levels within a 6-month
period, then this would be a significant advance. It could be that supplementation with gamma-linolenic acid actually effects improvements
which would not take place otherwise.

We are at present carrying out a further trial using a preparation
of fatty acids containing reduced amounts of the n-6 series but introducing n-3 series fatty acids, i.e. containing less GLA but wih a small
amount of eicosapentaenoic acid (EPA) as well as trace elements and
vitamins. Initial results, with 7 subjects for both the active preparation and the placebo show no difference between the EFA-supplemented and
the placebo groups over the 24-week period for the Perceptual Maze Test
or for Cogfun. However, the treated group's working memory deteriorated
significantly (p=0.03) in comparison with the placebo, whilst long-term
memory results showed no differences at any stage. For Little Men no
difference emerged at any stage. In Symbol-Digit the analysis of variance
shows no differences in changes over time in the two treatment groups,
but all the results differed from control values on every occasion. It is
notable however that, whereas results for the 1st 20 mean time improved
for both groups by 24 weeks, on 2nd and 3rd 20 mean time they all deteriorated. This was not the case in the replication trial reported here,
where all 3-week results were improved upon at 24 weeks.

The numbers analysed in this present trial so far are of course small but, even so, the contrast between supplementation of high n–6 and reduced n–6 is quite striking. It is also striking that the significant result achieved over the initial 3-week period for GGT, favouring high n–6 over the placebo (p<0.01; Active: n=24, Placebo: n=28), has not been found where the n–6 was reduced (Active: n=26, Placebo: n=29).

When more neuropsychological data become available analysis will determine whether a similar trend in neuropsychological results to that found with high n–6 supplementation also emerges when the amount of n–6 is reduced. The suggestion seems to be, however, that this is unlikely and thus that quantifiable benefits of GLA supplementation only emerge when a sufficiently large amount of GLA is taken: a suggestion which lends support to the hypothesis that damage to cell membranes caused by abuse of alcohol can in part at any rate, be repaired by GLA supplementation.

ACKNOWLEDGEMENTS

We are grateful to Dr A. Elithorn, Professor R.J. Draper and Mrs C. Acker for supplying test software and to Professor Draper and Mrs Acker for control data. Our thanks also go to Mr J. Miller for editorial advice and for typing the manuscript. The research was funded by Efamol Ltd., who also supplied the high n–6 supplements (Efamol) and the low n–6 supplements (Efamax) and the corresponding placebos.

REFERENCES

Acker, W. & Acker, C. (1982). Bexley-Maudsley Automated Psychological Screening and Bexley-Maudsley Category Sorting Test. Windsor: NFER-Nelson.

Acker, C., Jacobson, R.R. & Lishman, W.A. (1987). Memory and ventricular size in alcoholics. Psychological Medicine, 17, 343–348.

Alling, C., Gustavsson, L., Kristensson-Aas, A. & Wallerstedt, S. (1984). Changes in fatty acid composition of major glycero-phospho lipids in erythrocyte membranes from chronic alcoholics during withdrawal. Scandinavian Journal of Clinical Laboratory Investigation, 44, 283–289.

Besson, J., Glen, E., Glen, I., MacDonell, L. & Skinner, F. (1987). Essential fatty acids, mean cell volume and nuclear magnetic resonance of brains of ethanol-dependent human subjects. Alcohol and Alcoholism, Suppl.1, 577–581.

Brandt, J., Butters, N., Ryan, C. & Bayog, R. (1983). Cognitive loss and recovery in chronic alcohol abusers. Archives of General Psychiatry, 40, 435–442.

Draper, R., Manning, A., Daly, M. & Larragy, J. (1983). A novel cognitive function test for detection of alcoholic brain damage. Neuropharmacology, 22, 567–569.

Elithorn, A., Mornington, S. & Stavrou, A. (1982). Automated psychological testing: some principles and practice. International Journal of Man-Machine Studies, 17, 247–263.

Elithorn, A., Powell, J., Telford, A. & Cooper, R. (1980). An intelligent terminal for automated psychological testing and remedial practice. in: R.L. Grimsdale & H.C.A. Hankins (eds.). Human Factors and Interactive Displays. Buckingham: Network.

Glen, A.I.M., Glen, E.M.T., MacDonald, F.K., MacDonell, L.E.F., MacKenzie, J.R., Montgomery, D.J., Manku, M.S., Horrobin, D.F. & Morse, N. (1985). Essential fatty acids in the treatment of the alcohol dependence syndrome. in: G.G. Birch & M.G. Lindley (eds.). Alcoholic Beverages. Essex: Elsevier.

Glen, I., Skinner, F., Glen, E. & MacDonell, L. (1987). The role of essential fatty acids in alcohol dependence and tissue damage. Alcoholism: Clinical and Experimental Research, 11, 37–41.

Goldman, M.S. (1983). Cognitive impairment in chronic alcoholics: some cause for optimism. American Psychologist, 38, 1045–1054.

Horrobin, D.F. (1981). Clinical Uses of Essential Fatty Acids. Montreal: Eden Press.

Horrobin, D.F. (1987). Essential fatty acids, prostaglandins and alcoholism: an overview. Alcoholism: Clinical and Experimental Research, 11, 2–9.

Kleinknecht, R.A. & Goldstein, S.G. (1972). Neuropsychological deficits associated with alcoholism: a review and discussion. Quarterly Journal of Studies on Alcohol, 33, 999–1019.

Lieber, C.S. & Spritz, N. (1966). Effects of prolonged ethanol intake in man: role of dietary, adipose and endogenously synthesized fatty acids in the pathogenesis of the alcoholic fatty liver. Journal of Clinical Investigation, 45, 1400–1411.

MacDonell, L.E.F., Skinner, F.K. & Glen, E.M.T. (1987). The use of two automated neuropsychological tests, Cogfun and the Perceptual Maze Test, with alcoholics. Alcohol and Alcoholism, 22, 285–295.

Miller, W.R. & Saucedo, C.F. (1983). Assessment of neuropsychological impairment and brain damage in problem drinkers. in: C.J. Golden, J.A. Moses, J.A. Coffman et al. (eds.). Clinical Neuropsychology: Interface with Neurologic and Psychiatric Disorders. New York: Grune and Stratton.

Nervi, A.M., Peluffo, R.O., Brenner, R.R. (1980). Effect of ethanol administration on fatty acid desaturation. Lipids, 15, 263–268.

Parsons, O.A. (1983). Cognitive dysfunction and recovery in alcoholics. Substance and Alcohol Actions/Misuse, 4, 175–190.

Parsons, O.A. & Farr, S.P. (1981). The neuropsychology of alcohol and drug use. In S.B. Filskov & T.J. Boll (eds.). Handbook of Clinical Neuropsychology. New York: Wiley and Sons.

Parsons, O.A. & Lebev, W.R. (1981). The relationship between cognitive dysfunction and brain damage in alcoholics: causal, interactive, or epiphenomenal? Alcoholism: Clinical and Experimental Research, 5, 326–46.

Reitz, R.C. (1979). The effects of ethanol administration on lipid metabolism. Progress in Lipid Research, 18, 87–115.

Ron, M.A. (1977). Brain damage in chronic alcoholism: a neuropathological, neuroradiological and psychological review. Psychological Medicine, 7, 103–112.

Ryan, C. & Butters, N. (1980). Learning and memory impairments in young and old alcoholics: evidence for the premature-aging hypothesis. Alcoholism: Clinical and Experimental Research, 4, 288–293.

Sanchez-Craig, M. (1980). Drinking pattern as a determinant of alcoholics' performance on the trail making test. Journal of Studies on Alcohol, 41, 1082–1090.

Shaw, G.K. & Spence, M. (1985). Psychological impairment in alcoholics. Alcohol and Alcoholism, 20, 243–249.

Wilson, J.T.L., Brooks, D.N. & Phillips, W.A. (1982). Using a microcomputer to study perception, memory and attention after head injury. Poster Presentation, 5th INS European Conference, Deauville, France.

ESTIMATION OF PREMORBID INTELLIGENCE: A REVIEW OF RECENT DEVELOPMENTS

John R Crawford

INTRODUCTION

Whether for clinical, medico-legal or research purposes, the detection and quantification of intellectual impairment in the individual case is problematic. As there are substantial individual differences in intellectual ability in the general population, simply comparing a client's IQ test performance with the relevant test norms will be of little value. It is therefore necessary to compare current performance against an individualised comparison standard (Lezak, 1983). This standard is easily determined if test results are available from a period preceding the point at which neurological disorder or behavioural change raised the suspicion of impairment. However, such information is rarely available. It is therefore necessary to estimate an individual's 'expected' or 'premorbid' level of performance.

The most common approach to estimating premorbid IQ is to use tests of present ability which are considered to be relatively resistant to neurological and psychiatric disorder. A more recent approach involves building regression equations to estimate premorbid IQ from demographic variables known to be related to IQ test performance (e.g. education). These approaches will be evaluated in turn before finally examining a method which combines the two.

ESTIMATION OF PREMORBID IQ WITH TESTS OF PRESENT ABILITY

At the risk of overstating the obvious, a present ability measure must fulfil the following three criteria if it is to qualify as a valid means of estimating premorbid IQ. Firstly, it must have adequate reliability. Secondly, it must correlate highly with IQ (in the normal population). Finally, and most importantly, it must be largely resistant to the effects of neurological and psychiatric disorder. The Vocabulary subtest of the Wechsler scales (e.g. Wechsler, 1955; 1981) has probably been the test most commonly used to estimate premorbid IQ. The literature on Vocabulary will be reviewed below to determine the extent to which it meets the above requirements. This will provide a comparison standard for more recently advocated tests.

Vocabulary clearly fulfils the first two criteria. It has the highest split-half reliability of all the Wechsler Adult Intelligence Scale (WAIS) subtests; in the three age bands examined by Wechsler (1955, p15-17) reliability coefficients ranged between 0.94 and 0.96. Similarly, Vocabulary has the highest reliability of all Wechsler Adult Intelligence Scale - Revised (WAIS-R) subtests. The averaged split-half reliability across all age bands in the WAIS-R standardisation sample was 0.96 and the averaged test-retest reliability for the two age groups tested twice was 0.91 (Wechsler, 1981, p30-32). With regard to the second criterion, Vocabulary correlates very highly with both WAIS and WAIS-R Full Scale IQ. Wechsler (1955) reported correlations ranging between 0.86 and 0.87 for three age bands in the WAIS standardisation sample while a correlation of 0.85 was obtained when data from the full WAIS-R standardisation sample was analysed (Wechsler, 1981, p46). Factor analytic studies of the Wechsler scales, also using the standardisation data, have demonstrated that Vocabulary loads very highly on the first unrotated factor, which is regarded as representing general intelligence or 'g' (for reviews see Matarazzo, 1972; Leckliter, Matarazzo, & Silverstein, 1986). Similarly, high loadings on 'g' have been obtained in factor analytic studies of the WAIS and WAIS-R performance of non-clinical UK samples (Crawford et al., 1989d; Crawford et al., 1989a).

It can be seen that Vocabulary has both high reliability and high validity as a measure of intelligence. However, Vocabulary performance does not appear to be very resistant to cerebral dysfunction. A number of studies have reported that the Vocabulary performance of neurological or psychiatric groups was significantly lower than healthy subjects, or that, within clinical populations, neurological patients performed at a lower level than non-neurological patients. Before reviewing these studies, it is worth noting that a proportion of them suffer from a methodological problem common to much of the research in this area; a failure to take adequate account of premorbid demographic variables known to be related to IQ test performance (e.g. education, socio-economic level, age). As we shall see in a following section, these variables are capable of predicting a substantial proportion of IQ variance and have themselves been used as a means of estimating premorbid IQ. As most tests introduce a correction factor for age, the most important of these variables for the present purpose is probably educational level (see Matarazzo, 1972 for a review of the US literature on this topic). For the purposes of the current review, the present author examined the relationship between years of education and WAIS IQ in a UK sample of 155 non-clinical subjects. Education was highly correlated with WAIS Full Scale IQ (r=0.50, p<0.001) and Vocabulary age-graded scaled score (r=0.55, p<0.001). It can be seen that, if assessing the resistance of a test to dysfunction by comparing clinical and control subjects, it is important to match the groups on demographic variables. If such matching has not been achieved, some method of statistically controlling for their effects should be applied.

Russell (1972) calculated a biserial correlation coefficient between the presence or absence of brain damage and Vocabularly performance in a sample of 103 patients. A highly significant correlation was obtained suggesting that brain damage severely impaired Vocabulary performance. However, this study included congenitally brain damaged subjects and is therefore of little value in assessing the resistance of Vocabularly to adult-onset disorder (i.e. in patient groups who have enjoyed normal intellectual development). In addition, the non-brain-damaged group were of a significantly higher educational level (the author stated that this difference remained when the educational level of the congenital cases was removed from the analysis). In a study evaluating Wechsler's 'Hold-Don't Hold' index, Vogt and Heaton (1977) divided clinical subjects into 'impaired' and 'non-impaired' groups on the basis of their performance on the Halstead Impairment Index (Halstead, 1947). Comparison of the Vocabulary performance of these two groups (by t-test) revealed a highly significant difference in favour of the non-impaired; indeed the 't' value for Vocabulary was larger than that obtained for many of the other WAIS subtests. However, further analysis suggested that much of this difference was due to a between-group difference in educational level and indicated that Vocabulary was the second most resistant subtest.

Swiercinsky & Warnock (1977) administered the WAIS (and other cognitive measures that comprise the Halstead-Reitain Battery) to patients with and without brain damage. In order to asses how well these measures would differentiate between the presence and absence of brain damage, they carried out a stepwise discriminant function analysis. Vocabulary entered the analysis at step 4 and significantly increased discrimination between the groups (p<0.001). In a previous review of premorbid IQ estimates, Klesges, Wilkening & Golden (1981) interpreted this result as an indication that, 'Vocabulary scores deteriorate in brain-damaged patients as much as any other WAIS variable' (p35). However, two alternative explanations could be offered. Firstly, the groups may have differed in their <u>premorbid</u> intellectual level and the entry of Vocabulary was a reflection of this. Years of Education entered at step 6 of the analysis, but one would not argue that this variable deteriorated as a result of acquired brain damage. Secondly, Vocabulary and education may have acted as supressor variables (i.e. they did not differ between the two groups but did correlate with measures which entered the analysis at an earlier stage). In this interpretation Vocabulary and education entered because they partialled out the contribution of premorbid level to current test performance. It is unfortunately impossible to judge between these competing explanations on the evidence presented.

Nelson and McKenna (1975) built a regression equation to predict WAIS IQ from Vocabulary age-graded scaled scores in a sample of 98 subjects free of neurological disorder. These subjects obtained a significantly higher Vocabulary estimated IQ than a group of demented subjects (p<0.001) indicating that Vocabulary did not 'hold' in this latter group. Unfortunately, data on the educational level of the two groups were not presented. Hart, Smith and Swash (1986) used Nelson and McKenna's equation to compare the Vocabulary performance of patients with dementia of the Alzheimer type (DAT) and a control group of comparable age and education. The DAT patients obtained a significantly lower Vocabulary estimated IQ than controls (p<0.001). A further indication that organic disease can markedly impair Vocabulary performance was provided by Crawford, Besson and Parker (1988). They examined Vocabulary estimated IQ (again using Nelson and McKenna's equation) in groups of patients with DAT, multi-infarct dementia (MID), alcoholic dementia, Korsakoff's disease, Huntington's disease and closed head injury. Each clinical subject was individually matched for age, sex, and years of education with a healthy control. Despite the small sample sizes, all clinical groups obtained significantly lower Vocabulary estimated IQs than their respective control groups. The only exception was the closed head injured group. Using the same design, Crawford et al. (1987a) compared the Vocabulary performance of depressed patients and controls. The depressed group performed at a significantly lower level than controls indicating that impairment on Vocabulary can occur even in the absence of organic pathology. It can be concluded that, although Vocabulary is amongst the most resistant of the WAIS subtests, performance on the test is nevertheless markedly impaired in a range of clinical conditions. It is therefore liable to seriously underestimate premorbid intelligence.

Single Word Reading Tests

Clinicians who work with dementing patients will have observed that oral reading ability is commonly largely preserved until late on in the dementing process (although the ability to extract <u>meaning</u> from written text may well be severely impaired at a much earlier stage). On the basis of this clinical observation, Nelson and Mckenna (1975) suggested that oral reading tests could be used to estimate premorbid intelligence in dementia. They tested this hypothesis by administering the Schonell Graded Word Reading Test (Schonell, 1942) and the WAIS to a sample of demented patients and controls. In the control group, Schonell performance was highly correlated with WAIS IQ (pro-rated from seven subtests), thereby indicating that reading ability is a reasonable predictor of IQ in an adult population. Nelson and Mckenna (1975) reported that, as expected, mean scores on the WAIS scales were significantly lower in the demented group. However, there was no significant difference between the demented group and controls on the Schonell. Although, as noted, data on the educational level of the two groups were not reported, these results suggest that oral reading of single words can provide an estimate of premorbid IQ in dementia. Ruddle and Bradshaw (1982) in a cross-validation study, reported that Schonell performance was highly correlated (r=0.74) with WAIS IQ in a sample of healthy adult subjects confirming that the Schonell is a reasonable predictor of IQ. These authors also administered the Schonell and WAIS to three clinical groups - a group with neuroradiologically confirmed cortical atrophy, a group with 'suspected cognitive impairment', and a group of elderly patients with a clinical diagnosis of dementia. Mean WAIS FSIQ, VIQ and PIQ in these three groups were all significantly lower than their Schonell estimated IQ (the estimate being provided by regression equations generated from the healthy, normal sample). The only exception was the comparison between obtained VIQ and predicted VIQ in the 'suspected cognitive impairment' group. These results demonstrate that the Schonell is markedly more resistant to cerebral dysfunction than the WAIS.

The foregoing evidence suggests that single word reading tests have considerable potential as a means of estimating premorbid IQ. However, the Schonell was originally designed to assess reading ability in children and is therefore subject to a ceiling effect when used with adult subjects of above average IQ (the maximum WAIS IQ which can be predicted is 115). Partly because of this limitation, Hazel Nelson constructed what was initially termed the New Adult Reading Test (Nelson, unpublished). This test has subsequently been renamed and published as the National Adult Reading Test (NART; Nelson, 1982). The NART, like the Schonell, is a single word, oral reading test but consists of 50 words which are more appropriate for an adult population. The NART also differs from the Schonell in a further two, potentially important, respects. Firstly, the vast majority of words are short in length. Secondly, all words are irregular; that is, they do not follow normal grapheme-phoneme correspondence rules (e.g. ache, gauche). Because the words are short, subjects do not have to analyse a complex visual stimulus and because they are irregular, 'intelligent guesswork' will not provide the correct pronunciation. Therefore, it has been argued that successful test performance requires previous familiarity with the words but makes minimal demands on current cognitive capacity (Nelson & O'Connell, 1978).

The NART and a short-form WAIS were administered to a standardisation sample of 120 subjects free of neurological disorder. Regression equations were generated to predict WAIS IQ from NART errors. These are presented in the test manual along with tables to assess the probability of a particular size of discrepancy between NART estimated premorbid IQ and current WAIS IQ occurring in the normal population. Since publication of the test manual, the NART has rapidly become a widely used test for the estimation of premorbid IQ in clinical and research settings (e.g. Mckenna & Pratt, 1983; Kopelman, 1985, 1986; McCarthy et al., 1985; Oyebode et al., 1986; Acker et al., 1987). This usage has largely preceded research on the basic psychometric properties of the test. Recently, however, a number of studies have begun to address the necessary issues. These studies will be reviewed below to assess the exent to which the NART meets the three previously defined criteria for a valid psychometric measure of premorbid IQ.

Reliability of the NART

Nelson (1982) reported a split-half reliability of 0.93 for the NART based on the standardisation sample. As Crawford et al. (1988b) obtained a similarly high split-half reliability (0.90) in an additional sample of 201 non-clinical subjects, it can be safely concluded that the NART has high internal consistency. Crawford et al. (1989b) examined the test-retest reliability of the NART in a sample of 61 non-clinical subjects and reported a reliability coefficient of 0.98. A statistically significant practice effect was observed at retesting but this was of a very small magnitude (i.e. a mean change in NART error score of less than 1.0). O'Carroll (1987) conducted a pilot study of the NART's inter-rater reliabiity in which the NART performance of 12 subjects was rated by 10 clinical psychologists who routinely used the NART in their clinical practice. Pearson Product Moment correlations between all possible pairs of raters ranged between 0.89 and 0.99. Crawford et al. (1989b) have extended these findings by examining inter-rater reliability in a larger sample (n=40) with a wider range of NART scores. Correlations between all possible pairs of raters (n=10) ranged between 0.96 and 0.98. The higher correlations in this latter study were presumably due to the increased range of NART performance. Although all the raters in Crawford et al.'s study were clinical psychologists, five had no previous experience of the NART, the remainder used it routinely. It can be concluded that the NART has high inter-rater reliability, and that previous experience of the test is not a prerequisite for reliable scoring.

Validity of the NART as a Measure of Intelligence

In Nelson's (1982) original standardisation sample the NART predicted 55%, 60% and 32% of the variance in WAIS Full Scale, Verbal and Performance IQ respectively (WAIS IQ was prorated from seven subtests) suggesting that NART performance is a reasonable predictor of IQ. In order to examine the predictive ability of the NART in a cross-validation sample, Crawford et al. (1989b) administered the NART and a full WAIS to 151 subjects free of neurological, psychiatric or sensory disability. They reported that NART performance predicted 66%, 72% and 33% of the variance in WAIS FSIQ, VIQ and PIQ respectively. Normally, when regression equations are applied to cross-validation samples there is a shrinkage in predicted variance. The increase in predicted variance observed in Crawford et al.'s study was partly attributable to their use of a full WAIS. When WAIS IQ was prorated from the seven subtests used by Nelson (1982), predicted variance fell to a level consistent with her original findings. Provided that the shrinkage in predicted variance is not excessive in a cross-validation sample, it is desirable to combine this sample with the standardisation sample to generate new equations. These equations should have more stability than the originals (e.g. see Pedhazur, 1982). As this foregoing precondition was clearly met in the case of the NART, Crawford et al. generated new equations based on both samples (n= 271) and provided new discrepancy tables. As the NART predicted a larger proportion of IQ variance when the full WAIS was the criterion variable, and as a full WAIS is commonly administered in clinical practice, equations and discrepancy tables for the estimation of full WAIS IQ were also presented; these were necessarily based on the cross-validation sample alone.

Further evidence of the NART's construct validity as a measure of intelligence has been provided by a factor analytic study of the WAIS and NART (Crawford et al., 1989d). These authors reported that the NART loaded very highly (0.85) on 'g' (i.e. the first unrotated principal component). In many previous factor analytic studies of the Wechsler scales, the third factor to emerge after rotation has been identified as an 'attention/concentration' or 'freedom from distractability' factor (defined by high loadings from Digit Span and Arithmetic). This factor emerged in Crawford et al.'s study but encouragingly, the NART's loading was negligible.

It can be concluded that the NART is a powerful predictor of WAIS FSIQ and VIQ and 'g' but is relatively poor at predicting PIQ. Equations to predict WAIS-R IQ (Wechsler, 1981; Lea, 1986) have yet to be developed. However, reasonably encouraging results were obtained in a study by Crawford et al. (submitted for publication) in which a highly significant correlation (0.72) was observed between NART errors and WAIS-R IQ in a sample of 100 non-clinical subjects.

NART Performance and Normal Ageing

Before turning to an examination of NART performance in clinical groups it is important to ask if NART performance declines with increasing age in the normal population. Nelson (1982) reported that NART errors did not correlate significantly with age in the standardisation sample (r=0.14). Crawford et al. (1988b) reported a small but significant correlation between age and NART errors (r=0.18, p<0.01) in a sample of 201 normal subjects (age range 17-88). However, this correlation was no longer significant after partialling out either education or social class. For the purposes of this review the present author examined the relationship between age and NART errors in the additional adult general population sample (n=151) tested by Crawford et al. (1989b). The correlations between age and NART errors was non-significant (r=-0.06).

The above studies suggest that NART performance is unaffected by the normal ageing process. However, before this conclusion can be accepted with confidence it is necessary to exclude the possibility that a curvilinear relationship exists between NART performance and age in adult samples. Peformance may still be improving in early adulthood as the relevant word knowledge is acquired and may decline in old age. Such a relationship would render the use of correlation coefficients inappropriate. Crawford et al. (1988b) examined this issue by modelling the relationship between NART and age by multiple regression. NART performance was regressed on education and social class. Age and polynomial functions of age were then sequentially added to the model; none of these additions improved the fit of the model to the data by a statistically significant amount (p>0.10 in each case). Thus, there was no evidence of a curvilinear relationship between age and NART performance.

Two studies have examined NART performance in samples consisting exclusively of elderly subjects. Binks and Davies (1984) administered the NART and Millhill Vocabulary Scale (Raven, 1982) to 181 healthy elderly subjects living in the community. The sample had an age range of 64-84. They divided the ample into 4 age bands and reported that there was no significant main effect of age cohort on NART performance. In contrast, Millhill scores were significantly different across the age cohorts (p< 0.001). Brayne and Bearsdell (submitted for publication) examined NART performance in a sample of 358 elderly women (aged between 70 and 80). They divided the sample into two age bands (70-74 and 75-79) and reported a significant age effect for cognitive measures such as the Mini-Mental State Examination (Folstein, Folstein & McHugh et al., 1975) but not for the NART.

Is NART Performance Resistant to Neurological and Psychiatric Disorder?

Nelson and O'Connell (1978) compared the NART and WAIS performance of the NART standardisation sample with a group of patients (n=40) who had EMI scan evidence of cortical atrophy. Their results indicated that the atrophy group were severely impaired on the WAIS (p<0.001). In contrast, there was no significant difference in NART performance between the two groups. Although these results should be interpreted with caution because of the lack of demographic information on the samples (i.e. years of education), they do suggest that NART performance was unaffected by the presence of cortical atrophy. Following publication of these results, the NART has been used to estimate premorbid IQ in a diverse variety of clinical conditions. This practice could be viewed as dangerously premature as it is important to establish whether Nelson & O'Connell's results will hold for all conditions associated with cortical atrophy and whether similar results will be obtained in conditions with other neuropathological features. The currently available evidence on this issue is reviewed below.

As part of an examination of episodic and semantic memory in DAT, Nebes, Martin and Horn (1984) reported that the NART performance of DAT patients did not differ significantly from matched controls. In contrast, the NART performance of the DAT patients studied by Hart, Smith and Swash (1986) was significantly lower than matched controls (p<0.05). However, impairment on the NART was minimal compared with the severe impairment on WAIS summary measures and the Vocabulary subtest. As noted above, Crawford, Besson and Parker (1988) and Crawford et al. (1987a) compared the Vocabulary performance of clinical groups with matched controls. As in Hart, Smith and Swash's study, these groups were also administered the NART. In contrast to the disappointing results with Vocabulary, the NART 'held' in all groups examined (DAT, alcoholic dementia, MID, closed head injury, depression) with the exception of Korsakoff's disease and Huntington's disease. In these latter groups the NART produced a significantly higher premorbid IQ estimate than Vocabulary. The results in the patients with DAT were particularly striking as this group exhibited evidence of severe cognitive impairment (i.e. a mean Block Design age-graded scaled score of 1.9). They also exhibited severe cortical atrophy and ventricular dilation on nuclear magnetic resonance brain imaging and a marked reduction in cerebral blood flow (as measured by single photon emission tomography). It should be noted however that, because of the small sample sizes, Crawford, Besson and Parker (1988) study should be viewed as a preliminary investigation. Larger scale studies of NART performance in these clinical conditions are clearly required.

A further indication that NART performance is not entirely dementia-resistant has been provided by Stebbins and his colleagues (Stebbins et al., 1988; G.T. Stebbins, personal communication). They administered the NART to patients with dementia and healthy controls. Patients were classified as mildly, moderately or severely demented on the basis of their score on the Mini-Mental State Examination (Folstein, Folstein & McHugh, 1975). The NART performance of the moderately and severely demented patients was significantly lower than that of the mildly demented group and control group. However, the mild group did not differ significantly from controls. Crawford et al. (1988a) have reported encouraging preliminary results from a study of NART performance in idiopathic Parkinson's disease (IPD). Patients with IPD (n=72) were individually matched for age, sex, and years of education with a healthy subject. NART performance did not differ significantly between the two groups.

A second method of evaluating putative premorbid measures is to conduct longitudinal investigations of patients suffering from progressive conditions (e.g. DAT) to observe whether decline in these measures occurs. O'Carroll, Baikie and Whittick (1987) retested patients with dementia on the NART and other cognitive measures after a delay of one year. They reported a significant increase in measures of physical disability and severity of dementia at second testing. A significant decline was also observed on a Vocabulary test (the Millhill Synonyms Test; Raven, 1982) but not on the NART. It is to be hoped that additional longitudinal research on the NART will be forthcoming.

O'Carroll and Gilleard (1986) have adopted a third approach to evaluating the resistance of NART performance to dysfunction. These authors examined the correlation between NART performance and measures of dementia severity in a group of demented patients and reported that no significant correlations were obtained. This result suggests NART performance is largely dementia-resistant. In the previously cited study by Crawford et al. (1988a) a significant correlation was observed between NART performance and the Mini-Mental State Examination (MMSE) in a group of Parkinson's patients. This result highlights a problem with the correlational design. Although the absence of a significant correlation can be interpreted fairly unequivocally, the same cannot be said for the presence of a significant correlation. A correlation could arise because NART performance is sensitive to dysfunction but could also arise if the dementia measure was not distribution-free, i.e. differences in performance could partly reflect differences in (premorbid) intellectual level. To examine these competing possibilities Crawford et al. split their sample into those above and those below the MMSE cut-off for dementia. If the former explanation is correct then one would predict that a stronger correlation would be observed in the demented subgroup. The latter explanation would predict the reverse. Crawford et. al. (1988a) reported that the correlation was significant only in the non-demented subgroup. This pattern of results is consistent with the NART being relatively resistant to dysfunction and supports O'Carroll and Gilleard's (1986) original findings.

To summarise; the predominantly encouraging results reported in the above studies indicate that the NART is fairly resistant to the effects of neurological and psychiatric disorder. In those studies which also examined the more commonly used Wechsler Vocabulary subtest, the NART consistently proved to be the more resistant of the two tests. Given that the reliabilities and 'g' loadings of the two tests are very similar, the NART should therefore be considered the test of choice in estimating premorbid intelligence. However, it would be unrealistic to suppose that performance on any current ability measure would be entirely unaffected by severe cerebral dysfunction. Indeed, a number of the studies reviewed above have reported evidence of some deterioration in NART performance. The crucial question is to what extent this evidence undermines the clinical utility of the test. The major use of premorbid estimates is in the detection and quantification of cognitive impairment. It is reasonable to suggest that, where cerebral dysfunction is severe enough to markedly impair performance on a test as robust as the NART, comparison of the obtained IQ score with the premorbid estimate would be largely unnecessary as intellectual deterioration would be all too readily apparent.

Limitations of the NART and Future Research

The NART clearly cannot be used in dyslexic patients nor in clients with significant articulatory problems. The present format of the NART also limits its use to clients with reasonable visual acuity. This can be frustrating for the clinician as the NART is commonly used with the elderly. It would seem preferable that the words be organised in a booklet form so that they could be individually presented in a larger, more widely spaced typeface. As Crawford, Parker and Besson (1988) have noted, this would also serve to reduce attentional demands and would therefore be more in keeping with the test's aim of tapping previous word knowledge while minimising the demands on current cognitive capacity.

As with all currently available methods of estimation premorbid IQ, NART equations can only validly be used in their country of origin (the UK in the case of the NART). However, a study is currently underway to build equations for prediction of WAIS-R IQ in a Canadian sample (Ronan O'Carroll, personal communication). The results of UK research on the NART have been encouraging enough to justify building equations for use in other populations (e.g. the United States). Whether such attempts should use the same stimulus words or simply follow the general principles (i.e. employ short, irregular words) is a question best answered by local researchers. It will of course be impossible to develop an equivalent to the NART in languages (e.g. Italian) where there is a virtual absence of irregular words.

The most pressing research need is for a series of studies employing discriminant function analysis to compare a range of clinical conditions with controls. Such studies could determine the extent to which the NART improves discrimination between impaired and non-impaired subjects over the use of the WAIS alone, and determine in which clinical conditions the NART has maximum utility. They could also determine which of the three possible NART/WAIS comparisons (i.e. NART estimated FSIQ with obtained FSIQ, NART estimated VIQ with obtained VIQ etc.) achieves the maximum discrimination. As noted, the NART is a fairly poor predictor of PIQ. However, PIQ is commonly more sensitive to generalised dysfunction. The greater sensitivity of PIQ may therefore compensate for the poorer predictive ability of the relevant NART equation.

To date, all research on the NART has been conducted using the Wechsler scales as the criterion IQ measure. However, NART equations could be generated to estimate premorbid performance on a variety of other cognitive tests. A particularly good candidate for a criterion test would be the Raven's Progressive Matrices (Raven, 1982). Like Wechsler's PIQ, the Raven's is sensitive to impairment. However, it could be argued that, unlike the disappointing results with PIQ, NART equations will be capable of predicting a very substantial proportion of Raven's variance. In common with the NART, factor analytic studies of the Raven's have demonstrated that it has a very high loading on 'g' (e.g. Vernon, 1983). Further support for this suggestion comes from Ruddle and Bradshaw's (1982) demonstration that Schonell performance and age predicted 67% of Raven's variance in a sample of 78 healthy subjects (age was included in the equation because Raven's scores were not age-corrected). Pairing the Raven's and the NART is liable to create a very useful means of detecting cognitive impairment as it comes close to the ideal set of predictor and criterion variables; i.e. a sensitive criterion measure and a powerful but insensitive predictor.

ESTIMATING PREMORBID IQ WITH DEMOGRAPHIC VARIABLES

As already noted, a number of demographic variables have a reasonably strong relationship with measured IQ (Matarazzo, 1972). In attempting to identify intellectual impairment, clinicians examine IQ test performance to determine if it is consistent with a client's educational and occupational history. Wilson et al. (1978) attempted to make this process more systematic and objective by building regression equations to predict premorbid WAIS IQ from demographic variables. Using the WAIS (Wechsler, 1955) standardisation sample (n=1,700) they regressed WAIS FSIQ, VIQ and

PIQ on age, sex, race, education and occupation using a stepwise procedure. Education was the single best predictor of IQ for all the WAIS scales, although all three remaining demographic variables significantly improved predictive accuracy at subsequent steps of the analysis. The equations generated by this procedure predicted 54%, 53% and 42% of the variance in WAIS FSIQ, VIQ and PIQ respectively. Following publication of Wilson et al.'s study their equations have been used for a number of research purposes, e.g. as a means of determining the premorbid comparability of clinical groups (e.g. Bayles & Tomoeda, 1983; Weingartner, 1983) as a variable in the prediction of outcome in head-injured patients (Williams et al., 1984) and as a means of assessing the degree of intellectual deterioration (e.g. Hamsher & Roberts, 1985).

As demographic equations employ multiple predictor variables, the need to examine their predictive ability in cross-validation samples assumes an even greater importance than it does in the psychometric approach (where single predictors are used). Klesges, Sanchez and Stanton (1981) examined the correlations between demographically predicted IQ and obtained WAIS IQ in two 'neurologically unimpaired' clinical samples (an inpatient sample of 63, and an outpatient sample of 106). They reported highly significant correlations between predicted and obtained IQ in both groups. However, the proportion of IQ variance predicted was fairly low, i.e. 41% in the inpatient sample and 25% in the outpatient sample. These authors also reported that the equations significantly overestimated IQ in both samples and viewed this result as 'potentially discouraging' (p14). In a further study, Klesges et al. (1985) examined the relationship between demographically predicted IQ and obtained IQ in two groups of subjects referred for neuropsychological testing. One of these groups (n=125) had positive evidence of pathology on CAT scan the other (the 'normal' group) did not. These authors reported a non-significant correlation (0.15) between predicted and obtained FSIQ in the normal group (n= 73) and again found that the demographic equation significantly overestimated obtained IQ. Bolter et al. (1982) examined the correlation between predicted and obtained FSIQ in head injured patients at two test periods. Patients were divided into two groups on the basis of whether neuropsychological test results at second testing indicated that they had recovered (n=11) or were still impaired (n=11). A 'control' group of 'pseudoneurological' patients (n=24) was also examined. The correlations between predicted and obtained FSIQ in these groups ranged between 0.68 and 0.73. However, Bolter et al. reported that the demographic estimate misclassified the obtained IQ in a substantial proportion of patients (a misclassification was considered to have ocurred when the predicted IQ differed from obtained IQ by more than one standard error of estimate). They concluded that their study had 'revealed inadequacies in predicting premorbid IQs with the Wilson et al. (1978) equation among head trauma patients' (p174). A second study by this group (Gouvier et al., 1983) examined the same issues with the same patients but reported comparisons between predicted and obtained VIQ and PIQ (rather than FSIQ). Essentially similar results were obtained.

It is clear from the commentary of the above authors that they consider their results cast doubt on the validity of the demographic approach. It will be argued here that such a conclusion is unwarranted. In the present authors' view, an attempt to cross-validate Wilson et al's equation (or indeed cross-validate any method of estimating premorbid IQ) should have the following characteristics. Firstly, the sample should be of a reasonable size, otherwise misleadingly high or low correlations could easily be obtained by chance. This is particularly important in the case of the demographic method as it employs multiple predictor variables. The small sample sizes in the Gouvier et al. and Bolter et al. studies render it necessary to interpret their results with considerable caution. Secondly, the samples should reflect as much as possible the range in predictor and criterion variables observed in the general population. If the range of these variables is restricted, spuriously low estimates of the population correlation between predicted and obtained IQ will result. All of the above studies have problems in this regard. Thirdly, it would appear to be necessary to stress that the purpose of demographic equations is not to estimate the <u>current</u> IQ scores of clinical subjects but to estimate their <u>premorbid</u> IQ; i.e. the IQ level that would have been obtained had they not developed neurological or psychiatric disorder. As it is clearly impossible to compare estimates of premorbid IQ with the true premorbid IQ in clinical subjects (except in the very rare situation where previous test results are available) cross-validation should be carried out with healthy, normal subjects.

The major methodological problem with the studies reviewed above is their reliance on clinical cross-validation samples. The presence of intellectually impaired subjects in these samples cannot be ruled out and is in fact likely. All subjects were referred for neuropsychological assessment, presumably because there was reason to suspect cognitive deficits. Furthermore, in Klesges, Sanchez and Stanton's (1981) study a substantial proportion of subjects were schizophrenic. There is considerable evidence that schizophrenic illness (and anti-psychotic medication) is associated with intellectual impairment (e.g. see Aylward, Walker & Bettes, 1984). In Klesges et al. (1985) the normal group consisted of patients in whom CAT scanning had failed to detect cerebral lesions. However, a negative CAT scan can neither rule out the presence of cognitive impairment nor the presence of non-structural abnormalities which could produce such impairment. In fact, CAT scanning is not even a particularly sensitive means of detecting structural lesions. Where it has been compared with magnetic resonnance imaging it has commonly failed to detect lesions clearly visible with the latter technique (e.g. see Wiedmann & Wilson, this volume).

Perhaps the strongest grounds for concluding that many of the subjects in the above studies were intellectually impaired comes from simply examining the mean IQ scores. There are fairly compelling reasons to believe that the WAIS overestimates IQ in the contemporary US population by around 8 IQ points (see Flynn, 1984; 1986). If one takes a figure of 108 as an estimate of the population mean score on the WAIS, then the outpatient sample examined by Klesges, Sanchez & Stanton (1981) is around 1.5 standard deviation units below the population mean while the out-patient sample, and the sample examined by Klesges et al. (1985), is around 0.5 of a standard deviation unit below the mean. The presence of intellectually impaired subjects in a cross-validation sample would have two effects. Firstly, the correlation between estimated and current IQ would tend to be weaker than that obtained in the standardisation sample; current IQ would reflect not only variance associated with premorbid level but also variance arising from differences in the severity of impairment. Secondly, the demographic estimate of IQ would be higher than the IQ obtained by testing. It will be noted that this is exactly the pattern of results observed in the above studies. As it is impossible to determine whether such results reflect shortcomings of the demographic method or shortcomings of the samples, it can be concluded that these studies are of little value in assessing the predictive power and accuracy of the demographic method.

Fortunately, however, a large scale, methodologically sound, cross-validation study has been carried out by Karzmak et al. (1985). These authors compared demographically estimated IQ with obtained IQ in a sample of 491 healthy, normal subjects. Mean predicted FSIQ corresponded reasonably closely to obtained FSIQ (110.9 vs. 112.8). However, as one

would expect given the nature of regression, the lowest predicted IQs (<
90) were overestimates of obtained IQ and the highest predicted IQs ($\geq$
130) were underestimates. Karzmak et al. presented the mean differences
between predicted and obtained IQ at these levels and suggested they be
used to adjust the former (e.g. if the predicted IQ was $\geq$130 this would
be adjusted to 137).

Because of the low face validity of Wechsler's (1955) classification
system for occupation, Karzmak et al. recoded their subjects' occupation
using more sophisticated classification systems. Interestingly, when
these methods were substituted for Wechsler's in the regression runs,
there was a decrement in predicted variance. Although these methods were
more highly correlated with IQ than Wechsler's method, they also shared
more variance with education and therefore predicted less unique IQ variance. Although Karzmak et al.'s results were generally supportive of the
demographic equation they found that there was a shrinkage of 12% in predicted IQ variance; in the WAIS standardisation sample the equation predicted 54% of FSIQ variance whereas it predicted only 42% in the cross-
validation sample. As the authors note, this is not surprising given the
considerable number of intervening years between the testing of the
samples. During this time, one would expect there to have been some
changes in the inter-relationships between the predictor variables and
IQ.

In a further cross-validation study Goldstein, Gary and Levin (1986)
employed a variety of regression procedures to evaluate Wilson et al.'s
equations. The sample in this study consisted of patients referred for
neuropsychological or psychological/personality assessment (although
fairly rigorous attempts were made to exclude subjects liable to be
intellectually impaired). The range in predictor variables was also somewhat restricted. These characteristics of the sample are likely to produce results which underestimate the predictive accuracy of the demographic method. However, despite this, Goldstein, Gary and Levin concluded that the equations 'provided an adequate overall fit' to the subjects' IQ data.

Two studies have sought to determine whether Wilson et al.'s equations can aid discrimination between neurological and non-neurological
cases. Wilson, Rosenbaum and Brown (1979) examined the ability of
Wechsler's (1958) deterioration quotient to correctly classify patients
into neurological or non-neurological categories. The non-neurological
group comprised of healthy, normal subjects, schizophrenics and 'pseudoneurological' patients. An initial correct classification rate of 63.2%
was obtained. A second discriminant function analysis was performed in
which all subjects were randomly assigned to two groups. Cut-off scores
were derived from the first subsample and used to classify the second
sample and vice-versa. This resulted in a correct classification rate of
61.8%. Wilson, Rosenbaum and Brown then repeated the above procedures
with demographically estimated FSIQ substituted for Wechsler's 'Hold'
subtests. The correct classification rate was 71.8% on the first discriminant run and 72.8% on the second. This represents a gain over the deterioration quotient of 8.6% and 11% respectively. The authors noted that
the equations were particularly effective in reducing the rate of false-
positive errors (i.e. non-neurological patients incorrectly classified as
neurological).

In contrast to these moderately encouraging results, negative findings were reported in the previously discussed study by Klesges et al.
(1985). These authors calculated the discrepancy between demographically
estimated IQ and obtained IQ for each of their subjects. As previously
noted, the majority of these subjects had positive evidence of lesions on

CAT scan, the remainder did not. The biserial correlation coefficient between the presence or absence of identifiable lesions and the FSIQ discrepancy score was non-significant. In contrast, a low but significant correlation (0.21) was obtained with FSIQ scores. Although the methodological problems associated with this study would bias the outcome towards negative results, this finding nevertheless cast doubt on the utility of the Wilson et al. equations. The ability of the demographic method to aid in discriminating neurological cases from cases in whom investigations have proved negative is of considerable interest. However, a less ambitious and, it could be argued, more appropriate role for the demographic method is simply to aid in the detection of intellectual impairment. To evaluate the utility of the equations for this more modest purpose requires an unequivocally unimpaired group (i.e. healthy subjects) rather than a group which includes schizophrenics or other clinically referred cases. Unfortunately, studies incorporating such a group have not been conducted.

As Crawford et al. (1987b) have noted, the use of Wilson et al.'s equations are limited to the US as it cannot be assumed that the interrelationships between the predictor variables and IQ are the same in other countries. To the present author's knowledge there has only been one attempt outwith the US to predict premorbid IQ with this method. Crawford et al. (1989c) built demographic regression equations to predict WAIS IQ in the UK population. They administered the WAIS to a sample of 151 non-clinical subjects and recorded their demographic variables (age, sex, education and social class). Goodness of fit tests indicated that the sample was broadly representative of the UK population in terms of age and social class distribution. Using a stepwise procedure, WAIS IQ was regressed on the demographic variables. Crawford et al. reported that these variables predicted 50%, 50% and 30% of the variance in FSIQ, VIQ and PIQ respectively. It would appear, then, that the demographic method is a reasonable predictor of FSIQ and VIQ in the UK. However, it can be seen that the proportion of PIQ variance predicted was unimpressive. It should also be stressed that the predictive ability of these equations has not been investigated in a cross-validation sample.

The moderate success of the WAIS equations has prompted attempts to develop demographic equations for the estimaton of premorbid WAIS-R IQ. Demographic equations have also been developed to estimate premorbid IQ in children, using the Wechsler Intelligence Scale for Children - Revised (Wechsler, 1974) as the criterion measure (Reynolds & Gutkin, 1979). The current review is limited to an evaluation of adult premorbid indices; however, the reader may wish to consult the additional literature on the child equations (Klesges & Sanchez, 1981; Klesges, 1982a; 1982b; Reynolds & Gutkin, 1982).

Demographic Estimation of WAIS-R IQ

Barona & Reynolds (1984) have generated demographic equations from the WAIS-R standardisation sample for the estimation of premorbid WAIS-R IQ. The predictor variables employed were those used in the original WAIS equations (age, sex, race, education and occupation) plus a further three; urban/rural residence, geographical region and handedness. Despite these additional predictor variables, the WAIS-R equations predicted substantially less IQ variance than their WAIS counterparts (36%, 38% and 24% for FSIQ, VIQ and PIQ respectively) and had correspondingly larger standard errors of estimate.

Barona and Chastain (1986) suggested that the deletion of two subgroups from the standardisation sample would permit more accurate demographic estimation of IQ in the remaining subjects. The first subgroup consisted of subjects between 16 and 19 years of age. Occupational classification of these subjects was on the basis of their head of household because they were not yet steadily employed in full-time occupations. The second subgroup consisted of all races other than blacks or whites. Barona and Chastain argued that, because of the very small numbers of such subjects, coding them for inclusion in the analysis would produce meaningless results. Regression equations were generated from the remaining standardisation sample subjects (n=1,433). These equations predicted more IQ variance than the initial WAIS-R equations (43%, 47% and 28% for FSIQ, VIQ, and PIQ respectively) and should therefore be used in preference to the originals.

Studies employing the WAIS-R equations are now beginning to appear in the literature. In a study comparing the neuropsychological test performance of patients with classic and common migraine, Hooker and Raskin (1986) used the FSIQ equation to determine whether the groups were comparable in terms of premorbid IQ. Similarly, Levin et al. (1987) used the equations to compare head-injured samples and healthy controls.

To the present author's knowledge, there has been only one cross-validation study to date. Eppinger et al. (1987) examined demographically predicted WAIS-R IQ and obtained IQ in a sample of 163 patients; 80 patients were 'neurologically normal', the remainder (83) were 'brain-impaired'. These authors used the neurologically normal group to cross-validate Barona, Reynolds and Chastain's equations. Although this was a referred clinical sample, potential subjects were excluded if there was a history of substance abuse or psychotic disorder (presumably to remove patients in whom there was particularly strong grounds to suspect intellectual impairment). Mean estimated FSIQ was significantly higher than obtained IQ although the difference in mean IQs was slight (i.e. 101.5 vs. 98.4). As Eppinger et al. note, this result may have arisen because of mild intellectual deficit in the sample. Encouragingly, the discrepancy between estimated and obtained IQ was within one standard error of estimate in 69% of cases. Examination of the IQ variance predicted by the equations provided further encouraging, if surprising, results. For all three WAIS-R scales, the percentage of predicted variance was considerably larger than that obtained by Barona, Reynolds and Chastain in the standardisation sample (i.e. 58%, 61% and 36% of FSIQ, VIQ and PIQ respectively). To examine the clinical utility of the equations, discrepancy scores (between predicted and obtained IQ) were calculated for all 163 subjects. Mean discrepancy scores in the neurological group were significantly larger (p<0.0001) than in the non-neurological group. Eppinger et al. also conducted a more stringent test of clinical utility by examining whether the discrepancy scores would achieve greater discrimination than the WAIS-R alone. Although the discrepancy scores achieved a modest degree of discrimination (77%, 75% and 77% for FSIQ, VIQ and PIQ respectively), this represented an increase in accuracy of only 5% over the use of IQ scores alone. It is to be expected that further research on the WAIS-R equations will be forthcoming. A comparison of the predictive accuracy and discriminative ability of the original equations with Barona and Chastain's modified versions would be of particular interest.

NART AND DEMOGRAPHIC METHODS COMPARED

On present evidence (albeit very limited) the NART is liable to be a more powerful predictor of IQ test performance than demographic methods; i.e. it will predict more IQ variance and its equations will have smaller standard errors of estimate. A comparison of the two methods using their respective standardisation samples would be inappropriate for a variety of reasons. Firstly, there is a massive disparity in sample sizes. Secondly, the samples were of different nationalities. Thirdly, the NART was standardised with a short-form WAIS. However, the standardisation sample used to generate the UK demographic equations (Crawford et al., 1989c) was also used to cross-validate the NART (Crawford et al., 1989b). It is therefore possible to directly compare the two methods in the same sample. The percentage of predicted WAIS IQ variance and standard errors of estimate for both methods are presented in Table 1. It can be seen from Table 1 that there is little to choose between the two methods in terms of predicting PIQ as both produce fairly disappointing results. However the NART is markedly superior as a predictor of FSIQ and VIQ.

The lesser predictive ability of demographic methods is of course offset by their major advantage; they provide premorbid estimates that are entirely independent of a patient's current cognitive status. There-fore, unlike the NART, there is no danger of the premorbid estimates being subject to decline. The demographic method can also be used with patients for whom the NART would be inappropriate (e.g. dyslexic pati-ents). A final judgement on the relative clinical utility of the two methods must await future research. Studies directly comparing the ability of the two methods (when paired with current IQ measures) to discriminate between impaired and healthy subjects would clearly be very informative. At the present time, a sensible course would be to use both methods in clinical decision-making as neither are very time-consuming.

COMBINING PSYCHOMETRIC AND DEMOGRAPHIC APPROACHES

In a recent study, Crawford et al. (1989e) built a multiple regres-sion equation to predict WAIS IQ from the NART and demographic variables in the previously discussed sample of 151 non-clinical subjects. Their aim was to determine whether combining the psychometric and demographic approaches would predict more IQ variance than either method alone. In a previous study, Crawford et al. (1988b) demonstrated that there is con-siderable covariance between the NART and demographic variables (i.e. education, social class). Clearly, then, combining these variables will not have an additive effect on predicted IQ variance. However, Crawford et al. (1989e) hypothesised that a cumulative effect would be observed in that (1) unshared variance in the psychometric and demographic variables may still relate to IQ and (2) demographic variables may mediate the rel-ationship between the NART and IQ.

WAIS IQ was regressed on the NART and demographic variables (age,

TABLE 1

Percentage of WAIS IQ variance predicted by the NART
and the demographic method in a sample of 151 healthy subjects

	Full Scale IQ	Verbal IQ	Performance IQ
NART	66 (7.4)	72 (7.5)	33 (9.5)
Demographic equations	50 (9.1)	50 (10.2)	30 (9.8)

Note: standard error of estimate in parenthesis

sex, social class, and education) in a stepwise procedure. For all three WAIS scales, NART errors was the best predictor of IQ. All the demographic variables (except education) significantly increased predicted variance at subsequent steps. The resulting equations predicted 73%, 78% and 39% of the variance in FSIQ, VIQ and PIQ respectively. These figures compare very favourably with the results for either the NART or demographic methods alone (see Table 1). Although these equations have not been cross-validated the present results suggest that the combined method has considerable potential. The present author and his colleagues are currently developing similar equations to predict WAIS-R IQ.

CONCLUSIONS

In view of the considerable importance of premorbid IQ as a variable in neuropsychological research and practice there is a continuing need for research on this topic. However, it is clear that there has already been a number of significant developments in the field in recent years. We no longer need resort to purely subjective estimation from demographic variables nor to examination of the unsatisfactory 'Hold' subtests of the Wechsler scales. The more recent regression-based methods reviewed above are, of course, not without their own problems. In applying these methods in a clinical setting, it must be borne in mind that the estimates they provide are subject to a wide band of error (particularly in the case of the demographic approach). Furthermore, clinical judgement must be exercised to assess the appropriateness or likely accuracy of premorbid estimates in the individual case. For example, when using the demographic method, years of education should not be blindly entered into the equation as many atypical cases will be encountered (e.g. a proportion of a client's years of education may have been acquired because poor academic performance necessitated repeating years of schooling). Finally, although premorbid estimates constitute an important source of information in the neuropsychological assessment process, they are clearly only one of many sources that must be considered if this process is to be adequately performed.

REFERENCES

Acker, C., Jacobson, R.R. & Lishman, W.A. (1987). Memory and ventricular size in alcoholics. Psychological Medicine, 17, 343-348.
Aylward, E., Walker, E., & Bettes, B. (1984). Intelligence in schizophrenia: meta-analysis of the research. Schizophrenia Bulletin, 10, 430-459.
Barona, A., Reynolds, C.R. & Chastain, R. (1984). A demographically based index of premorbid intelligence for the WAIS-R. Journal of Consulting and Clinical Psychology, 52, 885-887.
Barona, A. and Chastain, R.L. (1986). An improved estimate of premorbid IQ for blacks and whites on the WAIS-R. International Journal of Clinical Neuropsychology, 8, 169-173.
Bayles, K.A. & Tomoeda, C.K. (1983). Confrontation naming impairment in dementia. Brain and Language, 19, 98-114.
Binks, M.G. & Davies, A.D.M. (1984). The early detection of dementia: a baseline from healthy community dwelling old people. in: D.B. Bromley (ed.). Gerontology: Social and Behavioural Perspectives. London: Croom Helm.
Bolter, J., Gouvier, W., Veneklasen, J. & Long, C.J. (1982). Using demographic information to predict premorbid IQ: a test of clinical validity with head trauma patients. Clinical Neuropsychology, 4, 171-174.
Brayne, C. & Bearsdell, L. Estimation of verbal intelligence in an

elderly community: an epidemiological study using NART. Submitted for publication.

Crawford, J.R., Allan, K.M., Besson, J.A.O., Cochrane, R.H.B. & Stewart, L.E. A comparison of the WAIS and WAIS-R in matched UK samples. Submitted for publication.

Crawford, J.R., Allan, K.M., Stephen, D.W., Parker, D.M. & Besson, J.A.O. (1989a). The Wechsler Adult Intelligence Scale - Revised (WAIS-R): factor structure in a UK sample. Personality and Individual Differences, in press.

Crawford, J.R., Besson, J.A.O. & Parker, D.M. (1988). Estimation of premorbid intelligence in organic conditions. British Journal of Psychiatry, 153, 178-181.

Crawford, J.R., Besson, J.A.O., Parker, D.M., Sutherland, K.M. & Keen, P.L. (1987a). Estimation of premorbid intellectual status in depression. British Journal of Clinical Psychology, 26, 313-314.

Crawford, J.R., Parker, D.M., Stewart, L.E., Besson, J.A.O. & De Lacey, G. (1989b). Prediction of WAIS IQ with the National Adult Reading Test: cross-validation and extension. British Journal of Clinical Psychology, 28, in press.

Crawford, J.R., Stewart, L., Calder, S., Ebmeier, K., Mutch, W., Besson, J. (1988a). Estimation of premorbid intelligence in idiopathic Parkinson's disease. 9th International Symposium on Parkinson's Disease. Israel, Book of Abstracts, 9.

Crawford, J.R., Stewart, L.E., Cochrane, R.H.B., Foulds, J. & Besson, J.A.O. (1987b). Predicting premorbid IQ from demographic variables: provisional results in a UK sample. British Journal of Clinical and Social Psychiatry, 5, 122-123.

Crawford, J.R., Stewart, L.E., Cochrane, R.H.B., Foulds, J.A., Besson, J.A.O. & Parker, D.M. (1989c). Predicting premorbid IQ from demographic variables: regression equations derived from a UK sample. British Journal of Clinical Psychology, in press.

Crawford, J.R., Stewart, L.E., Cochrane, R.H.B., Parker, D.M. & Besson, J.A.O. (1989d). Construct validity of the National Adult Reading Test: a factor analytic study. Personality and Individual Differences, in press.

Crawford, J.R., Stewart, L.E., Garthwaite, P.H., Parker, D.M. & Besson, J.A.O. (1988b). The relationship between demographic variables and NART performance in normal subjects. British Journal of Clinical Psychology, 27, 181-182.

Crawford, J.R., Stewart, L.E., Parker, D.M., Besson, J.A.O. & Cochrane, R.H.B. (1989e). Estimation of premorbid intelligence: combining psychometric and demographic approaches improves predictive accuracy. Personality and Individual Differences, in press.

Eppinger, M.G., Craig, P.L., Adams, R.L. & Parsons, O.A. (1987). The WAIS-R index for estimating premorbid intelligence: cross-validation and clinical utility. Journal of Consulting and Clinical Psychology, 55, 86-90.

Flynn, J.R. (1984). The mean IQ of Americans: massive gains 1932 to 1978. Psychological Bulletin, 95, 29-51.

Flynn, J.R. (1987). Massive IQ gains in 14 nations: what IQ tests really measure. Psychological Bulletin, 101, 171-191.

Folstein, M.F., Folstein, S.E. & McHugh, P.R. (1975). 'Mini-mental state': a practical method for grading the cognitive state of patients for the clinician. Journal of Psychiatric Research, 12, 189-198.

Goldstein, F.C., Gary, H.E. & Levin, H.S. (1986). Assessment of the accuracy of regression equations proposed for estimating premorbid intellectual functioning on the Wechsler Adult Intelligence Scale. Journal of Clinical and Experimental Neuropsychology, 8, 405-412.

Gouvier, W.D., Bolter, J.F., Veneklasen, J.A. & Long, C.J. (1983). Predicting verbal and performance IQ from demographic data: further findings with head trauma patients. Clinical Neuropsychology, 5, 119–121.

Halstead, W.C. (1947). Brain and Intelligence: A Quantitative Study of the Frontal Lobes. Chicago: University of Chicago Press.

Hamsher, K. deS. & Roberts, R.(1985). Memory for recent US Presidents in patients with cerebral disease. Journal of Clinical and Experimental Neuropsychology, 7, 1–13.

Hart, S., Smith, C.M. & Swash, M. (1986). Assessing intellectual deterioration. British Journal of Clinical Psychology, 25, 119–124.

Hooker, W.D., & Raskin, N.H. (1986). Neuropsychologic alterations in classic and common migraine. Archives of Neurology, 43, 709–712.

Karzmak, P. Heaton, R.K., Grant, I. & Matthews, C.G. (1985). Use of demographic variables to predict full scale IQ: a replication and extension. Journal of Clinical and Experimental Neuropsychology, 7, 412–420.

Klesges, R.C. (1982). Establishing premorbid levels of intellectual functioning in children: an empirical investigation. Clinical Neuropsychology, 4, 15–17.

Klesges, R.C. (1982). Confusing clinical and statistical significance? A reply to Reynolds and Gutkin. Journal of Consulting and Clinical Psychology, 50, 772–774.

Klesges, R.C., Fisher, L., Vasey, M. & Pheley, A. (1985). Predicting adult premorbid functioning levels: another look. International Journal of Clinical Neuropsychology, 7, 1–3.

Klesges, R.C., Sanchez, V.C. & Stanton, A.L. (1981). Cross validation of an adult premorbid functioning index. Clinical Neuropsychology, 3, 13–15.

Kleges, R.C., Wilkening, G.N., & Golden, C.J. (1981). Premorbid indices of intelligence: a review. Clinical Neuropsychology, 3, 32–39.

Kopelman, M.D. (1985). Multiple memory deficits in Alzheimer-type dementia: implications for pharmacotherapy. Psychological Medicine, 15, 527–541.

Kopelman, M.D. (1986). Clinical tests of memory. British Journal of Psychiatry, 148, 517–525.

Lea, M. (1986). A British Supplement to the Manual for the Wechsler Adult Intelligence Scale – Revised. San Antonio: Psychological Corporation.

Leckliter, I.N., Matarazzo, J.D. & Silverstein, A.B. (1986). A literature review of factor analytic stdies of the WAIS-R. Journal of Clinical Psychology, 42, 332–342.

Levin, H.S., Mattis, S., Ruff, R.M., Eisenberg, H.M., Marshall, L.F., Tabaddor, K., High, W.M. & Frankowski, R.F. (1987). Neurobehavioural outcome following minor head injury. Journal of Neurosurgery, 66, 234–243.

Lezak, M.D. (1983). Neuropsychological Assessment (2nd Edit.). New York: Oxford University Press.

Matarazzo, J.D. (1972). Weschler's Measurement and Appraisal of Adult Intelligence (5th Edit.). Baltimore: Williams & Wilkins.

McCarthy, R., Gresty, M. & Findlay, L.J. (1985). Parkinson's disease and dementia. Lancet, i, 407.

McKenna, P. & Pratt, R.T.C. (1983). The effect of unilateral non-dominant ECT on memory and perceptual functions. British Journal of Psychiatry, 142, 276–279.

Nebes, R.D., Martin, D.C. & Horn, L.C. (1984). Sparing of semantic memory in Alzheimer's disease. Journal of Abnormal Psychology, 93, 321–330.

Nelson, H.E. (1982). National Adult Reading Test (NART): Test Manual. Windsor: NFER Nelson.

Nelson, H.E. & McKenna, P. (1975). The use of current reading ability in the assessment of dementia. British Journal of Social and Clinical Psychology, 14, 259–267.

Nelson, H.E. & O'Connell, A. (1978). Dementia: the estimation of premorbid intelligence levels using the new adult reading test. Cortex, 14, 234-244.

O'Carroll, R.E. (1987). The inter-rater reliability of the National Adult Reading Test (NART): a pilot study. British Journal of Clinical Psychology, 26, 229-230.

O'Carroll, R.E., Baikie, E.M. & Whittick, J.E. (1987). Does the National Adult Reading Test hold in dementia? British Journal of Clinical Psychology, 26, 315-316.

O'Carroll, R.E. & Gilleard, C.J. (1986). Estimation of premorbid intelligence in dementia. British Journal of Clinical Psychology, 25, 157-158.

Oyebode, J.R., Barker, W.A., Blessed, G., Dick, D.J. & Britton, P.G. (1986). Cognitive functioning in Parkinson's disease: in relation to prevalence of dementia and psychiatric diagnosis. British Journal of Psychiatry, 149, 720-725.

Pedhazur, E.J. (1982). Multiple Regression in Behavioural Research, Explanation and Prediction (2nd Edit.). New York: Holt, Rinehart & Winston.

Raven, J.C. (1982). Revised Manual for Raven's Progressive Matrices and Vocabulary Scale. Windsor: NFER Nelson.

Reynolds, C.R. & Gutkin, T.B. (1979). Predicting the premorbid intellectual status of children using demographic data. Clinical Neuropsychology, 1, 36-38.

Reynolds, C.R. & Gutkin, T.B. (1982). Clinical samples of children with below average IQs are not 'unimpaired': comment on Klesges and Sanchez. Journal of Consulting and Clinical Psychology, 50, 576-577.

Ruddle, H.B. & Bradshaw, C.M. (1982). On the estimation of premorbid intellectual functioning: a validation of Nelson & McKenna's formula and some new normative data. British Journal of Clinical Psychology, 21, 159-165.

Russell, E.W. (1972). WAIS factor analysis with brain-damaged subjects using criterion variables. Journal of Consulting and Clinical Psychology, 39, 133-139.

Schonell, F. (1942). Backwardness in the Basic Subjects. London: Oliver & Boyd.

Stebbins, G.T., Wilson, R.S., Gilley, D.W., Bernard, B.A. & Fox, J.H. (1988). Estimation of premorbid intelligence in dementia. Journal of Clinical and Experimental Neuropsychology, 10, 63-64.

Swiercinsky, D.P. & Warnock, J.K. (1977). Comparison of the neuropsychological key and discriminant analysis approaches in predicting cerebral damage and localisation. Journal of Consulting and Clinical Psychology, 45, 808-814.

Vernon, P.A. (1983). Speed of information processing and general intelligence. Intelligence, 7, 53-70.

Vogt, A.T. & Heaton, R.K. (1977). Comparison of Wechsler Adult Intelligence Scale indices of cerebral dysfunction. Perceptual and Motor Skills, 45, 607-615.

Wechsler, D. (1955). Manual for the Wechsler Adult Intelligence Scale. New York: Psychological Corporation.

Wechsler, D. (1958). The Measurement and Appraisal of Adult Intelligence (4th Edit.). Baltimore: Williams & Wilkins.

Wechsler, D. (1974). Manual for the Wechsler Intelligence Scale for Children - Revised. New York: Psychological Corporation.

Wechsler, D. (1981). Manual for the Wechsler Adult Intelligence Scale - Revised. New York: Psychological Corporation.

Weingartner, H. (1983). Forms of memory failure. Science, 221, 380-382.

Williams, J.M., Gomes, F., Drudge, O.W. & Kessler, M. (1984). Predicting outcome from closed head injury by early assessment of trauma severity. Journal of Neurosurgery, 61, 581-583.

Wilson, R.S. & Rosenbaum, G. (1979). The problem of premorbid intelligence in neuropsychological assessment. Journal of Clinical Neuropsychology, 1, 49-53.

Wilson, R.S., Rosenbaum, G., Brown, G., Rourke, D., Whitman, D. & Grisell, J. (1978). An index of premorbid intelligence. Journal of Consulting and Clinical Psychology, 46, 1554–1555.

LANGUAGE IN DEMENTIA OF THE ALZHEIMER TYPE

Edgar Miller

INTRODUCTION

In reviewing the psychological research into dementia a little over a decade ago it was evident that most of the systematic work had been directed at examining the memory impairment (Miller, 1977). There was then very little work directed at any other psychological functions. Since that time the psychological literature relating to dementia, and Alzheimer type dementia in particular, has increased considerably. Not only has it grown in volume but it has also extended much more deeply into other functions aside from memory. The purpose of this review is to consider what has been achieved in exploring the nature of language impairment in Alzheimer type dementia.

Almost all authorities who have written on Alzheimer's disease agree that people with this disorder will exhibit some impairment in language in the course of the disease. Although decline in memory is typically the first manifestation of early dementia to be noticed, there are cases where apparent dysphasia is the presenting sign (Wechsler, 1977). The question of interest is therefore not whether language impairments exist, since the evidence is overwhelmingly in favour of this assumption, but their nature or characteristics.

Before moving to consider the evidence in any detail some preliminary points need to be made. Firstly, the concern is with Alzheimer type dementia but Alzheimer's disease is a diagnosis that can only be made with any certainty at autopsy. This means that in life a diagnosis can only be presumptive. On top of this, not all studies make use of criteria for the selection of subjects that could be regarded as the most optimal. In the investigations to be considered here the diagnostic accuracy cannot therefore be considered to be anything approaching perfection. For present purposes the term 'dementia' as used below will refer to subjects who seem to have been selected with a view to being cases of the Alzheimer type of dementia although the degree to which this selection can be considered satisfactory varies from study to study.

Secondly, it is probably naive to assume that dementia (even of the Alzheimer type) produces a single type of impairment in language. The disturbance in language varies during the course of the illness. The first manifestation is most commonly a mild impoverishment of speech and the language impairment will gradually progress until it becomes a total, or near total loss of communicative ability in the final stages. It is also possible that there may be variations in the pattern of language impairment even across cases at the same stage of the illness. Age of onset of the disorder could well be a relevant variable in determining the degree or nature of the language impairment (Seltzer & Sherwin,

1983). With very few exceptions, such sources of variation have not been taken into account in the work that has been published so far.

Thirdly, it is difficult to say where language ends and other functions begin and this is complicated by the fact that the same or very similar test procedures can often be used with different goals in mind. For example, tests of verbal fluency have been used both as a means of studying language (e.g. Miller & Hague, 1975) and as ways of tapping semantic memory (e.g. Ober et al., 1986). For the most part this review has been conservative and only considered work from investigations that have been explicitly directed at language functioning. No attempt has been made to include work overtly concerned with other psychological processes but which might be interpreted as having implications for language as well.

Finally, the approach taken to the study of language in dementia has been relatively atheoretical in that it has centred around a number of investigative procedures rather than being driven by particular psycholinguistic theories. This review will follow in this tradition and present the material in terms of the type of test or methodology primarily employed. In doing so no assumptions are being made as to this being the ideal way to consider language impairment in dementia or that the various headings used will comprehensively cover the whole range of linguistic behaviour.

USE OF APHASIA BATTERIES

One common approach has been to use batteries of tests which are either specifically designed, or similar to, those used to investigate and classify patients with aphasia due to focal lesions. Possibly the first investigation of this type was that of Ernst et al. (1970) who applied the system of examination pioneered by the well-known Russian neuropsychologist, A.R. Luria. They were able to identify no clear cut pattern of aphasia in their demented subjects. However, they felt that all showed poverty of vocabulary in narrative speech and many had difficulties in naming. These conclusions do not fit in with most other investigations of this type but might be explicable on the basis of Ernst et al. using rather early cases or a system of examination which does not force all manifestations of language impairment into one or other of the possible categories of aphasia.

The most common outcome has been for demented subjects to be claimed to exhibit the pattern of language malfunctioning typical of transcortical sensory aphasia. This conclusion was reached by both Cummings et al. (1985) and Murdoch et al. (1987) using different batteries of tests. In a series of reports, Kertesz and his colleagues (e.g. Appell et al., 1982; Kertesz et al., 1986) used the Western Aphasia Battery with demented patients. They agreed with Cummings et al. (1985) in regarding all their subjects as having some degree of language impairment with word fluency being the particular subtest which discriminated best between demented and normal subjects. The most common of the aphasia patterns that they observed were the more posterior types being transcortical sensory, Wernicke's and global aphasia. The more anterior forms of aphasia, i.e. transcortical motor and Broca's aphasias, were much less frequently encountered. This group were also concerned to examine the progression in the type of language impairment with increasing severity of dementia. The sequence they suggested is that dementia starts with anomia and then moves through transcortical sensory and Wernicke's aphasias before eventually arriving at global aphasia. Whilst these conclusions from the Kertesz group are interesting it should be noted

76

that the whole edifice is built on only 25 cases with differing lengths of illness in a cross-sectional study.

Studies of this type lead to a number of conclusions. These are that the most commonly reported aphasia patterns are those of the more posterior forms of aphasia, especially transcortical sensory aphasia. In addition many of these reports have also stressed that demented subjects have particular difficulties with naming and word fluency. These two latter aspects of language will be dealt with in the next two sections. In a very similar kind of study to that described in this section, Bayles (1982) also reached the conclusion that it was the semantic aspects of language that were most affected with the phonolgical and syntactical aspects being relatively well preserved. This is a theme that will also be encountered later.

The major problem with this group of studies is that, for the most part, they tend to beg the question. Many of the aphasia batteries used will tend to force any subject with some form of language impairment into one of the categories of aphasia that the battery is designed to assess. As indicated already, it could be because the method of assessment used by Ernst et al. (1970) was less likely to force the issue in this way that resulted in their report being the one that found no clear pattern of aphasia in demented subjects. In this respect it can also be noted that some studies that have specifically compared demented subjects with those suffering from aphasia due to focal lesions have found differences between the two (e.g. Rochford, 1971; Schwartz et al., 1979).

NAMING

Naming is probably the most commonly encountered language impairment, both in dementia and in subjects with aphasia due to focal lesions. However, the basis of the naming problem in dementia has been in dispute with some making claims that would deny that it is a reflection of a genuine linguistic impairment.

Stengel (1964) was one of the first to report detailed clinical observations of naming in demented subjects. According to Stengel the errors shown by those with dementia were not the same as those exhibited by subjects with aphasia due to focal lesions. The truly aphasic patients gave the impression of knowing what the object was but being unable to provide the name. In contrast the errors made by demented patients appeared to be the consequence of misperceiving the nature of the object.

This conclusions was followed up more systematically by Rochford (1971) who studied naming in samples of elderly demented subjects and those with aphasia due to focal lesions (the latter also being younger than the former). Analysing the errors in naming led Rochford to a similar conclusion to that offered by Stengel (1964). Moving on from this, Rochford argued that a naming task which reduced any difficulties in identifying the object to be named should have a beneficial effect on the naming of demented subjects but make little or no difference to those with aphasia. Using parts of the body as the easily recognised stimuli, Rochford confirmed his prediction.

Other experiments have yielded results in agreement with the views of Stengel and Rochford. For example, Kirschner et al. (1984) varied the perceptual difficulty involved in identifying the objects to be named. He used the actual objects themselves, photographs, line drawings, etc., with the assumption that they represented a progression in the ease of identification. This manipulation of perceptual difficulty affected the naming of their demented subjects in the expected way.

The evidence considered so far strongly suggests that there is a perceptual element in the naming disorder. Equally there is evidence that is difficult to reconcile with the idea that perceptual difficulties can account for all of the problem in naming. Others have also examined the kinds of error made by demented patients on naming tasks and contradicted Stengel and Rochford by suggesting that these were mainly semantic in nature rather than being explicable on the basis of perceptual difficulties (e.g. Bayles & Tomoeda, 1983; Martin & Fedio, 1983). However, as Huff et al. (1986) have pointed out, evidence based on the analysis of errors is not wholly convincing because errors can be difficult to interpret. For example, if the subject is shown a picture of a donkey and then says 'horse' does this indicate a perceptual or a semantic error?

More impressive evidence of findings difficult to fit into a perceptual hypothesis is easy to find. In a set of studies of naming Barker and Lawson (1968) and Lawson and Barker (1968) showed that demented subjects were not only much less accurate in naming objects than controls but were also worse at naming when the word concerned was less frequently encountered in the language. A similar finding has since been reported by Skelton-Robinson and Jones (1984). This word frequency effect on naming is difficult to account for on a purely perceptual basis unless it is further assumed that pictures of objects with the more rarely encountered names are also more difficult to perceive. In a rather different kind of study, Huff et al. (1986) first used a test of visual discrimination and retained for the second part of the study only those demented subjects who scored within the normal range on this test. Examining the naming of this restricted group with normal perceptual ability still revealed clear evidence of a naming impairment.

Further information about the basis of the naming difficulty has come from Schwartz et al. (1979) and Williams et al. (1987) who have both carried out very similar experiments. The subject is shown a picture and has to select the word that goes with the picture from a set of alternatives. In addition to the correct word, this set of alternatives includes distractors which are both semantically and phonologically related to the correct name, as well as unrelated words. Both of these experiments agree in showing that when errors do occur the demented subject shows a strong tendency to opt for the semantically related word. Schwartz et al. (1979) was in fact a detailed study of a single case and they also show how their subject with Alzheimer type dementia used the word 'dog' to apply to cats as well. This seems to be an example of a broadening of semantic boundaries. As indicated by these two experiments, phonology remains intact.

So far investigations of naming indicate that naming breaks down for at least two reasons. In the first place, there is evidence which indicates that perceptual problems may underlie some naming difficulties. On the other hand, perceptual failures cannot provide the whole explanation and it does appear that there is a truly linguistic component as well. To date the indications are that this relates to a breakdown in the semantic aspects of language. Just what is the nature of the semantic breakdown remains to be determined. The clue that comes from Schwartz et al's. (1979) single case study is of a broadening of semantic boundaries but whether this will hold up under further scrutiny remains to be seen.

It is tempting to try to speculate as to the degree to which naming impairments are due to truly linguistic impairments as opposed to perceptual inadequacies. Martin (1987) has come down very firmly on the side of the semantic breakdown being the most significant. This could be the case for most subjects under most circumstances, but there are objections to making general statements of this kind. It is obvious that if the stimuli to be named are indistinct, or otherwise difficult to identify, then this will increase the relative importance of the perceptual aspect in determining naming errors or failures. It also could well be the case that individuals with dementia may vary in the degree to which they are perceptually or linguistically affected. Some caution is therefore required in trying to determine the relative importance of the two causes of the naming impairment that have been identified so far.

FLUENCY

As noted in an earlier section, subjects with dementia are often impaired on fluency tasks. Here word fluency is being assessed by requiring the subject to provide as many words as possible from a given category within a set time period. The categories involved can be words beginning with a given letter, classes of objects such as the names of trees or flowers, or even, in one instance, items that can be found in a supermarket. The time interval used is often one minute but may be as long as five minutes. Before going further it should also be noted that impaired word fluency is found in other types of disorder besides dementia, and especially in subjects with lesions in the frontal lobes of the brain (e.g. Miller, 1984a; Milner, 1964).

Rosen (1980) used a number of different fluency tests and confirmed that subjects with dementia are impaired on this type of measure. In addition they showed that their group with dementia were better differentiated from controls where the fluency task used words beginning with a set letter rather than if the words had to belong to categories such as the names of animals. She suggested that this differential effect might occur because the category of 'animals' will break down hierarchically into subgroups like felines, farm animals, and so on, whereas words beginning with a given letter do not subcategorize in a similar way. She then claimed some weak support for this view by examining the way in which the recalled words were distributed over the time span available for their recall.

Ober et al. (1986) also carried out a detailed examination of word fluency. They used words beginning with given letters, words belonging to set categories (like names of animals) and things that could be found in a supermarket. They hypothesized that demented subjects would be selectively impaired in accessing low-dominance semantic category members. For the most part their results gave little support for this hypothesis and what little support there was came from the words recalled in the category of things found in a supermarket. There was not even any evidence that the demented group had a selective difficulty in accessing less frequent words in general. This latter observation fits in with the findings of an earlier study by Miller and Hague (1975) who concluded that there was no selective loss of access to rarer words; it was just that all words appeared to be less accessible.

One study looking at fluency in dementia has, amongst other things, produced results which raise an important underlying issue for the study of fluency and, by implication, of other aspects of language in dementia. Miller (1984a) used a version of the word fluency task (producing as many words as possible in one minute beginning with each of the letters F, A and S). Fluency as measured in this way was appreciably lowered as compared to control subjects in both demented subjects and those with frontal lesions of the brain. However, a measure of verbal intelligence was also applied to all subjects. Using the relationship between the measure of intelligence and fluency in the control group, it was then possible to re-examine the other groups to see whether their fluency score was reduced as compared with that expected on the basis of their verbal intelligence. For subjects with frontal lesions fluency still seemed impaired. In the case of the group with dementia, the fluency scores were not any lower than would have been predicated on the basis of their verbal intelligence.

This finding has certain possible implications. If intelligence is regarded as an overriding, superordinate capacity then it is possible to just see impaired fluency (and possibly other language impairments in dementia as well) as merely being a manifestation of a decline in general intelligence. It might be argued that no other explanation is then required. On the other hand, if a more fragmented view of intelligence is taken with it reflecting a number of discrete functions which just happen to correlate to a modest degree, then some other explanation is required. There is, as yet, very little indication of what such an explanation might be. All that is established is that fluency declines and in line with the decline in verbal intelligence.

COMPREHENSION

There has been very little work on comprehension in aphasia. The studies which have used aphasia batteries (as described in an earlier section) and which have concluded that those suffering from dementia commonly show the more posterior forms of aphasia imply that there is a comprehension difficulty. One of the best established tests of comprehension is the Token Test (De Renzi & Vignolo, 1962) and the present writer has used this in an unsystematic way in examining patients with dementia. These certainly do not do well on this test. The difficulty is that poor memory might also affect performance on the Token Test. In addition, it is difficult to distinguish between lack of verbal comprehension and general intellectual decline.

Schwartz et al. (1979) have described one of the very few studies of comprehension in dementia. Their single subject was compared with three cases of Broca's aphasia (due to focal lesions) on a task in which subjects had to select the picture which best illustrated a sentence. The Broca's aphasics managed quite well with sentences where purely lexical information without lexical cues were adequate (e.g. 'boy eats apple') because once the words are correctly identified the boy has to be eating the apple rather than the apple eating the boy. The aphasic subjects had difficulty where syntax was also important in determining meaning, thus responding to a sentence such as 'boy helps girl' by often selecting a picture showing the girl helping the boy. In contrast, the demented subject tended to show the reverse pattern with errors that were predominantly lexical in nature. Errors indicating a faulty appreciation of syntax were largely avoided.

SPONTANEOUS SPEECH

Yet another approach to analysing the use of language in dementia is to examine the spontaneous speech of subjects. This is generally based on studies which involve engaging the subject in conversation or conducting an open ended interview in order to collect an adequate sample which can then be recorded for analysis. Miller and Hague (1975) took samples of conversational speech and looked at the statistical characteristics of the words used. Specifically they were concerned with whether demented subjects would rely on a smaller range of words each of which would then have to be used more frequently within a sample of a given length. Comparison of early cases of dementia with normal controls revealed no differences of this type. Hutchinson and Jensen (1980) engaged elderly patients with dementia and control subjects in conversation for 45 minutes and used a form of discourse analysis. The group with dementia emitted fewer utterances and produced fewer utterances per 'turn' in the conversation. Somewhat surprisingly the demented group initiated more topics within their utterances but further analysis revealed that these tended to violate the normal rules of conversation (e.g. by introducing obviously irrelevant issues). This might be because they had lost track of the conversation or misunderstood what the other person had said.

Hier et al. (1985) reported a similar study. Cases with Alzheimer type dementia used a much more simple sentence structure (e.g. had fewer subordinate clauses). These authors also concluded that their subjects showed lexical rather than syntactical defects and suggested that they might have difficulty in accessing the mental lexicon. Again they regarded the appreciation of syntax as remaining intact. This report by Hier et al. (1985) differs from that of Miller and Hague (1975) in that the latter found no evidence of impaired lexical access. However, this discrepency might be more apparent than real in that Miller and Hague's cases were probably at an earlier stage in the disease process. Also Hier et al. used a much more structured conversational situation which might have produced heavier demands on the subjects (e.g. by making it more difficult to follow the track of the conversation and by the need to discuss prescribed topics thus forcing subjects to try to access particular vocabulary items).

In summary, there is general agreement that the speech of demented subjects is impoverished and there are descriptions of the kinds of disturbances that appear in more spontaneous forms of speech. However, there is little in the way of any detailed analysis although access to the lexicon may be a specific problem. The evidence again suggests that appreciation of syntax remains intact.

PERSEVERATION

A commonly encountered feature of the speech of demented subjects is that it is often perseverative, although it must also be recognised that perseveration is often not something that is confined to language behaviour. Motor movements may be perseverated as well. This could also mean that perseveration is not a unitary phenomenon. Possibly the first investigation of perseveration in demented subjects was that of Freeman and Gathercole (1966). Unfortunately, the only other group studied in this experiment was a much younger sample of schizophrenic patients. A variety of different tasks designed to elicit perseveration were utilised. The demented group appeared to perseverate to a similar degree to the schizophrenics. However, the authors had invented a taxonomy of perseverative errors. The demented group were particularly prone to the type of perseveration that Freeman and Fathercole described as 'impaired switching' (where a response given to one stimulus is inappropriately repeated to another, later stimulus). In contrast the schizophrenic group indulged more in 'compulsive repetition' as when an action, word or phrase is repeated over and over again in succession. 'Ideational perseveration', where the same theme crops up repeatedly in speech, did not discriminate between the two groups.

Bayles et al. (1985) studied perseveration in a wide range of disorders including dementia with a modification of Freeman and Gathercole's taxonomy. Again subjects with dementia failed to show an excess of what Freeman and Gathercole (1966) described as 'compulsive repetition'. They also failed to make greater use of what Bayles et al. described as 'carrier phrases' (e.g. 'well......', 'let's see......'). The kind of perseveration most elicited from their demented subjects was a tendency to repeat ideas or phrases after an intervening response (e.g. when asked to say what a nail is, the subjects says 'it's sharp,.....it's long, ...it's sharp'). It is possible that this type of perseveration might be linked to memory failure in that, having gone on to give a second characteristic of a nail, the subject returns to saying that it is sharp having forgotten that this had already been mentioned.

As already indicated, perseveration is a commonplace observation in demented subjects and the two investigations described have gone a little way in defining the nature of the perseverative responses that are most commonly encountered. Just why it occurs has yet to be elicited, although the fact that perseveration is not just confined to speech may mean that it is not primarily a linguistic phenomenon. Alternatively, it could be the case that linguistic perseveration owes its basis to a quite different mechanisms from that which underlies motor perseveration. Perseveration is therefore a phenomenon that might repay more detailed attention.

DISCUSSION

A number of issues arise from this review of investigations of language in dementia. As will be apparent, the work so far has tended to cluster around a number of fairly basic paradigms and the level of analysis achieved so far is not very impressive as compared with the considerably greater sophistication of many studies of aphasia now being published. Nevertheless a start has been made on the problem. There is also some justification in the claim that, whilst not a great deal of consequence has yet been established, the key issues demanding a much more detailed analysis are now starting to be identified. Given the relatively small amount of attention that the area has received so far, this state of affairs is probably to be expected.

One fundamental issue that has arisen is whether the language impairment in dementia can be considered as if it were a form of aphasia as this is encountered in those who have suffered focal brain lesions. The common line of research that approaches language in dementia through the use of aphasia batteries appears to assume that this is the case. The advantages of accepting this assumption lie in the fact that research on aphasia has progressed considerably and a wide range of theoretical ideas and methods of investigation are thereby more obviously opened up to the investigation of language in dementia.

On the other hand, there are quite strong reasons why assuming that the language impairment in dementia is a form of aphasia could be misleading. In the first place, as pointed out earlier, studies which have directly compared language behaviour in demented subjects with that in subjects with aphasia due to focal lesions have often revealed differences between the two (e.g. Rochford, 1971; Schwartz et al., 1979). It might be countered that differences would not have emerged between the groups if the demented subjects had been compared with the right kind of aphasia. This is possible but is not a convincing way to explain all the differences that might be cited.

Of greater importance to this issue is the fact that aphasia due to focal lesions is typically studied in subjects for which the language disorder is the predominant neuropsychological impairment. The subjects may have other impairments as well but these are typically not anything like as pronounced as the language deficit. In dementia the situation is quite different. Dementia by its very nature is a protean disturbance that has very wide ranging effects on all aspects of psychological functioning. The occasional very early case that may present with a language impairment as the most obvious manifestation is quite atypical and, in any case, the presence of significant impairments in other functions will soon become obvious as the condition progresses. This means that poor performance on language related tests could be at least partially the consequence of deficits in other functions such as memory and perception. In fact, the discussion of naming provided above has presented evidence that naming deficits in dementia are partly the consequence of a failure to identify accurately the object or picture to be named. The general point that what, on the face of it, is linguistic behaviour might be influenced by other things was made some time ago by de Ajuriguerra and Tissot (1975) and has been confirmed experimentally. This is a complication that does not arise in studies of aphasia due to focal lesions or, at least, to nothing like the same degree.

If this line of argument is correct it is therefore naive to consider language in dementia as being too closely similar to some form of aphasia. This of course does not mean that certain ideas and techniques used in the study of aphasic language cannot be fruitfully exploited in dementia. Indeed the study of language in dementia can probably use some work on aphasia as a model to great advantage. What is important is that it is also realised that the two lines of research are also inevitably going to diverge simply because the potential influences on language behaviour in dementia are much more diverse.

One conclusion that emerges from a number of different types of study considered in this survey is that it is certain aspects of language that are most prone to disturbance in dementia. The evidence appears to indicate that phonology and the appreciation of syntax remain intact whilst it is the semantic/lexical aspects that are obviously affected. This dissociation between phonology and syntax on the one hand, and the semantic/lexical aspects on the other, may well not be as clear cut as many of the results of the reported investigations seem to suggest. This is because it is always possible that more sensitive indices of phonology and syntax might reveal some impairment in these aspects of language. Also, given the pervasive nature of the effects of dementia, it would be a little surprising if phonology and syntax remained wholly unaffected throughout all stages of the disease. Nevertheless, there is no doubt that the evidence so far indicates that more specific analyses of language in dementia need to concentrate on the semantic aspects of language and on lexical access. To date there is little indication as to what might be specifically wrong in these aspects other than a few speculations such that semantic categories might be unduly broadened (e.g. Schwartz et al., 1979). This is one specific area where progress might be enhanced by borrowing from work on aphasia by using similar models and techniques to those employed by students of aphasia in analysing the same aspects of language in aphasia.

One of the most obvious characteristics of dementia is that it is a slowly progressive disorder. The fact that the severity of any impairment, and probably its nature as well, changes over time means that looking at the development or evolution of deficits is important in understanding any kind of impairment in dementia; whether it be memory, language or anything else. Longitudinal studies whereby a sample of early cases is taken and followed throughout the course of the illness are therefore of particular value. To date this is something that has only received, at best, token acknowledgement. As described above, Kertesz et al. (1986) have commented on the progression of language impairment in dementia but their observations are cross-sectionally based on a single assessment of a relatively small sample with different lengths of illness. Longitudinal studies are difficult and take a long time to complete. Nevertheless they are probably essential if a complete understanding of the impact of dementia on language is ever to be achieved.

As indicated in the introduction, the study of language in dementia has been relatively atheoretical. There has been very little attempt to go beyond simple experimental paradigms or to incoporate theoretical ideas derived from linguistics or psycholinguistics. As more detailed work on such things as lexical access gets under way such theoretical sterility will be less and less possible. Even if investigators manage to remain relatively atheoretical in an overt sense it will be more difficult to avoid implicit theoretical assumptions in terms of the detailed lines of investigation that are chosen. In effect it will become increasingly implausible and counterproductive to try to study language in dementia in isolation from other aspects of research on language whether in normal or abnormal populations.

Finally, the fact that dementia is a major social and medical problem should not be forgotten. Dementia is not just a source of interesting academic problems that are difficult to resolve. Those who suffer and those who care for them, the latter mainly being relatives in the community, are faced with considerable difficulties that demand a response. The fact that communication between carer and sufferer becomes difficult, and eventually can be almost impossible, can be one of the greatest sources of distress. It is therefore important that one significant thrust in the study of language impairment in dementia should be directed towards the question of doing something to resolve communication difficulties. It is unlikely that psychology will arrive at means of restoring basic communicative abilities once these have been lost (c.f. Miller, 1984b), but some worthwhile amelioration of the practical problems that these impairments create may eventually prove possible.

REFERENCES

Ajuriguerra, de J. & Tissot, R. (1975). Some aspects of language in various forms of senile dementia (comparisons with language in childhood). in: E.H. Lenneberg & E. Lenneberg (eds), Foundations of Language Development. New York: Academic Press.

Appell, J., Kertesz, A. & Fishman, M. (1982). A study of language functioning in Alzheimer patients. Brain and Language, 17, 73-91.

Barker, M.G. & Lawson, J.S. (1968). Nominal aphasia in dementia. British Journal of Psychiatry, 114, 1351-1356.

Bayles, K.A. (1982). Language function in senile dementia. Brain and Language, 16, 265-280.

Bayles, K.A. & Tomoeda, C.K. (1983). Confrontation naming in dementia. Brain and Language, 19, 98-114.

Bayles, K.A., Tomoeda, C.K., & Kazniak, A.W. (1985). Verbal perseveration in dementia patients. Brain and Language, 25, 102-110.

Cummings, J.L., Benson, D.F., Hill, M.A. & Read, S. (1985). Aphasia in dementia of the Alzheimer type. Neurology, 35, 394-397.

De Renzi, E. & Vignolo, L.A. (1962). The token test: a sensitive test to detect receptive disturbances in aphasics. Brain, 85, 665-678.

Ernst, B., Dalby, M.A., & Dalby, A. (1970). Aphasic disturbances in presenile dementia. Acta Neurologica Scandinavica, Supplement, 43, 99-100.

Freeman, T. & Gathercole, C.E. (1965). Perseveration — the clinical symptoms — in chronic schizophrenia and organic dementia. British Journal of Psychiatry, 112, 27–32.

Hier, D.B., Hagenlocker, K. & Shindler, A.G. (1985). Language disintegration in dementia: effects of etiology and severity. Brain and Language, 25, 117–133.

Huff, F.J., Corkin, S. & Growdon, J.H. (1986). Semantic impairment and anomia in Alzheimer's disease. Brain and Language, 28, 235–249.

Hutchinson, J.M. & Jensen, M. (1980). A pragmatic evaluation of discourse communication in normal and senile elderly in a nursing home. in: L.K. Obler & M.L. Albert (eds), Language and Communication in the Elderly. Lexington, Mass: Lexington Books.

Kertesz, A., Appell, J. & Fisman, M. (1986). The dissolution of language in Alzheimer's disease. Canadian Journal of Neurological Science, 13, 415–418.

Kirschner, H.S., Webb, W.G. & Kelly, M.P. (1984). The naming disorder of dementia. Neuropsychologia, 22, 23–30.

Lawson, J.S. & Barker, M.G. (1968). The assessment of nominal dysphasia in dementia. British Journal of Medical Psychology, 41, 411–414.

Martin, A. (1987). Representation of semantic and spatial knowledge in Alzheimer's patients: implications for models of preserved learning in amnesia. Journal of Clinical and Experimental Neuropsychology, 9, 191–224.

Martin, A. & Fedio, P. (1983). Word production and comprehension in Alzheimer's disease: the breakdown of semantic knowledge. Brain and Language, 19, 124–141.

Miller, E. (1977). Abnormal Ageing. Chichester: John Wiley & Sons.

Miller, E. (1984a). Verbal fluency as a function of a measure of verbal intelligence and in relation to different types of cerebral pathology. British Journal of Clinical Psychology, 23, 53–57.

Miller, E. (1984b). Recovery and Management of Neuropsychological Impairments. Chichester: John Wiley & Sons.

Milner, B. (1964). Some effects of frontal lobectomy in man. in: J.M. Warren & K. Akert (eds), The Frontal Granular Cortex and Behaviour. New York: McGraw-Hill.

Ober, B.A., Dronkers, N.F., Koss, E., Delis, D.C. & Friedland, R.P. (1986). Retrieval from semantic memory in Alzheimer-type dementia. Journal of Clinical and Experimental Neuropsychology, 8, 75–92.

Rochford, G. (1971). A study of naming errors in dysphasic and in demented patients. Neuropsychologia, 9, 437–443.

Rosen, W.G. (1980). Verbal fluency in aging and dementia. Journal of Clinical Neuropsychology, 2, 135–146.

Schwartz, M.F., Marin, O.S.M. & Saffran, E.M. (1979). Dissociations of language function in dementia: a case study. Brain and Language, 7, 277–306.

Skelton-Robinson, M. & Jones, S. (1984). Nominal dysphasia and the severity of senile dementia. British Journal of Psychiatry, 145, 168–171.

Stengel, E. (1964). Psychopathology of dementia. Proceedings of the Royal Society of Medicine, 57, 911–914.

Wechsler, A.F. (1977). Presenile dementia presenting as aphasia. Journal of Neurology, Neurosurgery and Psychiatry, 40, 303–305.

PATTERNS OF HEMISPHERIC ASYMMETRY SET AGAINST CLINICAL EVIDENCE

Ziyah Mehta, Freda Newcombe and Graham Ratcliff

INTRODUCTION

The notion of hemispheric asymmetry has provided a convenient and productive framework for the study of brain-behaviour relationships. The morphology of the brain encourages this 'sagittal' viewpoint. Hypotheses vary from those envisaging a relatively sharp division of function to those allocating a more equal partnership to the left and right hemisphere. Evidence for a right/left hemisphere dichotomy abounds in the neuropsychological literature of the last three decades and can be traced to classical Greece. Thus, Soranus: 'there are two brains in the head, one of which gives understanding, and another which provides sense perception. That is to say, the one which is lying on the right side is the one that perceives; with the left one, however, we understand' (Lokhorst, 1982). Advocates of the partnership notion can be found in the nineteenth century. Gall envisaged the brain as 'a double organ with integrant parts - symmetrical, duplicate, and subject to genetic and ontogenetic influences' (cited by Harrington, 1985). The imaginative physician, Wigan (1844) considered the hemispheres to be 'two perfect organs of thought and volition - each, so to speak, a sentinel and a check on the other.' Although the hemispheres were thought to duplicate their intrinsic cognitive capacities, there were nevertheless slight inequalities of form, energy and function: thus in Wigan's view, the left hemisphere was 'superior in power' - hence 'the superior efficacy of the right hand as an instrument of volition.' Perhaps the two approaches are not as discordant as may at first appear.

Evidence for the dichotomous view is at first overwhelming. The salient, if not exclusive, role of the left hemisphere in core linguistic functions (language comprehension, word-finding, and segmental phonology), verbal memory, and the programming of skilled motor sequences is not at issue: studies of aphasia, ideational apraxia, and the sequelae of left temporal-lobe epilepsy are unambiguous. The role of the right hemisphere has proved somewhat more impervious to clear-cut definition. Nevertheless, Jackson's (1876) deduction (from an insightful case study of spatial derangement and topographical memory loss) that the posterior right hemisphere might be the 'leading side' for 'visual ideation' (the presumptive role of the posterior areas of the brain), has been fleshed out by clinical studies, temporal lobectomy data, and split-brain research.

It has to be conceded, however, that a satisfactory taxonomy of right hemisphere functions has not yet been achieved and in a recent survey of the literature, Young and Ratcliff (1983) emphasise the lack of a satisfactory conceptual framework. Elsewhere, Ratcliff (1982) has suggested three broad groups of ability that may be (differentially) perturbed by right hemisphere lesions as deduced from the processing demands of the tasks concerned. One group of tasks is characterised by perceptual difficulty, with superimposed stimuli (Kimura, 1963; De Renzi & Spinnler, 1966; Faglioni, Scotti & Spinnler, 1969), reduced information (De Renzi & Spinnler, 1966; Warrington & James, 1967a; Lansdell, 1968; Newcombe & Russell, 1969; Orgass et al., 1972; Wasserstein et al., 1984), or objects viewed from an unusual angle (Warrington & Taylor, 1973). A second group involve more elaborate cognitive processing (Patterson & Zangwill, 1944; McFie, Piercy & Zangwill, 1950; Ettlinger, Warrington & Zangwill, 1957), including the mental rotation of figures in two or three dimensions (Ratcliff, 1979). A third group involve an appreciation of spatial relationships as required by, for example, maze tasks (Benton et al., 1963; Newcombe & Russell, 1969). De Renzi's (1982) valuable recent survey of studies on space exploration reflects both a substantial corpus of data and the need for a heuristic theoretical framework.

As Hardyck (1983) has pointed out, attempts to encapsulate the quiddity of left and right hemisphere characteristics in terms of a 'perfect pair of polar descriptive adjectives' have not been particularly successful. The candidate pairs - verbal versus non-verbal, sequential versus simultaneous, digital versus analog, analytic versus holistic - have not been sufficient or even accurate for a variety of reasons that have been cogently discussed by Moscovitch (1979), Bertelsen (1982) and Hannay (1986). Moreover, they are not invariably tempered by such powerful factors as ontogenetic change and individual difference. As Marshall (in press) observed, 'their primary vice, as currently stated, is vagueness: their application to data-bases thus permits unconstrained, posthoc "strategic" fudges that allow almost any pattern of results to fall under whatever label the theoretician chooses'.

A more judicious approach to the topic was presented more than two decades ago by Piercy (1964). His seminal article touched on several issues that remain of central interest for the study of brain organisation. He considers different but coexisting patterns of hemispheric organisation in relation to ontogenetic factors, pathophysiological evidence and complementary research on infrahuman species. Among the possible modes of hemispheric interaction, he singles out contralateral control, undifferentiated bilateral representation (such that a bilateral lesion produces an additive effect - 'a special instance of Lashley's principle of mass action'), interhemispheric duplication of function (such that a unilateral lesion produces no deficit - 'a special instance of Lashley's principle of equipotentiality'), and a hierarchical or 'dominant' relationship. He adds the rider that bilaterally corresponding brain regions may serve qualitatively different functions.

FOCAL INJURY AND HEMISPHERE FUNCTION

Our objective now is to consider to what extent we can fractionate some of the 'non-verbal deficits' conventionally associated with right hemisphere lesions and envisage their implications for theories of hemispheric organisation within the framework outlined above. For reasons of space, we will focus almost exclusively on data derived from our studies of the long-term consequences of chronic, focal missile injury to the brain. This experimental population is especially valuable in that the lesions were incurred in young, healthy adult brains and that the experimental groups are closely matched for a number of important variables: aetiology of injury, age of injury and interval of time between injury and examination. Moreover, their scores on general intelligence tests do not differ from those of the normal, uninjured population of the same age group. This provides a unique opportunity to compare specific deficits in unilateral and bilateral groups. In other pathologies, the latter groups tend to be more diffusely impaired. In the missile injury population, therefore, selective cognitive disabilities can be studied against a background of well-preserved intelligence and the capacity to sustain attention for long and regular test sessions – conditions that do not invariably obtain in the study of acute neurological populations.

Our early studies of this population suggested that selective impairments, associated with left or right hemisphere lesions and measurable more than 25 years after injury, could be classified respectively under the loose rubric of verbal/non-verbal (Newcombe, 1969). The two tasks which provided the most compelling evidence of right hemisphere, non-verbal deficits were visual closure (Mooney Faces – Mooney, 1960) and maze-learning (Newcombe & Russell, 1969). Subsequent findings did not conform to the expected pattern. There were a number of tasks on which both unilateral groups performed equally poorly: visual recognition (after a brief delay) or irregular dot patterns and contours (Ratcliff, 1970; Newcombe & Ratcliff, 1979), visual memory for geometrical patterns and nonsense figures (Newcombe, 1969, using Kimura's 1963 test material), and spatial visualisation (Newcombe, unpubished data – using the NFER Form Relations test). Unexpectedly, one of the spatial tasks – the locomotor maze (Semmes et al., 1955; 1963) – elicited a highly significant deficit peculiar to the group with bilateral lesions. These data, taken in conjunction with our other work on functional hemispheric asymmetries, led us to propose a variety of patterns of hemispheric organisation which could be interpreted in the light of Piercy's (1964) framework. First, contralateral control was the most plausible explanation for the data on localisation within the peripheral visual field (Ratcliff & Davies-Jones, 1972). Second, an additive effect was suggested by the short-term visual memory impairment (Newcombe & Ratcliff, 1979) (see Figure 1). Third, the possibility of duplication: a unilateral lesion, regardless of laterality, did not produce a deficit, as on the locomotor maze (Ratcliff & Newcombe, 1973) (Figure 2). Perhaps the notion of duplication requires to be qualified here. It is feasible that qualitative differences exist between the hemispheres such that alternative but equally efficient strategies are available for solving the locomotor task. Fourth, the mode of 'dominance' is strongly suggested by the object-naming (Newcombe et al., 1971) and the stylus maze data (Ratcliff & Newcombe, 1973) in the case of left and right hemisphere lesions respectively (see Figure 3).

The next long-term objective was a fractionation of the visuospatial domains, to identify component systems and their processing modes. This

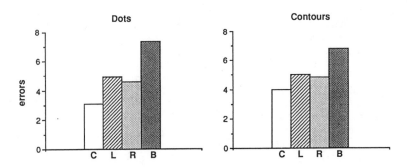

Figure 1. Performance on short-term visual memory tasks (Dots and Contours) of men with bilateral (B), left (L) or right (R) hemisphere missile injury compared with that of age-matched male control subjects (C).

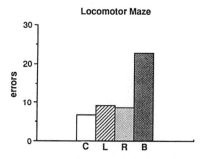

Figure 2. Performance on the locomotor maze task of men with bilateral (B), left (L) or right (R) hemisphere missile injury compared with that of age-matched male control subjects (C).

is a large endeavour, not helped by the apparent absence of coherent conceptual models. In terms of mechanism, even such plausible notions that right and left hemisphere constructional apraxia is qualitatively different and can be ascribed respectively to perceptual and constructional deficits has not been consistently demonstrated (Dee, 1970). One of the few attempts to provide a 'process' hypothesis is to be found in an unpublished work of Greene (1971). While conceding that factorial studies based on complex tasks had been disappointing, he extracted two of Thurstone's (1944) factors (A: speed and strength of closure and E: flexibility in dealing with competing configurations) which were subsequently 'identified' in other studies (Vernon, 1947; Cohen, 1952). There seemed to be empirical support for the failure of the perceptual integration hypothesis in right hemisphere disease (Kimura, 1963; Meier & French, 1965; De Renzi & Spinnler, 1966; Lansdell, 1968). But failure of perceptual differentiation, assuming that this process was measured by such tasks as Gottschaldt figures and the Ghent-Poppelreuter overlapping figures, were less clearly tied to the right hemisphere (compare Kimura, 1963 and De Renzi & Spinnler, 1966).

Greene's own experiments were based on 40 patients: 20 with left and 20 with right hemisphere disease, mainy 'fairly circumscribed, surgically confirmed, space occupying lesions'. The exceptions were four patients with abscesses and two with intracerebral haematomas. To be sure, these lesions were not 'localised' satisfactorily (given the inadequate imaging facilities of the day) but Greene attempted to find lesions confined to the temporo-parietal area and ensured that the two groups were matched as carefully as possible in terms of age, presence or absence of visual field defects and sensorimotor loss. Despite the limitations of his patient sample, he was able to suggest some dissociations: hints of 'modular' organisation. The predicted failure of perceptual integration (as measured by tachistoscopic recognition of fragmented figures and dot subitising) in association with right hemisphere lesions was significant. The predicted failure of perceptual differentiation in association with left hemisphere lesions was disconfirmed: both experimental groups were impaired on tasks requiring the detection of overlapping or embedded figures (Gottschaldt figures). A centroid analysis of his data, with the two factors specifically predicted in advance, seemed to confirm their presence and that of a third factor, which - propter hoc - Greene deduced to represent spatial ability. Several earlier studies had suggested such a factor. Guilford and Zimmerman (1948) had indeed envisaged the underlying process as that of 'imagining movement, transformations and other changes in visual objects, for which purpose the clear perception of the spatial arrangement of the elements is necessary'.

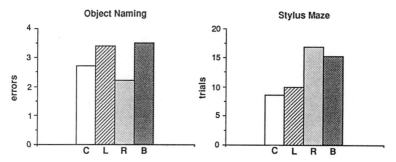

Figure 3. Performance on the object naming task and the stylus maze of men with bilateral (B), left (L) or right (R) hemisphere missile injury compared with that of age-matched male control subjects (C).

Greene's second series of experiments suggested that impairments in spatial ability were more significant in right than left hemisphere lesions and more associated with parietal than temporal lesions. He went on to speculate that perceptual integration and differentiation were two complimentary processes which may be differentially organised in the brain: namely, that the differentiation of the field into parts is more globally represented whereas the ability to organise these parts into wholes is a function of the right hemisphere. He did not speculate at length on the representation of spatial ability.

The factorial techniques exploited by Greene are, to be sure, no longer fashionable, if not ruled out of court. Nevertheless, in his work can be found an attempt to distinguish the dissociable processes involved in higher-order' perceptual loss: that is, a preliminary search in the direction of modular organisation of visual processing.

Subsequent research, as indicated earlier, has certainly strengthened the claim for the association between right hemisphere dysfunction and failures of perceptual 'integration' and related these to occipito-temporal dysfunction. Failures of 'differentiation', if that is indeed the operation measured by, for example, the Gottschaldt figures, is certainly observed in association with lesions of either hemisphere (Russo & Vignolo, 1967) and has been related to severity of lesion (Corkin, 1979). Regarding the third factor 'spatial ability' - this seemed to be compromised by right hemisphere lesions in Greene's study. This innovative but apparently little-known study has the rare virtue of testing plausible process hyotheses; it deserves wider recognition. Given the limitations of neuro-imaging at that time, it is remarkable that such clear differences in relatively small, acute neurological patient groups could be observed.

Clearly, however, the over-general concept of 'spatial ability' needs to be dissected. But one has only to consider the plurality of space-systems (Paillard, 1986) and the panoply of spatial abiities (De Renzi, 1982) to be aware of the magnitude of the problem. As a first approach, it may be possibe to detach biologically 'meaningful' segments of behaviour that can be operationally dissociated. The distinction between egocentric (body-centred) and allocentric (extracorporal) space represents one dimension that has yielded suggestive differences between frontal and parietal lesions in both human (Semmes et al., 1963; Teuber,

1964; Butters, Soeldner & Fedio, 1972) and primate research (Pohl, 1973).

The study reported here is focussed on predominantly <u>allocentric</u> visual and spatial perception within the <u>central</u> visual field. Our starting point was the double dissociation between visuoperceptual and visuospatial skills suggested by our earlier data (Newcombe & Russell, 1969). Of the current research, we shall focus on four tasks: two visuoperceptual – visual closure (Mooney, 1960) and unfamiliar face matching (Benton & Van Allen, 1973); and two visuospatial – Line Orientation (Benton, Varney & Hamsher, 1978) and the Vandenberg rotation task (1983) (based on Shepard's paradigm). We could confidently predict, on the basis of our previous findings, a right hemisphere deficit on the closure task and we expected, on the basis of the literature (Benton et al., 1983) a similar hemispheric difference on unfamiliar face matching. Regarding the spatial tasks, again the literature (summarised by De Renzi, 1982) would suggest a significant right hemisphere deficit on line orientation (Benton, Hannay & Varney, 1975). The prediction for the rotation task was less obvious. A right hemisphere deficit on Benson and Gedye's (1963) Mannikin task had been reported by Ratcliff (1979) although not found on an adapted version of the same task by Kim et al. (1984). Our earlier unpublished data on three dimensional pattern-matching (NFER Form Relations task) had not shown a hemispheric difference and recent suggestions that the left hemisphere was involved in the evocation of mental imagery (Farah, 1984) increased the uncertainty of prediction. The results (see Figure 4) reflected this difference in predictive confidence. Again, there was a clear-cut difference on the closure task, a finding consistent with research on patients with temporal lobe epilepsy (Milner, 1968)

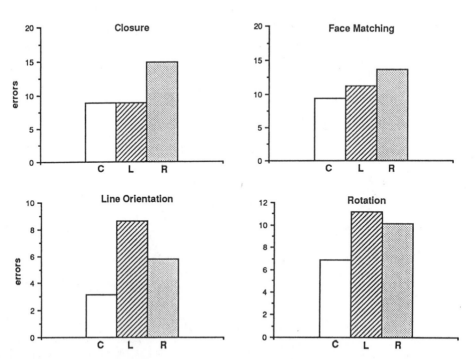

Figure 4. Performance on two visuoperceptual tasks (Closure and Face Matching) and two visuospatial tasks (Line Orientation and Rotation) of men with left (L) or right (R) hemisphere missile injury compared with that of age–matched male control subjects (C).

and those with temporo-parietal lesions due to cerebrovascular disease (Wasserstein et al., 1984). The findings were less clear-cut for Benton's unfamiliar face-matching task. The right hemisphere group were significantly inferior to the control group. The mean score of the left hemisphere group fell between that of the right hemisphere group and the control subjects and did not differ significantly from either. In contrast, on the two spatial tasks, it was the left and not the right hemisphere group who were significantly impaired in relation to the age-matched control subjects; comparison of the two experimental groups did not show a significant difference.

We have already discussed these findings (Mehta, Newcombe & Damasio, 1987) in terms of a potential left hemisphere contribution to visuospatial processing. We have additional evidence of a left hemisphere deficit as severe as that of the right hemisphere, on other visuospatial tasks including Corsi's short-term, spatial span task (Milner, 1971), Thurstone's Flags and a task requiring the recall of object location, the Montreal adaptation of Kim's game (Smith & Milner, 1981).

Clearly, these findings await replication. But we emphasise that they cannot be discounted in terms of sampling bias in relation to age, intelligence, or neuroanatomy. As they stand, however, they argue for complex and shifting patterns of hemispheric organisation of the type envisaged by Piercy (1964). We can therefore propose that the right hemisphere is 'leading' (to use Jackson's phrase) for complex, non-verbal pattern recognition, specifically face recognition whether of familiar (Warrington & James, 1967b) or unfamiliar faces (Benton & Van Allen 1968). But the left hemisphere clearly has the capacity to support these skills as demonstrated by the fact that the isolated left hemisphere in split brain studies can recognise faces and that a bilateral lesion is usually required to produce a frank prosopagnosia (Damasio, Damasio & Van Roesen, 1982). We might even speculate that the area in the right hemisphere, homologous to Wernicke's area in the left, has evolved as a face and pattern processing system at a comparable level of complexity to that required for recognising words.

As far as spatial processing is concerned, we could envisage considerable duplication in the two hemispheres which could serve the need to chart and scan a wide extrapersonal spatial universe. Parietal cortex provides the organism with an ideal subtrate for the visual monitoring of body and eye movements in extrapersonal space. It receives input from all the major sensory systems that contribute to the maintenance and updating of spatial reference systems. The cellular machinery of posterior parietal cortex collates somatosensory information about body-centred (egocentric) space with that derived, mainly visually, from extrapersonal (allocentric) space for the efficient steering of movement in a coherent, stabiised visual world, under the influence of intentional and motivational processes (Hyvarinen, 1962; Mountcastle et al., 1975). It seems to us plausible that both parietal cortices play a substantial role in these basic biological requirements.

The problem remains as to whether the contribution of the two hemispheres to spatial processing is qualitatively different. Young (1962) has suggested that 'bilaterality was originally a necessity for nervous systems that operate by means of a map-like analog system' although 'the more complex computing sections of nervous systems, such as the human one, are less dependent on topographic mapping and, therefore, bilaterality becomes less important.' From the philogenetic point of view, Nauta (1962) suggested that 'those systems that did capitalise on the bilateral symmetry of the brain have in common that they all have to do, in one way or another, with the stability of the organism in its spatial environment'. This requirement initially must rely on isomorphic mapping. But as recent physiological research on vision has shown, this mapping becomes progressively more elaborate and more abstract (Cowey, 1978; 1982; Ungerleider & Mishkin, 1982; Pandya & Ungerleider, 1985) as the organism is required to perceive, recognise, and act. Asymmetry would appear to have developed most sharply in man although it is increasingly apparent in infrahuman species (Denenberg, 1984). The biological advantage of asymmetry must be intimatey connected with the comparatively recent development of language in our species and with the need for a single central control mechanism for the expression of speech and the planning of skilled motor sequences (Kimura, 1982; Heilman & Gonzalezz Rothi, 1985; see also Nottebohm, 1970). For the detection of movement, however, and the location of events in extracorporal space, there would appear to be no clear advantage in marked asymmetry and an obvious requirement for wide scanning of the visual field. The paradoxical phenomenon of unilateral spatial neglect, frequent in acute right posterior lesions and rare in comparable lesions of the left hemisphere, is at first blush difficult to accommodate within such a framework. Mesulam and Geschwind's (1978) attentional hypothesis is one of the more plausible candidates for interpreting this marked asymmetry in spatial perception.

An acceptable, coherent, and comprehensive model of 'non-verbal' processing and hemispheric organisation remains elusive but at least its absence must stimulate contemporary neuropsychology. Unarguably, a heuristic scheme has to be shaped within the demands and constraints of ontogenetic and biological factors. It calls for theoretial input of the power that formal linguistics (e.g. Chomsky, 1986) has supplied to the study of language and aphasia.

REFERENCES

Benson, A.J. & Gedye, J.L. (1963). Logical processes in the resolution of orientation conflict. R.A.F. Institute of Aviation Medicine Report No.259. London: Ministry of Defence (Air).
Benton, A.L., Elithorn, A., Fogel, M.L. & Kerr, M. (1963). A perceptual maze test sensitive to brain damage. Journal of Neurology, Neurosurgery and Psychiatry, 26, 540-544.
Benton, A.L. & Van Allen, M.W. (1968). Impairment in facial recognition in patients with cerebral disease. Cortex, 4, 344-358.
Benton, A.L. & Van Allen, M.W. (1973). Manual: Test of Facial Recognition. Neurosensory Center Publication No. 287, Department of Neurology, University Hospitals, Iowa City, Iowa.
Benton, A.L., Hamsher, K. DeS., Varney, N.R. & Spreen, O. (1983). Contributions to Neuropsychological Assessment: A Clinical Manual. New York: Oxford University Press.
Benton, A.L., Hannay, J. & Varney, N.R. (1975). Visual perception of line direction in patients with unilateral brain disease. Neurology, 25, 907-910.
Benton, A.L., Varney, N.R. & Hamsher, K. DeS. (1978). Visuo-spatial judgement: a clinical test. Archives of Neurology, 35, 364-367.
Butters, N., Soeldner, C. & Fedio P. (1972). Comparison of parietal and frontal lobe spatial deficits in man: extrapersonal vs. personal (egocentric) space. Perceptual and Motor Skills, 34, 27-34.
Chomsky, N. (1986). Knowledge of Language: Its Nature, Origin and Use. New York: Praeger.
Cohen, J. (1952). Factors underlying Wechsler-Bellevue performance of three neuropsychiatric groups. Journal of Abnormal and Social Psychology, 47, 359-365.
Corkin, S. (1979). Hidden-figures-test performance: lasting effects of unilateral penetrating head injury and transient-effects of bi-

lateral cingulotomy. Neuropsychologia, 17, 585–605.

Cowey, A. (1978). Cortical visual maps and visual perception. The Grindley Memorial Lecture. Quarterly Journal of Experimental Psychology, 31, 1–17.

Cowey, A. (1982). Sensory and non-sensory visual disorders in man and monkey. Philosophical Transactions of the Royal Society of London, B 298, 3–13.

Damasio, A.R., Damasio, H. & Van Hoesen, G.W. (1982). Prosopagnosia: anatomical basis and behavioural mechanisms. Neurology, 32, 331–341.

Dee, H.L. (1970). Visuoconstructive and visuoperceptive deficits in patients with unilateral cerebral lesions. Neuropsychologia, 3, 305–314.

Denenberg, V.H. (1984). Behavioral asymmetry. in: N. Geschwind & A.M. Galaburda (eds.). Cerebral Dominance: The Biological Foundations, Cambridge, Mass.: Harvard University Press.

De Renzi, E. (1982). Disorders of Space Exploration and Cognition. Chichester and New York: John Wiley.

De Renzi, E. & Spinnler, H. (1966). Visual recognition in patients with unilateral cerebral disease. Journal of Nervous and Mental Disease, 142, 515–525.

Desimone, R., Schein, S.J., Moran, J. & Ungerleider, L.G. (1985). Contour, colour and shape analysis beyond the striate cortex. Vision Research, 25, 441–452.

Ettlinger, G., Warrington, E.K. & Zangwill, O.L. (1957). A further study of visual-spatial agnosia. Brain, 80, 335–361.

Faglion, P., Scotti, G. & Spinnler, H. (1969). Impaired recognition of written letters following unilateral hemisphere damage. Cortex, 5, 120–133.

Farah, M.J. (1984). The neurological basis of mental imagery: a componential analysis. Cognition, 18, 245–272.

Greene, J.G. (1971). A factorial study of perceptual function in patients with cerebral lesions. Unpublished Ph.D. Thesis, University of Glasgow.

Guildford, J.P. & Zimmerman, W.S. (1948). The Guildford-Zimmerman Aptitude Survey. Journal of Applied Psychology, 32, 24–34.

Hannay, J. (1986). Some issues and concerns in neuropsychological research: an introduction. in: J. Hannay (ed.). Experimental Techniques in Human Neuropsychology. New York: Oxford University Press.

Hardyck, B. (1983). Research Publication of the Association for Research in Nervous and Mental Disease, 42, 270–283.

Harrington, A. (1985). Nineteenth century ideas on hemispheric differences and 'duality of mind'. Behavioral and Brain Sciences, 6, 617–660.

Heilman, K.M. & Gonzalez Rothi, L.J. (1985). Apraxia. in: K.M. Heilman & E. Valenstein (eds.). Clinical Neuropsychology. New York & Oxford: Oxford University Press.

Hinshelwood, J. (1899). Letter-, Word- and Mind-Blindness. London: H.K. Lewis.

Hyvärinen, J. (1962). Posterior parietal lobe of the primate brain. Psychological Review, 62, 1060–1129.

Jackson, H. (1876). Case of large cerebral tumour without optic neuritis and with left hemiplegia and imperception. Royal London Ophthalmic Hospital Report, 8, 434–444.

Kim, Y., Morrow, L., Passafiume, D. & Boller, F. (1984). Visuoperceptual and visuomotor abilities and locus of lesion. Neuropsychologia, 2, 177–185.

Kimura, D. (1963). Right temporal lobe damage: perception of unfamiliar stimuli after damage. Archives of Neurology, 8, 264–271.

Kimura, D. (1982). Left-hemisphere control of oral and brachial movements and their relation to communication. Philosophical Transactions of the Royal Society, London, B 298, 135–149.

Lansdell, H. (1968). Effect of extent of temporal lobe ablations in two lateralised deficits. Physiology and Behaviour, 3, 271-273.

Lokhorst, G.J. (1982). An ancient Greek theory of hemispheric specialisation. Cliomedica, 17, 33-38.

Marshall, J.C. (1989) Cerebral Laterality: Rube Goldberg at the Bauhaus. in: A. Glass (ed.). Individual Differences in Hemispheric Specialisation, in press.

McFie, J., Piercy, M.F. & Zangwill, O.L. (1950). Visual-spatial agnosia associated with lesions of the right cerebral hemisphere. Brain, 73, 167-190.

Mehta, Z., Newcombe, F. & Damasio, H. (1987). A left hemisphere contribution to visuospatial processing. Cortex, 23, 447-461.

Meier, M.J. & French, L.A. (1965). Lateralised deficits in complex visual discrimination and bilateral transfer of reminiscence following unilateral temporal lobectomy. Neuropsychologia, 3, 261-272.

Mesulam, M-M & Geschwind, N. (1978). On the possible role of neocortex and its limbic connections in the process of attention and schizophrenia: clinical cases of inattention in man and experimental anatomy in monkey. Journal of Psychiatric Research, 14, 249-259.

Milner, B. (1968). Visual recognition and recall after temporal-lobe excision in man. Neuropsychologia, 6, 191-209.

Milner, B. (1971). Interhemispheric differences in the localisation of psychological processes in man. British Medical Bulletin, 27, 272-277.

Mooney, C.M. (1960). Recognition of ambiguous and unambiguous visual configurations with shorter and longer exposures. British Journal of Psychology, 51, 119-125.

Moscovitch, M. (1979). Information processing and the cerebral hemispheres. in: M.S. Gazzaniga (ed.). Handbook of Behavioral Neurobiology, Vol.2, Neuropsychology. New York: Plenum.

Mountcastle, V.B., Lynch, J.C., Georgopoulos, A., Sakata, H. & Acuna, C. (1975). Posterior parietal association cortex of the monkey: command functions for operations within extrapersonal space. Journal of Neurophysiology, 38, 871-908.

Nauta, W.J.H. (1962). Discussion of J.Z. Young's chapter 'Why do we have two brains'. in: V.B. Mountcastle (ed.). Interhemispheric Relations and Cerebral Dominance. Baltimore: The John Hopkins Press.

Newcombe, F. (1969). Missile Wounds of the Brain: A Study of Psychological Deficits. Oxford: Oxford University Press.

Newcombe, F., Oldfield, R.C., Ratcliff, G.G. & Wingfield, A. (1971). Recognition and naming of object-drawings by men with focal brain wounds. Journal of Neurology, Neurosurgery and Psychiatry, 34, 329-340.

Newcombe, F. & Ratcliff, G. (1979). Long-term consequences of cerebral lesions. in: M. Gazzaniga (ed.). Handbook of Behavioral Neurology. New York: Plenum Press.

Newcombe, F. & Russell, W.R. (1969). Dissociated visual perceptual and spatial deficits in focal lesions of the right hemisphere. Journal of Neurology, Neurosurgery and Psychiatry, 32, 73-81.

Nottebohm, F. (1979). Origins and mechanisms in the establishment of cerebral dominance. in: M. Gazzaniga (ed.). Handbook of Behavioral Neurobiology. New York: Plenum.

Orgass, B., Poeck, K., Kerschensteiner, M. & Hartje, W. (1972). Visuocognitive performance in patients with unilateral hemispheric lesions. Zeitschrift für Neurologie, 202, 177-195.

Paillard, J. (1986). Cognitive versus sensorimotor encoding of spatial information. in: P. Ellen & C. Thinus-Blanc (eds.). Cognitive Processes and Spatial Orientation in Animal and Man. Dordrecht: Martinus Nijhoff.

Pandya, D.M. & Yeterian, E.H. (1984). Proposed neural circuitry for spatial memory in the primate brain. Neuropsychologia, 22, 109-122.

Patterson, A. & Zangwill, O.L. (1944). Disorders of visual space perception associated with lesions of the right cerebral hemisphere. Brain, 67, 331–358.

Phillips, C.G., Zeki, S. & Barlow, H.B. (1984). Localisation of function in the cerebral cortex: past, present and future. Brain, 107, 328–361.

Piercy, M. (1964). The effects of cerebral lesions on intellectual function: a review of current research trends. British Journal of Psychiatry, 110, 310–352.

Pohl, W. (1973). Dissociation of spatial discrimination deficits following frontal and parietal lesions in monkeys. Journal of Comparative and Physiological Psychology, 82, 227–239.

Ratcliff, G. (1970). Aspects of disordered space perception. Unpublished D.Phil. Thesis, University of Oxford.

Ratcliff, G.G. (1979). Spatial thought, mental rotation and the right cerebral hemisphere. Neuropsychologia, 17, 49–54.

Ratcliff, G. (1982). Disturbances of spatial orientation associated with cerebral lesions. in: M. Potegal (ed.). Spatial Abilities: Development and Physiological Foundations. New York: Academic Press.

Ratcliff, G. & Davies-Jones, G.A.B. (1972). Defective visual localisation in focal brain wounds. Brain, 95, 49–60.

Ratcliff, G. & Newcombe, F. (1973). Spatial orientation in man: effects of left, right and bilateral posterior cerebral lesions. Journal of Neurology, Neurosurgery and Psychiatry, 34, 448–454.

Russo, M. & Vignolo, L.A. (1967). Visual figure-ground discrimination in patients with unilateral cerebral disease. Cortex, 3, 113–127.

Semmes, J., Weinstein, S., Ghent, L. & Teuber, H.-L. (1955). Spatial orientation in man after cerebral injury: I. analysis by locus of lesion. Journal of Psychology, 39, 227–244.

Semmes, J., Weinstein, S., Ghent, L. & Teuber, H.-L. (1963). Correlates of impaired orientation in personal and extrapersonal space. Brain, 86, 747–772.

Smith, M.L. & Milner, B. (1981). The role of the right hippocampus in the recall of spatial location. Neuropsychologia, 6, 781–793.

Teuber, H.-L. (1964). The riddle of frontal lobe function in man. in: J.M. Warren & K. Akert (eds.). Frontal Granular Cortex and Behavior. Pennysylvania State University: McGraw Hill.

Thurstone, L.L. (1944). A Factorial Study of Perception. Chicago: University of Chicago Press.

Ungerleider, L.L. & Mishkin, M. (1982). Two cortical visual systems. in: D.J. Ingle, M.A. Goodale & R.J.W. Mansfield (eds.). Analysis of Visual Behaviour. Cambridge, Mass: MIT Press.

Vandenberg, S.G. (1983). Vandenberg's Test of three-dimensional spatial visualisation. in: J. Eliot & I. Macfarlane Smith (eds.). An International Directory of Spatial Tests. Windsor: NFER-Nelson.

Vernon, M.D. (1947). Different types of perceptual abilities. British Journal of Psychology, 38, 79–89.

Warrington, E.K. & James, M. (1967b). An experimental investgation of facial recognition in patients with unilateral cerebral lesions. Cortex, 3, 317–326.

Warrington, E.K. & Taylor, A.M. (1973). The contribution of the right parietal lobe to object recognition. Cortex, 9, 152–164.

Wasserstein, J., Zappulla, R., Rosen, J. & Gerstman, L. (1984). Evidence for differentiation of right hemisphere visual-perceptual functions. Brain and Cognition, 3, 51–56.

Wigan, A.L. (1844, reprinted in 1985). A New View of Insanity: the duality of Mind proved by the structure, functions, and diseases of the brain and by the phenomena of mental derangement, and shown to be essential to moral responsibility. USA: Joseph Simon.

Young, A.W. & Ratcliff, G. (1983). Visuospatial abilities of the right hemisphere. in: A.W. Young (ed.). Functions of the Right Hemisphere. London: Academic Press.

Young, J.Z. (1962). Why do we have two brains? in: V.B. Mountcastle (ed.). Interhemispheric Relations and Cerebral Dominance. Baltimore: The Johns Hopkins Press.

INTERHEMISPHERIC TRANSMISSION TIMES

A David Milner and Michael D Rugg

INTRODUCTION

Post-war interest in the functional properties of the corpus callosum in normal human subjects grew out of the dramatic animal studies of
Myers and others in the 1950s, followed by the even more striking work of
Sperry and his collaborators in the 1960s on the effects of commissurotomy in man (Ettlinger & Blakemore, 1969). In the twenty years following
the first report on those patients, there was an explosion of research
aimed at investigating cerebral asymmetries in normal individuals, generally by the use of lateralised visual stimulation; and there was much
discussion of the role of the commissures in mediating performance of
such tasks. Such discussion led to the reintroduction of a simple technique, first used by Poffenberger (1912), designed to measure the time
taken for an elementary sensory message to be transmitted from one hemisphere to the other. The task requires a subject to make an invariant
finger movement, as rapidly as possible, in response to an unstructured
visual stimulus which may be located in either the ipsilateral or the
contralateral visual hemi-field. Some studies randomised the side of
presentation (e.g. Jeeves, 1969) whilst others used a blocked method of
testing (e.g. Berlucchi et al., 1971); in either case steady ocular
fixation was required, and both left and right hands were given equal
numbers of test trials. In some studies, subjects responded concurrently
with both hands on each trial (e.g. Jeeves, 1969).

The logic of these studies is straightforward, given that each hemifield sends its inputs to the opposite cerebral hemisphere. Individual
finger movements are believed to be controlled strictly contralaterally
through the corticospinal tract (Kuypers, 1978); therefore an ipsilateral
light should be responded to manually without the need for commissural
transmission, whilst a contralateral one could not be. The difference
between these 'uncrossed' and 'crossed' reaction times (RTs) should
provide an estimate of interhemispheric transmission time. To avoid
question-begging, and for the sake of generality, we shall refer to these
observed (crossed minus uncrossed) differences as CUDs. In normal subjects they generally average out at between 2 and 3 milliseconds.

It is important to emphasise, as have previous reviewers (Berlucchi,
1978; Rizzolatti, 1979; Bashore, 1981), that CUDs cannot be seriously
regarded as interhemispheric transmission-time (ITT) estimates where the
RT task incorporates an element of choice. This applies not only to
discriminative tasks where different hands (or fingers) are used for
different stimuli, but even to those where the choice is between responding and not responding ('go, no-go' tasks). In all these cases, the
interhemispheric transmission latency becomes swamped by 'compatibility'
differences between crossed and uncrossed reactions. Such tasks will not
be reviewed here.

Jeeves (1969) and Berlucchi et al. (1971) followed up Poffenberger's investigation in order to determine whether the CUD reflected the inter-hemispheric transmission of a sensory message, as might be assumed prima facie. They in fact provided evidence in favour of interhemispheric transmission but against its sensory nature. Firstly, Jeeves found that in two patients with congenital absence (agenesis) of the corpus callosum, the CUD in a two-handed response task reached a mean of 39.2 msec, in contrast with 1.6 msec for two groups of normal subjects. Such elevated CUDs have generally been confirmed in studies of other acallosal patients (Kinsbourne & Fisher, 1971; Reynolds & Jeeves, 1974; Milner, 1982; Milner et al., 1985), though not in all (Ettlinger et al., 1972). The best estimate of acallosal CUDs may perhaps be calculated by weighting all the published values by the numbers of RT observations contributing to them. For the six patients that have been documented, the mean figure using single-handed responding comes to 17.2 msec; for the four who have been tested using the double-handed technique the figure is 25.2 msec.

With the recent publication of comparable data on two commissuro-tomised patients (CUDs averaging 39.6 msec: Sergent & Myers, 1985) it may then be concluded that an intact corpus callosum does seem to be a pre-requisite for the normal 2-3 msec CUD. Hence that CUD in normal subjects may plausibly be taken to be an estimate of a callosal transmission time. The second question was 'what sort of information is transmitted?'

CALLOSAL ROUTES

If the CUD measures a sensory conduction latency, then it should be possible to manipulate it by manipulating sensory variables. In particular, Berlucchi et al. (1971) pointed out that callosal neurons originating in the primary visual cortex are especially responsive to stimuli presented in the close vicinity of the vertical meridian of the field. Even those which emanate from secondary cortical visual areas have receptive fields weighted towards that midline region (Berlucchi, 1981). Hence they expected that stimuli further from the midline should yield greater CUDs. However they found that varying the eccentricity of the visual stimuli between 5° and 35° had no effect upon the CUD. In a similar vein, Milner & Lines (1982) varied the intensity of the visual stimulus; they reasoned that a stronger neural signal would traverse synapses on to callosal neurons more rapidly than a weak one, just as seems to be the case for the passage of signals from eye to cortex (Tepas & Armington, 1962; Lennie, 1981; Vaughan, Costa & Gilden, 1966). However they too found that the CUD remained unchanged across their stimulus variations.

Somewhat disappointingly then, the evidence points to a nonsensory origin of the CUD; perhaps a motor command or trigger passes via neuronal collaterals through the more anterior (nonvisual) corpus callosum, so as to mediate a crossed simple reaction. If so, the CUD as a measure of callosal latency tells us little of relevance to an understanding of visual processing asymmetries. Nonetheless, it could tell us something about the efficiency of one callosal pathway, and indeed about its functional integrity in cases of brain damage.

Clearly however it would be more valuable, and of broader neuropsy-chological interest, if a way of measuring transmission latencies between the visual cortices could be devised. Following from some work by Kleinman et al. (1976), Milner and Lines (1982) used a simple vocal RT technique, to explore whether this could yield a solution. If only the left hemisphere (at least in most subjects) is capable of initiating a rapid spoken response, then the difference between left and right hemi- field RTs should provide a measure of callosal latency. Furthermore if a vocal response could not be triggered from the right hemisphere directly, then the brain might be forced to respond to left hemifield stimuli on the basis of a visual message passing from right to left hemisphere. Milner and Lines excluded subjects who did not exhibit a clear right hemifield advantage in the task, and in the remaining subset did observe a trend for the hemifield latency difference to vary inversely with the stimulus light intensity. They therefore proposed that these subjects were indeed using a visual callosal relay in responding to left hemifield stimulation, which was slower and more variable in latency than the route evidently underlying the manual CUD. Their assumption that the corpus callosum was implicated was supported by the observation that an acal- losal patient (KC) showed an elevated hemifield difference on the task of 17.8 msec. This is comparable with her mean manual CUD value of 20.2 msec using the same stimuli and apparatus (Milner, 1982).

Others have questioned the validity of Milner and Lines' selective use of subjects (Tassinari, Morelli & Berlucchi, 1983). However it is unlikely that their results were based, as Tassinari et al. suggest, on the use of subjects who happened to have a right hemifield RT advantage due simply to an attentional preference. First, this seems an unlikely explanation of the elevated difference observed in patient KC (Milner, 1982). Secondly, it cannot explain the finding of a significant inter- action between stimulus intensity and hemifield. When field differences are brought about experimentally by manipulating attentional bias (Graham, 1983; Hughes, 1984), variations of stimulus intensity have no effect upon the latency difference values. Thirdly, Milner and Lines' finding of a significant right-hemifield advantage for simple vocal RTs among right-handers has since been replicated in an extensive study by St John et al. (1987). Their subjects showed no main hemifield effect upon manual RTs. However it was found that the vocal RT difference was relat- ively unstable across sessions. This might explain the failure of Tassinari et al. (1983) to find a significant effect.

However, irrespective of the validity of their experimental logic, Milner and Lines' vocal RT procedure clearly could not be applied uni- versally. Furthermore RT methods in general require several hundreds of measurements for reliable differences of these magnitudes to be achieved (Milner, 1986). Consequently we have looked to the use of event-related potentials (ERPs) as an alternative approach to the measurement of visual ITTs, in the hope of devising a more readily-applicable technique.

EVENT-RELATED POTENTIALS

The use of averaged ERPs in both experimental and clinical investi- gations of the geniculostriate visual system has been extensive for many years (see e.g. Regan, 1972; Halliday, 1982). With small flash stimuli, the earliest deflections which can be recorded from electrodes over posterior brain areas consist of a positive-going peak with a latency of around 100-130 msec (often known as 'Pl'), followed by a negative peak with a latency around 150-170 msec ('Nl'). While the distribution of Pl is confined to posterior scalp regions, suggesting a generator in visual cortex, Nl can also be recorded from central and frontal electrodes. The anterior Nl has a peak latency which is typically some 10-15 msec shorter than that recorded posteriorly (e.g. Rugg, Lines & Milner, 1984). This suggests that anterior and posterior Nl deflections do not arise from the same intra-cranial generators.

There are several previous studies where the latencies of the P1 and/or N1 deflections have been compared between homologous sites on the two sides of the head in response to lateralised visual stimulation (Rugg, 1982). The logic of such comparisons is that the directly stimulated hemisphere (contralateral to the visual hemifield stimulated) should evince these ERP components at a shorter latency than the other hemisphere, which would be dependent on an additional interhemispheric transmission time. Assuming then that electrodes placed on one side of the scalp actually do pick up the electrical activity from that same side of the brain, then latency measurements of the P1 and N1 peaks should provide relatively direct estimates of the transmission time.

Although some of the earlier studies can be criticised on their methodology (Rugg, 1982), others do afford presumably valid estimates of transmission latency. Thus Andreassi, Okamura & Stern (1975) and Ledlow, Swanson and Kinsbourne (1978) found that simple stimuli (a small cross at varying eccentricities, or a small square with or without a cross in it, respectively) yielded latency differences of 19.3 msec and 18 msec for P1. In a study using more complex stimuli (upper-case letters), Rugg and Beaumont (1978) observed a difference of 15.2 msec. In all cases the electrodes were placed over the homologous occipital regions of the head. Clearly these estimates, whilst internally consistent, are quite incompatible with the transmission times inferred from manual RT experiments, where CUDs of the order of 2-3 msec are observed. However they would be compatible with the model proposed by Milner and Lines (1982), because they could reflect an occipital (visually-coded) relay which is too slow to mediate crossed manual reactions; those might always be determined by a faster motoric relay.

We set out to test this idea by recording not only from occipital electrodes but also from the central sites C3 and C4 (Jasper, 1958; approximately over the motor cortex hand area). In our first study (Rugg, Lines & Milner, 1984) we used two pairs of occipital electrodes, the second of which (LO1 and LO2) were situated laterally to the 'standard' O1 and O2. The subject was required to fixate a dim LED during a series of trials in which a bright light (at 4° out to left or right) was flashed either for 10 msec or 90 msec. The task was to detect the brief (target) stimuli and to make a finger response using the ipsilateral hand.

We were not surprised to find a behavioural CUD far in excess of the values typical for simple RTs, since we were using a choice RT task (cf Anzola et al., 1977). Of more direct interest however was our finding of ipsi/contralateral latency differences in the prominent N1 (henceforth referred to by its modal latency, as N160) at the O1/O2, LO1/LO2 and C3/C4 sites, of 15.7, 12.4 and 3.7 msec respectively. In separate ANOVAs, the hemifield-by-site interaction was significant only for the two occipital electrode pairs. We also found in all comparisons between homotopic electrodes that the amplitude of the N160 was significantly greater over the contralateral than the ipsilateral hemisphere.

These findings were replicated in two further experiments (Lines, Rugg & Milner, 1984), in which we examined the effects of visual stimulus intensity upon the putative callosal transmission times. In the first (see Fig. 1), we found that at the occipital sites (only LO1 and LO2 were used) the latency difference increased from 12.5 msec to 18.9 msec with the less intense stimuli, whilst at the central sites it remained essentially constant at a mean value of 3.2 msec. An ANOVA on these ITT estimates yielded a significant intensity x site interaction (see Fig.2). In the second experiment we used a simple RT task, and also a larger difference in light intensity between the two stimulus conditions employed.

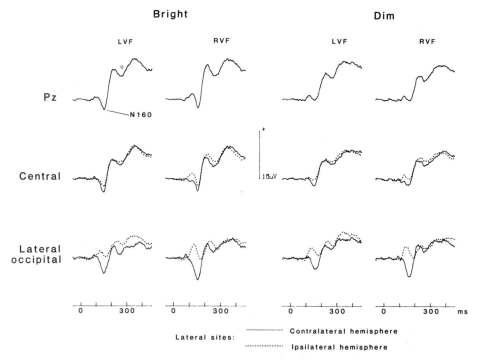

Figure 1. Grand average ERP waveforms derived from the 'NOGO' trials of Experiment 1 of Lines, Rugg and Milner (1984). The ERPs are time-locked to the onset of a flashed LED, at time zero on the abscissae.

Although 7 out of 15 subjects tested had to be excluded because their ERPs were not measurable in the dim condition, the remaining eight yielded ITT estimates at both O1/O2 and LO1/LO2 electrodes which were large and again intensity-dependent (O: 8.4 and 15.1 msec for the bright and dim conditions respectively; LO: 10.9 and 17.6 msec). At the C3/C4 electrodes, the ITT estimate remained constant at about 2.6 msec, which compares with the mean behavioural CUD of 1.8 msec. In this study the hemifield-by-site effect was significant for the N160 latencies at the central as well as at the occipital electrodes in separate ANOVAs.

These three experiments provide strong support for our contention that two distinct callosal pathways of relevance to visual RT experiments exist and can be chronometrically investigated. Not only are transmission-time estimates derived from occipital-site ERPs consistently greater than those from centrally-recorded ERPs, but also they vary in a manner predicted from our assumption that they alone reflect the transmission of sensory information.

In the final study in this series, we looked at the influence of both stimulus, eccentricity and reference electrode site on our results. We therefore replicated the basic experiment on a further group of subjects using a non-cephalic (chest) electrode as well as our usual linked-mastoid reference electrodes, and secondly used two different visual eccentricity conditions (4° and 10°). Neither factor had any appreciable effect upon the results (Rugg, Lines & Milner, 1985). The fact that stimulus eccentricity had no effect on the latency difference strongly

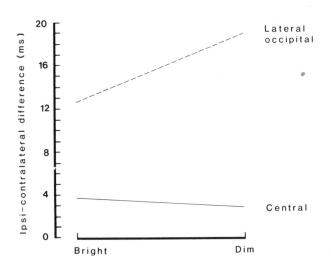

Figure 2. Mean latency differences between homotopic N160 peaks recorded ipsilateral and contralateral to a flashed LED in the GO/NOGO reaction time task. The data are collapsed over visual hemifields, separately shown in Figure 1.

opposes any suggestion that light scatter from the stimulated into the non-stimulated hemifield could be the cause of the observed ipsilateral N160 (or the occipital P120, which yielded similar latency data in this experiment). In addition, the 10° stimuli could not possibly have stimulated that small subset of retinal ganglion cells which lie close to the vertical meridian of the retina and send their axons to the 'wrong' side of the brain (Bunt, Minckler & Johanson, 1977). Indeed the latency difference at 10° derived from the N160 deflection at the LO electrodes remained at about 10 msec, just as had been the case with the identical higher luminance stimuli used in the first experiment of Lines et al. (1984). Consequently the suggestion by Marzi (1986) that the relatively low occipital ERP latency difference when high intensity lights are used, could be due to the stimulation of cells in the retina's nasotemporal overlap region is untenable.

The above series of studies on normal subjects successfully conformed to the predictions we made from the two-route model of Milner and Lines (1982). Nonetheless, like the behavioural RT studies, it provides no direct evidence that what is being measured really is a callosal transmission relay. Therefore, an important test (as in the behavioural domain) was to repeat the experiments using patients who, either due to agenesis or surgery, lack the corpus callosum. We have done this with our two acallosal patients KC and BF (Rugg, Milner & Lines, 1985).

We found that both patients gave us ERPs which, when recorded from electrodes contralateral to the stimulated hemifield, were essentially normal. However, the ipsilateral N160 was not clearly identifiable in either patient on either side (Fig. 3). It is possible that there could be visual information arriving at the ipsilateral cortex (e.g. through the anterior commissure) which in theory could be picked up at scalp electrodes. Our methods may have failed to detect such information either because it arrived with a high temporal variance, or perhaps because our electrodes were located too posteriorly. (The anterior commissure in nonhuman primates has its cortical projection field entirely in the

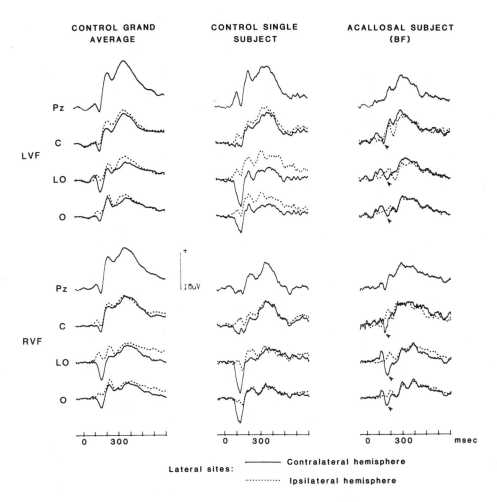

CONTROL GRAND AVERAGE   CONTROL SINGLE SUBJECT   ACALLOSAL SUBJECT (BF)

LVF

Pz

C

LO

O

RVF

Pz

C

LO

O

10uV

0   300   0   300   0   300   msec

Lateral sites: ————— Contralateral hemisphere

.... Ipsilateral hemisphere

Figure 3. Averaged waveforms recorded from an acallosal patient (BF), a typical normal control, and a group of controls, elicited by a flashed LED during a GO/NOGO task. The cortralateral N160 deflection in BF's data is indicated by arrows. C, LO and O refer to C3/C4, LO1/LO2, and O1/O2 electrode sites respectively.

temporal lobe: Jouandet & Gazzaniga, 1979). In any event, the absence of a detectable ipsilateral N160 in our acallosal ERP data would appear to rule out noncallosal mechanisms in its generation, such as volume conduction from the directly activated hemisphere, and therefore provides support for our interpretation of the normal data in terms of callosal transmission.

A final point about the waveforms illustrated in Figs. 1 and 3 should be briefly discussed. In much of our data, we find a larger positive deflection (P1) at **ipsi**lateral occipital electrodes. This may be partly due to activity emanating from the medial surface of the contralateral occipital cortex (Barrett et al., 1976). This is known to occur with VEPs elicited by checkerboard reversal, but has not been demonstrated to our knowledge with unstructured flash stimuli. Such an effect

105

could have two consequences on the ipsilateral N160 peak: firstly an apparent reduction (through linear summation) in the amplitude of the deflection, and secondly an apparent increase in its latency.

These possibilities are however unlikely for the following reasons: firstly, the P1 has a posterior distribution, yet N160 amplitude asymmetries are reliably found between central as well as occipital pairs of electrodes. Secondly, it is possible to find subjects in whom both the contralateral P1 and contralateral N1 are larger than their ipsilateral counterparts, suggesting that P1 and N1 amplitude asymmetries are dissociable. Finally, appeal to a 'paradoxically' lateralising P1 cannot account for the data obtained with our acallosal patients. As the ipsilateral P1 is supposed to arise as a result of volume conduction to the contralateral hemisphere, rather than neurally-mediated transfer, it should be in evidence at the ipsilateral occipital electrodes of acallosal subjects. As illustrated in Fig. 3, while both our patients do indeed show evidence of a positive deflection at ipsilateral electrodes, this is considerably delayed compared to the controls' ipsilateral P1 component, in marked contrast to the normal latencies of the acallosals' contralateral N160s. Our favoured explanation for the P1 amplitude asymmetries observed in many normal subjects is that they arise because of asymmetries in the onset and amplitude of the overlapping N160. Thus, the contralateral P1 is depressed in amplitude in comparison to P1 on the ipsilateral side because of summation with an earlier and larger N160.

In conclusion, we believe that the ERP technique we have developed does provide a method for studying interhemispheric transmission latencies, through two routes (a visual one and an anterior nonsensory route), in normal subjects. Future studies could examine the effects of other stimulus variables (e.g. complexity: cf Rizzolatti, 1979) as well as of putative individual differences in callosal anatomy. A significant sex difference in manual CUDs has in fact been recently reported (St John et al., 1987).

At the present stage little more can be said about the two routes we have hypothesised. However one possible explanation of the much greater apparent ITT that we (and other investigators) have observed at occipital electrodes has been proposed by Marzi (1986). He has argued that information takes about 11-12 msec to pass from primary visual cortex (V1) to the prestriate areas MT or V4 in the monkey brain (Maunsell & Schiller, 1984). Consequently the typical differences of 14-15 msec measured at occipital sites between ipsilateral and contralateral ERP latencies could be the sum of two times: a forward (intrahemispheric) transmission plus a quick (2 msec) axonal transfer across the callosum. This account implies that the contralateral N160 is being generated in V1, whilst the ipsilateral peak is generated more anteriorly. However the former suggestion is most improbable given the scalp distribution; the evidence seems clear from P100 studies that a V1 generator (being medially located in the hemisphere) would give a paradoxically lateralised ERP. On the other hand Marzi (1986) is surely correct, that callosal neurons in the striate cortex, which have a very narrow retinal range abutting the vertical meridian, are an unlikely source of the ipsilateral ERPs (cf Rugg, Lines & Milner, 1985).

NONCALLOSAL ROUTES

The very fact that crossed reactions are possible, albeit slowed, in the absence of the corpus callosum, shows that other neural routes must be able to mediate such reactions. Broadly there have been two hypotheses as to the nature of the route traversed in patients with callosal agenesis. Some have argued that a noncallosal commissure such as the anterior commissure (Ettlinger et al., 1974) or the commissure of the superior colliculus (Jeeves, 1965; Ettlinger et al., 1972) could provide the means for a visual signal to reach contralateral motor mechanisms. Others (Kinsbourne & Fisher, 1971) have proposed that crossed reactions might be brought about without the need for commissural tansmission at all; instead ipsilateral motor pathways could provide a direct output from the stimulated hemisphere. According to the former class of theories, the elevated CUD in acallosal subjects results from a less efficient, circuitous commissural route; according to the latter theory it results from an increased vulnerability in some individuals and/or tasks to the stimulus-response incompatibility inherent in crossed reactions (see also Broadbent, 1974). The data reported by Jeeves (1965) could be interpreted as supporting such a raised susceptibility in acallosal subjects.

We have investigated the nature of the acallosal CUD by manipulating stimulus luminance using levels identical to those used by Milner & Lines (1982), in a simple RT paradigm. The results were similar in both of the patients we tested (Milner, 1982; Milner et al., 1985), and are shown in Figure 4. There was a significant inverse relationship between stimulus intensity and CUD in both subjects. It is difficult to see how this result could have been predicted from the ipsilateral-control hypothesis of Kinsbourne and Fisher; in fact the only simple explanation is to assume that transmission through a visually-coded neuronal system underlies the CUD.

In one of these experiments (Milner et al., 1985) we also manipulated stimulus-response ('S-R') compatibility, by having the subject (BF) responding either with a finger switch on the ipsilateral side of space as the arm being used or with the switch located in contralateral space. If crossed reactions in the former ('normal') case suffer through spatial incompatibility, then the reverse should be the case in the latter test condition. That is, the CUD should change from a large positive to large negative value. In practice, we found no reduction whatever in the CUD in the second condition. This result argues against any role of S-R incompatibility in bringing about the large CUD in callosal agenesis; in this respect such individuals appear to resemble normal subjects (Anzola et al., 1977; Berlucchi et al., 1977).

Thus there is evidence in favour of the visual-commissural hypothesis and also evidence against the ipsilateral-control hyothesis.

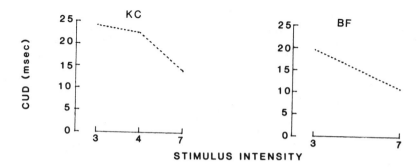

Figure 4. Mean crossed-uncrossed differences in simple reaction time to a light flash in two acallosal patients, under different conditions of flash luminance. Data taken from Milner (1982) and Milner et al. (1985).

However there is no direct evidence as to which of the two noncallosal commissures known to carry visually-coded information is the more likely candidate. The electrophysiological evidence would tend to favour the anterior commissure (Gross, Bender & Mishkin, 1977) rather than the commissure of the superior colliculus; this latter tract normally may interconnect nonvisual cells (Antonini et al., 1979). However these arguments, since they are based on normal brains, are not entirely compelling.

The most direct evidence would be to compare the CUDs of acallosal subjects known to possess an intact anterior commissure (as most do: Loeser & Alvord, 1968) with those of patients who do not. The advent of MRI techniques (see the chapter by Besson, later in this book) may permit such a study in the future. At present we only have the indirect evidence that commissurotomised patients (in whom the anterior commissure is cut along with the corpus callosum and psalterium) seem to evince even larger CUDs than acallosal patients (Sergent & Myers, 1985). If Sergent & Myers are correct in their interpretation that the midbrain route is being used by these commissurotomised patients, then this route would presumably be available also to acallosal subjects. Yet the shorter CUDs in callosal agenesis suggest that in practice, it is not being exploited: at least not in those who are able to use an anterior commissure. There is also an indication in the data of Sergent & Myers (albeit based on very few RT observations) that stimulus intensity does not influence the CUDs of commissurotomised patients; this too would support the idea that our acallosal subjects (though maybe not all such patients) use a different route. However another possible route for the surgical patients would be the use of ipsilateral motor control systems (Gazzaniga, 1970). In that case, the data of Sergent & Myers would provide no means for narrowing the alternatives in callosal agenesis.

In any event it seems likely that the anterior commissure must be necessary for the more complex visual cross-integration that at least some patients are capable of (Ettlinger et al., 1974; Milner & Jeeves, 1979; Jeeves & Milner, 1987).

CLINICAL IMPLICATIONS

Callosal pathology can come about both as the result of head trauma (e.g. Adams, Gennarelli & Graham, 1982) and a a result of cerebral disease (e.g. Geschwind & Kaplan, 1962). In some cases of closed head injury the neuropsychological consequences of this callosal lesion may be well-defined (e.g. Rubens et al., 1977 Schott et al., 1969), whilst in others they may be obscured by the presence of widespread pathology elsewhere in the brain. Nonetheless even in such latter cases a measure of callosal dysfunction could have diagnostic and prognostic value as an index of white-matter damage. In cases of more localised cerebral lesions it could provide a test of suspected or hypothesised callosal involvement where behavioural signs point in that direction.

We have thus far only tested one patient (SP) who has a known callosal lesion without associated traumatic damage. SP received an anterior callosotomy for the relief of intractable epilepsy in April 1986, and we were able to see her in September 1987. In this instance, the ERP data were disappointing in that the waveforms from contralateral electrodes did not yield identifiable Pl or Nl deflections. Therefore no assessment could be made of abnormalities in SP's ipsilateral waveforms. This problem, not uncommonly encountered in patient populations in our experience, presently places constraints on the clinical utility of the ERP technique. However we also tested SP's manual reaction times using a simple RT procedure similar to our previously-published paradigm, at two levels of stimulus luminance. The prediction from the Milner & Lines' (1982) model would be that a CUD approximating the 12-15 msec ipsilateral/contralateral occipital ERP difference should be found. The quick nonsensory route should have been blocked, and the visual route used instead; thus the CUD should be both larger than normal and also subject to variation as a function of stimulus luminance. Our results have only partially confirmed these expectations; a higher-than-normal mean CUD of 8.4 msec was found, which did not however differ beteen the two light-intensity conditions. The patient's RTs and their variance were both high, as is often the case with neurological patients (Milner, 1986; Benton, 1987) making the absolute CUD magnitude unreliable.

Although loose ends remain, we believe that by combining behavioural and electrophysiological techniques, we have achieved more than we could have by the use of either technique alone. With the advent of MRI, and the ability with this third technique to visualise small lesions in the callosum, we are hopeful that still further progress can be achieved.

ACKNOWLEDGEMENTS

The authors wish to thank a number of clinicians, especially Mr I Jacobson (Dundee Royal Infirmary) for their co-operation and help. They also are eternally grateful for the patience and co-operation of all those patients who gave of their time, especially KC, BF and SP.

REFERENCES

Adams, J.H., Gennarelli, T.A. & Swash, M. (1986). Brain damage in non-missile head injury: observations in man and subhuman primates. in: W.T. Smith & J.B. Cavanagh (eds.). Recent Advances in Neuropathology. Edinburgh: Churchill Livingstone.

Andreassi, J.L., Okamura, H. & Stern, M. (1975). Hemispheric asymmetries in the visual cortical evoked potential as a function of stimulus location. Psychophysiology, 12, 541-546.

Antonini, A., Berlucchi, G., Marzi, C.A. & Sprague, J.M. (1979). Importance of corpus callosum for visual receptive fields of single neurons in cat superior colliculus. Journal of Neurophysiology, 42, 37-52.

Anzola, G.P. Bertoloni, G., Buchtel, N.A. & Rizzolatti, G. (1977). Spatial compatibility effects and anatomical factors in simple and choice reaction time. Neuropsychologia, 15, 295-302.

Barrett, G., Blumhardt, L., Halliday, A.M., Halliday, E. & Kriss, A. (1976). A paradox in the lateralisation of the visual evoked response. Nature, 261, 253-255.

Bashore, T.R. (1981). Vocal and manual reaction time estimates of interhemispheric transmission time. Psychological Bulletin, 89, 352-368.

Benton, A. (1987). Reaction time in brain disease: some reflections. Cortex, 22, 129-140.

Berlucchi, G. (1978). Interhemispheric integration of simple visuomotor responses. in: P.A. Buser & A. Rougeul-Buser (eds.). Cerebral Correlates of Conscious Experience. Amsterdam: North Holland.

Berlucchi, G. (1981). Recent advances in the analysis of the neural substrates of interhemispheric communication. in: O. Pompeiano & C.A. Marsan (eds.). Brain Mechanisms and Perceptual Awareness. New York: Raven Press.

Berlucchi, G., Crea, F., Di Stefano, M. & Tassinari, G. (1977). Influence of spatial stimulus-response compatibility on reaction time of ipsilateral and contralateral hand to lateralized light stimuli. Journal of Experimental Psychology: Human Perception and Performance, 3, 505-517.

Berlucchi, G., Heron, W., Hyman, R., Rizzolatti, G. & Umilta, C. (1971). Simple reaction times of ipsilateral and contralateral hand to lateralized visual stimuli. Brain, 94, 419–430.

Broadbent, D.E. (1974). Division of function and integration of behavior. in: F.O. Schmitt & F.G. Worden (eds.). The Neurosciences: Third Study Program. Cambridge: MIT Press.

Bunt, A.H., Minckler, D.S. & Johanson, G.W. (1977). Demonstration of bilateral projection of the central retina of the monkey with horseradish peroxidase neuronography. Journal of Comparative Neurology, 171, 619–630.

Ettlinger, G. & Blakemore, C.B. (1969) The behavioral effects of commissure section. in: A.L. Benton (ed.). Contributions to Clinical Neuro psychology. Chicago: Aldine.

Ettlinger, G., Blakemore, C.B., Milner, A.D. & Wilson, J. (1972). Agenesis of the corpus callosum: a behavioural investigation. Brain, 95, 327–346.

Ettlinger, G., Blakemore, C.B., Milner, A.D. & Wilson, J. (1974). Agenesis of the corpus callosum: a further behavioural investigation. Brain, 97, 225–234.

Gazzaniga, M.S. (1970. The Bisected Brain. New York: Appleton-Century-Crofts.

Geschwind, N. & Kaplan, E. (1962). A human deconnection syndrome. Neurology, 12, 675–685.

Graham, L.C.M. (1983). The effect of attentional bias on reaction time under three conditions of light intensity. Unpublished B.Sc. Honours Thesis, University of St. Andrews.

Gross, C.G., Bender, D.B. & Mishkin, M. (1977). Contributions of the corpus callosum and the anterior commissure to visual activation of inferior temporal neurons. Brain Research, 131, 227–239.

Halliday, A.M. (1972).Evoked Potentials in Clinical Testing. London: Churchill Livingstone.

Hughes, H.C. (1984). Effects of flash luminance and positional expectancies on visual response latency. Perception and Psychophysics, 36, 177–184.

Jasper, H.H. (1958). The ten twenty electrode system of the International Federation. Electroencephalography and Clinical Neurophysiology, 10, 371–375.

Jeeves, M.A. (1965). Psychological studies of three cases of congenital agenesis of the corpus callosum in man. in: G. Ettlinger (ed.). CIBA Foundation Study Group No.20. Functions of the Corpus Callosum. London: Churchill.

Jeeves, M.A. (1969). A comparison of interhemispheric transmission times in acallosals and normals. Psychonomic Science, 16, 245–246.

Jeeves, M.A. & Milner, A.D. (1987). Specificity and plasticity in interhemispheric integration: evidence from callosal agenesis. in: D. Ottoson (ed.). Duality and Unity of the Brain. London: Macmillan.

Jouandet, M.L. & Gazzaniga, M.S. (1979). Cortical field of origin of the anterior commissure of the rhesus monkey. Experimental Neurology, 66, 381–397.

Kinsbourne, M. & Fisher, M. (1971). Latency of uncrossed and of crossed reaction in callosal agenesis. Neuropsychologia, 9, 471–473.

Kleinman, K.M., Carron, R., Cloninger, L. & Halvachs, P. (1976). A comparison of interhemispheric transmission times as measured by verbal and manual reaction-time. International Journal of Neuroscience, 6, 285–288.

Kuypers, H.G.J.M. (1978). From motor control to conscious experience. in: P.A. Buser & A. Rougeul-Buser (eds.). Cerebral Correlates of Conscious Experience. Amsterdam: North Holland.

Ledlow, A., Swanson, J.M. & Kinsbourne, M. (1978). Differences in reaction times and average evoked potentials as a function of direct and indirect neural pathways. Annals of Neurology, 3, 525–530.

Lennie, P. (1981). The physiological basis of variations in visual latency. Vision Research, 21, 815–824.

Lines, C.R., Rugg, M.D. & Milner, A.D. (1984). The effect of stimulus intensity on visual evoked potential estimates of interhemispheric transmission time. Experimental Brain Research, 57, 89–98.

Loeser, J.D. & Alvord, E.C. (1968). Agenesis of the corpus callosum. Brain, 91, 553–570.

Marzi, C.A. (1986). Transfer of visual information after unilateral input to the brain. Brain and Cognition, 5, 163–173.

Maunsell, J.H.R. & Schiller, P.H. (1984). Evidence for the segregation of parvo- and magnocellular channels in the visual cortex of the macaque monkey. Society for NEUROSCIENCE Abstracts, 10, 520.

Milner, A.D. (1982). Simple reaction times to lateralized visual stimuli in a case of callosal agenesis. Neuropsychologia, 20, 411–419.

Milner, A.D. (1986). Chronometric analysis in neuropsychology. Neuropsychologia, 24, 115–128.

Milner, A.D. & Jeeves, M.A. (1979). A review of behavioural studies of agenesis of the corpus callosum. in: I.S. Russell, M.W. van Hof & G. Berlucchi (eds.). Structure and Function of Cerebral Commissures. London: Macmillan.

Milner, A.D. & Lines, C.R. (1982). Interhemispheric pathways in simple reaction time to lateralized light flash. Neuropsychologia, 20, 171–179.

Milner, A.D., Jeeves, M.A., Silver, P.H., Lines, C.R. & Wilson, J. (1985). Reaction times to lateralized visual stimuli in callosal agenesis: stimulus and response factors. Neuropsychologia, 23, 323–331.

Poffenberger, A.T. (1912). Reaction time to retinal stimulation with special reference to time lost in conduction through nerve centers. Archives of Psychology, 3 (Serial no. 23), 1–73.

Regan, D. (1972). Evoked Potentials in Psychology, Sensory Physiology and Clinical Medicine. London: Chapman and Hall.

Reynolds, D.M. & Jeeves, M.A. (1974). Further studies of crossed and uncrossed pathways responding in callosal agenesis: a reply to Kinsbourne and Fisher. Neuropsychologia, 12, 287–290.

Rizzolatti, G. (1979). Interfield differences in reaction times to lateralised visual stimuli in normal subjects. in: I. S. Russell, M.W. van Hof & G. Berlucchi (eds.) Structure and Function of Cerebral Commissures. London: Macmillan.

Rubens, A.B., Geschwind, N., Mahowald, M.W. & Mastri, A. (1977). Post-traumatic cerebral hemispheric disconnection syndrome. Archives of Neurology, 34, 750–755.

Rugg, M.D. (1982). Electrophysiological studies. in: J.G. Beaumont (ed.). Divided Visual Field Studies of Cerebral Organisation. London: Academic Press.

Rugg, M.D. & Beaumont, J.G. (1978). Interhemispheric asymmetries in the visual evoked response: Effects of stimulus lateralisation and task. Biological Psychology, 6, 283–292.

Rugg, M.D., Lines, C.R. & Milner, A.D. (1984). Visual evoked potentials to lateralised visual stimuli and the measurement of interhemispheric transmission time. Neuropsychologia, 22, 215–225.

Rugg, M.D., Lines, C.R. & Milner, A.D. (1985). Further investigation of visual evoked potentials elicited by lateralized stimuli: effects of stimulus eccentricity and reference site. Electroencephalography and Clinical Neurophysiology, 62, 81–87.

Rugg, M.D., Milner, A.D. & Lines, C.R. (1985). Visual evoked potentials to lateralized stimuli in two cases of callosal agenesis. Journal of Neurology, Neurosurgery and Psychiatry, 48, 367–373.

Schott, B., Michel, F., Michel, D. & Dumas, R. (1969). Apraxie ideomotrice unilaterale gauche avec main gauche anomique: syndrome de deconnexion calleuse? Revue Neurologique, 120, 359–365.

Sergent, J. & Myers, J.J. (1985). Manual, blowing, and verbal simple reactions to lateralized flashes of light in commissurotomised patients. Perception and Psychophysics, 37, 571–578.

St. John, R, Shields, C., Krahn, P. & Timney, B. (1987). The reliability of estimates of interhemispheric transmission times derived from unimanual and verbal response latencies. Human Neurobiology, 6, 195–202.

Tassinari, G., Morelli, M. & Berlucchi, G. (1983). Interhemispheric transmission of information in manual and verbal reaction time tasks. Human Neurobiology, 2, 77–85.

Tepas, D.I. & Armington, J. (1962). Properties of evoked visual potentials. Vision Research, 2, 449–461.

Vaughan, H.G., Costa, L.D. & Gilden, L. (1966). The functional relation of visual evoked response and reaction time to stimulus intensity. Vision Research, 6, 645–656.

DIVIDED VISUAL FIELD STUDIES IN SCHIZOPHRENIA

Anthony S David

INTRODUCTION

Ever since Hippocrates, physicians have been trying to locate the origin of madness somewhere in the brain. It was not until 1844, that Wigan (1844) suggested that insanity might be due to the failure of the two cerebral hemispheres to work in harmony. Such a thesis remained ignored until the 1960's when a generation of psychologists produced an impressive body of research illuminating the role of the corpus callosum (CC) in integrating brain function. They did this by studying individuals who had undergone surgical division of the CC (see for example Gazzaniga, et al. (1965)), or had become 'disconnected' by lesions from other sources (Geschwind, 1965). The function of this broad band of more than 200,000,000 myelinated fibres was inferred from the effects of its transection which led to speculation regarding the unity of conscious experience, the unconscious and the mind-body problem (see Sperry, 1968). Psychiatry tends to lag behind psychology by about a decade and so it was not until the early 1970's that questions were raised as to whether this new knowledge might be relevant to the understanding of abnormal mental phenomena (Lishman, 1971; Galin, 1974).

A report of thickening of the CC in the post-mortem brains of 10 chronic schizophrenics (Rosenthal & Bigelow, 1972) provided further impetus to study interhemispheric transmission (IHT) in schizophrenia. The late Stuart Dimond a neuropsychologist who had studied 'split brain' patients in the U.S.A. and his colleague, Graham Beaumont were the first to apply divided visual field (DVF) techniques to psychiatric patients (Beaumont & Dimond, 1973). Their paper, brief and inconclusive as it was (see later) stimulated a minor explosion of studies using these and other techniques. Ten years later, Beaumont warned psychologists that 'the findings in commissurotomy patients should not be overrated' (Beaumont, 1982), and this coincided with a falling off of psychiatric research in the area. The 1980's has witnessed more reviews of cerebral laterality in relation to psychopathology (Wexler, 1980; Newlin, Carpenter & Golden, 1981; Walker & McGuire, 1982; Colbourn, 1982; Gruzelier, 1983; Beaton, 1985; Cutting, 1985; Robertson & Taylor, 1987) than original work. Despite this, DVF (or 'tachistoscopic') studies, which allow hemispheric and interhemispheric function to be examined in detail, non-invasively and relatively inexpensively, continue to nourish a fertile area of psychiatric exploration.

DIVIDED VISUAL FIELD STUDIES: METHODOLOGICAL CONSIDERATIONS

The basic principle underlying DVF studies is that visual inform-ation in one hemifield is projected entirely to the opposite cerebral hemisphere. To take advantage of this, presentation duration must be short (<150msec) so as to avoid reflex visual scanning, and stimuli should be outside the foveal region (>2°) where there may be bilateral cerebral connections (see Young, 1982 for a recent review). Numerous studies (see Beaumont, 1982; Beaton, 1985) have shown that verbal stimuli (e.g. letters, words, letter strings) are better recognised, named and matched when presented to the right visual field/left hemisphere (RVF/-LH). Non-verbal stimuli (e.g. dot location, line orientation, form and facial recognition) tend to produce a left visual field/right hemisphere (LVF/RH) advantage, but results are less consistent. Whatever dichotomy is invoked, be it verbal/nonverbal, analytic/gestalt, serial/parallel, lateralisation of function is perhaps best viewed as a dimensional rather than categorical concept (Bradshaw & Nettleton, 1981).

The above generalisations must be tempered by an acknowledgement of the complexity of brain function whereby cognitive strategy, response bias, attention and task demands may all affect the outcome of an apparently simple experiment. It is simplistic to assume that a 'verbal test' (precisely what this constitutes is debatable) is synonymous with a 'left hemisphere test'; both hemispheres may cooperate in subtle processes involving many synapses (Moscovitch, 1986). Sergent (1983) has examined the effects which the psychophysical properties of visual input (e.g. stimulus duration, luminance, retinal eccentricity, stimulus size) as well as task difficulty and familiarity (Ross-Kossak & Turkewitz, 1984), have on hemispheric asymmetries. Subject differences including sex, age, handedness and intelligence are also potentially confounding variables. These methodological problems are especially relevant when DVF techniques are applied to psychiatric populations. This will now be discussed.

METHODOLOGICAL PROBLEMS PERTAINING TO STUDIES OF SCHIZOPHRENIC PATIENTS

Differential Deficit

There is a truism: 'give any test to a schizophrenic and he will perform it more poorly than a normal control.' Further, the more difficult the test the worse he will do. This leads to the 'differential deficit problem' whereby an apparently specific deficit is due to a failure to match tests on difficulty and hence discriminating power (Chapman & Chapman, 1973). A spurious deficit may not only emerge in a comparison of schizophrenics and controls but also between hemispheres within the patient group if say, the 'LH task' is more difficult than that of the RH. Another general problem is the variability and by implication, unreliability of schizophrenics' performance both individually and as a group. So often a promising finding in one study, fails to be replicated in another for this reason.

Normal Controls

Selection of control groups is highly problematic. Chapman and Chapman (1977) have argued that psychiatric controls as well as normals should be used so that factors pertaining to hospitalization may be controlled, a view which has much to commend it. However the matter does not end there. Cognitive tests should be given to subjects (including normals) matched for IQ which for schizophrenics often means low-normal. The deleterious effect schizophrenia has on IQ (Goldstein, 1986) may be obviated by using tests which appear to tap premorbid abilities (Nelson & O'Connell, 1978), or by including data on education attainment. Despite taking pains to select appropriately matched controls, it may still prove impossible to design a test which avoids reaching the schizophrenics' performance 'ceiling' whilst remaining firmly on the controls' 'floor'.

One appealing way round this, used in DVF studies, is to determine a threshold level for each subject by altering the presentation time (Gur, 1978; Colbourn & Lishman, 1979). Although greatly enhancing the sensitivity of the test, alteration in exposure duration may have differing effects on each hemisphere's efficiency, so confounding the results. Using multiple exposure times for all groups would help to clarify this issue.

Psychiatric Controls

Which psychiatric patients should be used as controls? The study of 'typical' hospitalized affective disorder patients may be fruitful in its own right but in comparison to schizophrenics they will tend to be older, predominantly female (inpatient schizophrenics are more often male) and are likely to have been in hospital for a shorter time (Wing & Wing, 1982). Therefore, accurate matching may lead to the inclusion of atypical cases. Attempts to match groups for degree of psychopathology creates another problem due to the lack of reliability and validity of clinical diagnosis. As non-schizophrenic controls approach schizophrenics on degree or even nature of psychopathology, for example schizoaffectives, so they are bound to include 'true' schizophrenics wrongly classified. As a result the control group's performance will begin to approximate that of the schizophrenics' (see Shenton et al., 1987). This emphasises the need to improve the reliability of diagnoses by using standardized assessments and criteria supplemented by quantitative and qualitative ratings of symptoms.

An alternative strategy may be to compare groups on the basis of specific symptoms alone rather than their diagnoses, such as patients with hallucinations, affective and schizophrenic, versus those without. This may prove rewarding in determining possible psychological mechanisms for those symptoms. Along the same lines, dividing schizophrenic patients into subgroups according to symptoms e.g. with or without hallucinations (Alpert et al., 1976); Schneiderian first rank symptoms (David, 1987) may be informative, given the accepted heterogeneity of 'the schizophrenias' (Bleuler, 1911). One a priori subdivision popular with many psychologists is the paranoid-nonparanoid distinction (Magaro et al., 1981). The Maine Scale used for this purpose groups auditory hallucinations with thought disorder and cognitive impairment to form the nonparanoid dimension, separating them from various delusions which form the paranoid dimension. This is flawed on two counts. Firstly, clinicians have demonstrated that hallucinations and delusions cluster together under the heading, 'positive symptoms' whereas 'negative symptoms' tend to go with cognitive impairment (Andreasen, 1987), with thought disorder perhaps forming a third cluster (Liddle, 1987). Secondly, these groupings are not mutually exclusive with many patients experiencing paranoid and nonparanoid phenomena. Nevertheless, the more clinically familiar categorisations may yet prove to reflect lateralised cerebral dysfunction (Gruzelier, 1984). Subdivisions in terms of acute and chronic may reveal qualitative differences in hemispheric function but the latter group of patients tends to have more severely and globally impaired performance (see Cutting, 1985).

Medication

Medication is a potential source of unsystematic bias in studies of psychiatric populations. Most schizophrenics available for testing will be on neuroleptic drugs. Those who are not, are by definition atypical and are likely to be less severly disturbed or so disturbed as to be untestable. There are exceptions such as those admitted to specialized research units or patients who though symptomatic and in psychiatric care, have refused medication or defaulted from treatment. Some chronically ill patients with affective disorder may be treated with neuroleptics but these too are somewhat atypical. Although parkinsonism and other neuroleptic induced extrapyramidal side effects may significantly hamper motor speed (David et al., 1987), overall performance, including speed of visual information processing (Braff & Saccuzzo, 1982) is improved by neuroleptics. Eaton et al., (1979) found that neuroleptics improved both left and right hemisphere performance but not uniformly for different cognitive tasks. Hammond & Gruzelier (1978) showed that left hemisphere functioning was differentially improved compared to right. Caution must be exerted in interpreting these claims: if an experimental design has revealed an LH deficit, it is predictable that after treatment, it may be attenuated. Such a result is not necessarily proof of a specific LH drug effect. Also, 'state dependant' abnormalities may disappear with clinical improvement regardless of whether the improvement is spontaneous or pharmacologically mediated. Testing patients during the acute illness and again after a period of treatment, whether or not the patient has responded might shed light on this (see Wexler, 1986; Johnson & Crockett, 1982).

Fixation

Accurate fixation can be achieved in a variety of ways from simply urging the patient to look straight ahead (Clooney & Murray, 1977; David, 1987), to requiring the subject to recall a central digit (Gur, 1978; Magaro & Page, 1983) or by visual monitoring (Eaton et al., 1979). Though ensuring fixation is important in preventing information entering the 'wrong' visual field, it has been suggested that the central stimulus may interfere with the cognitive processing of the test stimulus so that direct or video monitoring is the preferred method (Young, 1982). Poor fixation will result in unreliable data though it should not give rise to error in one visual field rather than the other, unless perhaps asymmetries in the direction of gaze exert an effect.

Another methodological problem appertaining to DVF studies is the use of masking techniques. Two studies have used a backward mask (Colbourn & Lishman, 1979; Gur, 1978) which may have had a particularly adverse effect on the schizophrenic groups' performance (Holtzman, 1987).

Divided visual field studies in schizophrenia will now be reviewed with these general comments in mind.

RESULTS

Clinical Variables

Of the 16 studies reviewed (see Table 1), only 7 included a psychiatric control group. Explicit, standardized diagnostic criteria were used in 11 studies. Handedness and sex were usually controlled for. Few studies attempted to match individuals on an estimate of IQ in addition to a record of length of schooling. Of those that did, 2 were able to match the schizophrenics with the normal controls (George & Neufeld, 1987; David, 1987) against 2 that did not (Colbourn & Lishman, 1979; Magaro & Page, 1983). Only 2 projects recruited unmedicated patients (Eaton et al., 1979; Connolly et al., 1983) the results of which do not point to dramatic drug-induced lateralized differences of cerebral function as they are consistent with similar studies of medicated patients.

Left Hemisphere Abnormality

The results of DVF studies in schizophrenia have been interpreted as

Table 1. Summary of divided visual field studies of schizophrenic patients

Investigators	Subjects (medication) Diag criteria	Controls	Experimental Task (dependent var - response mode)	Results	Comment
Beaumont & Dimond (1973)	12 Sz (M) "active" No criteria	12 mixed psych pts 12 general hospital pts	Matching: letters shapes and digits Across & within VFs (accuracy - vocal)	Poor X matching of shapes & letters Sz vs Cs	Poor LH letter matching Sz vs Cs; poor RH digit & shape matching, Sz vs psychiatric patients
Clooney & Murray (1977)	12 para Sz 12 non para (M) No criteria	12 normals	Matching: letter combinations (LJU) Across & within VFs (R & L manual RT)	Poor matching across & within, Sz vs Cs LH=RH	Para Sz with ↑ RT with ↑ number of letters for 'same' judgment only (R hand response)
Gur (1978)	12 para Sz 12 nonpara (M) No criteria	24 normals	Dot location & syllable recognition within VFs (accuracy - vocal)	Sz ↓ on syllable test vs Cs. Sz RH advantage for dots preserved	Sz ↓ on dot location vs Cs. RH verbal task scores relatively good vs Cs
Colbourn & Lishman (1979)	13 Sz (M) PSE	9 affectives 11 psych pts-non-psychotic 19 normals	Word & complex shape recognition within VFs (accuracy - vocal)	No LH ↓ for word task in male Sz only. No RH deficit.	No RH ↑ shown by Sz or Cs in non-verbal task. Only 5 male Sz showed abnormal laterality
Connolly et al., (1979)	15 Sz (M) PSE	6 affectives 14 psych pts-non-psychotic 20 normals	Dot pattern & alphanumeric recognition in R or L VF (vocal RT)	LH deficit for lexical & spatial tasks, Affs & Sz vs other Cs.	Sz and Affs poor overall. Lexical task failed to produce LH advantage in Cs
Hillsberg (1979)	5 Sz (M)	10 normals-5 students 5 hospital workers	Matching of arrow directions Across & within VFs (bimanual RT)	LH slower than RH in Sz. All slower in bilateral vs single VF matches	Sz much slower vs Cs. Trend for Sz across VFs match to be most ↓ of all

(Continued)

117

Table 1. Summary of divided visual field studies of schizophrenic patients (cont.)

Investigators	Subjects (medication) Diag criteria	Controls	Experimental Task (dependent var – response mode)	Results	Comment
Eaton (1979) & Eaton et al., (1979)	51 Sz RDC 24 Sz Feighner	18 normals (pre/post treatment)	Matching: letters digits and shapes Across & within Vfs (manual RT/accuracy)	Sz less accurate on verbal task, Poor X matching of shapes	General improvement posttreatment, LH ↑ more for digit task, RH ↑ for verbal task
Pic'l et al., (1979)	10 para Sz 10 nonpara Chronic (M) No criteria	10 psych in-patients 10 normals	Dot enumeration & identification of 4 letter strings (accuracy – vocal)	LH ↑ for lexical task in all groups, Nonpara RH ↓ for dot task	All pts poorer vs normals on LH (& RH) tasks. Nonparanoids worst of all
Schweitzer (1982)	16 Sz (M) DSM-III	16 normals	Shape/word STM matching, within R or L VF (accuracy – vocal)	LH shape task performance=Cs. RH shapes task vs Cs	Word task accuracy Sz=Cs, regardless of VF
Connolly et al., (1983)	12 Sz (no M)	16 normals	Identification of dot patterns and letters, R or L VF (R & L manual RT)	LH ↓ (RH ↑) for letters, Sz vs Cs RH ↑ for dots Sz & Cs. Normal IHTT	Sz ↓ on all tasks. R hand ↑ for dots. Weak LH advantage on verbal task in Cs
Margaro & Page (1983)	8 para Sz 8 nonpara (M) DSM-III/RDC	8 mixed psych in-pts 8 normals	Matching: letters shapes and faces Across & within VFs (accuracy – vocal)	Nonpara ↓ for all RVF stimuli & X matching of letters	Para Sz poor at X matching of shapes. RH ↓ for matching in all subjects
Shelton & Knight (1984)	12 Sz (M) DSM-III	12 mixed psych in-pts	Identification of inverted U R or L VF (R & L manual RT)	Sz=Cs for IHTT. No VF or hand advantage in either group	No reliable estimate of IHTT obtained in Sz or Cs, RHd reponse poor in Sz

Investigators	Subjects (medication) Diag criteria	Controls	Experimental Task (dependent var – response mode)	Results	Comment
Schwartz et al., (1984)	10 Sz Chronic (M) DSM-III & Feighner	9 normals	Temporal discrimination of 2 dots (SDA) Across & within VFs (vocal)	LH ↑ for Sz & Cs Slower IHTT for Sz vs Cs	Sz responses slower throughout. No difference for bi vs uni-lateral, Sz & Cs
George & Neufeld (1987)	14 para Sz 14 nonpara (M) RDC	14 mixed psych in-pts 14 students 14 normals	Matching: target (face/word) followed by stimulus in VF (manual RT/accuracy)	LH ↑ for words & RH ↑ for faces, Sz and Cs, Sz ↓ generally vs Cs	Nonpara Sz most ↓ & affected by increased cognitive load. Effect different in R & L VFs
Merriam & Gardner (1987)	16 Sz Chronic (M) DSM-III	16 normals	Matching: bilateral word/dots followed by same in R or L VF (manual RT/accuracy)	Poorer matching X VFs in Sz & Cs. Sz slower & less accurate than Cs	LH ↑ for word & dot matching accuracy in Sz & Cs. Within VF matches, Sz ↓ vs Cs
David (1987)	22 Sz (M) RDC	14 affective 16 normals	Naming of colors in R or L VF. Matching Across & within VFs (vocal - accuracy)	Poorer LVF color naming Sz vs Cs. Sz ↓ matching of colours across VFs	R & L VF matching and RVF color naming not ↓ Sz vs Cs. Suggests ↓ callosal transmission

Key to abbreviations:

Sz: schizophrenics; RT: reaction time; X Matching: matching across visual fields; LH: left hemisphere; RH: right hemisphere; RHd: right hand; para: paranoid schizophrenics; nonpara: non paranoid schizophrenics; Cs: controls; Affs: affectives; Feighner: Feighner Diagnostic Criteria (1972); psych: psychiatric; pts: patients; STM: short term memory; SOA: stimulus onset asynchrony; VF: visual field; PSE: Present State Examination (1974); VF: visual field; RDC: Research Diagnostic Criteria (1975); (M): medication; DSM-III: Diagnostic & Statistical Manual of the American Psychiatric Association, Vol III (1980); IHTT: interhemispheric transmission time.

showing hemisphere overactivation, underactivation and/or dysfunction; altered or reduced asymmetry, lack of integration or impaired interhemispheric transfer. Sometimes a superiority in one hemisphere is interpreted as abnormal overactivation in that hemisphere or an abnormal underactivation of the opposite hemisphere. Such explanations may suit almost any hypothesis and are therefore irrefutable. At this stage in our understanding of models of hemisphere interaction, it is perhaps wiser to resist unbridled speculation on the basis of equivocal data and instead confine ourselves to modest statements about the nature of the abnormality we believe we have uncovered.

An LH abnormality in the broadest sense has been found in the majority of DVF studies to date (see Table 1). This has manifested in: (1) impaired RVF matching of letters (Beaumont & Dimond, 1973; Magaro & Page, 1983); (2) impaired RVF identification of letters, in schizophrenics and manic depressives (Connolly et al., 1979) and unmedicated schizophrenics (Connolly et al., 1983); (3) impaired RVF identification of 3-letter syllables, arranged vertically (Gur, 1978), and 4-letter nouns (Colbourn & Lishman, 1979). However, the remaining studies which claim to show an RH abnormality or no lateralized deficit, also show generally poor performance on tasks including those presented to the RVF/LH. In other words, the LH abnormality has not been an isolated finding. The pattern of asymmetry was the same in both schizophrenics and controls in Clooney and Murray's study (1977), and schizophrenics showed the anticipated LH advantage for verbal tests in studies by Pic'l et al. (1979), George and Neufeld (1987) and Merriam and Gardner, (1987). In an effort to be more specific about the nature of the LH abnormality workers have examined the accuracy and/or speed of processing of 'non-verbal' stimuli presented to the RVF/LH. There is a hint that RVF/LH performance on non-verbal tasks may be less impaired than on verbal tasks (Pic'l et al., 1979; Connolly et al., 1979; Connolly et al., 1983; Gur, 1978; Eaton et al., 1979). Connolly et al. (1979) argue that this indicates intact RH along with CC functioning, in that spatial percepts must be transferred to the RH for processing. Given the dimensional nature of hemisphere asymmetries already mentioned (Bradshaw & Nettleton, 1981) relative sparing of LH non-verbal processing is an equally plausible explanation. Hillsberg (1979) found an RVF/LH deficit in a non-verbal matching task which is somewhat contradictory, but her schizophrenic group were considerably slower than controls overall so that this plus the small sample size raises the possibility of a Type I error.

Failure to find an expected hemisphere advantage in normal controls has undermined the basic assumptions of many studies since the presence of just such an asymmetry or its opposite in the patient group is almost impossible to interpret. In 2 studies, the 'lexical' task revealed only minimal asymmetry in normal subjects (Connolly et al., 1979; Connolly et al., 1983; Magaro & Page, 1983) in this case LH superiority, and in other studies, an RH advantage for shapes (Colbourn & Lishman, 1979) and faces (Magaro & Page, 1983) was not elicited in controls. Merriam & Gardner (1987) in an across VF matching paradigm found an LH advantage for both words and dots, the latter being contrary to prediction. One reason for the inconsistency in determining lateral advantages may be that the 'verbal' and 'non-verbal' tasks may differ considerably in difficulty (see Gur, 1978; Connolly et al., 1979) as discussed earlier.

In summary there is support for a left sided intrahemispheric abnormality in most schizophrenics but further comparisons with psychiatric controls and more careful matching of tasks on level of difficulty is required before definitive statements can be made.

Right Hemisphere Abnormality

A degree of impairment in the processing of stimuli presented to the LVF/RH is shown in the majority of DVF studies though, as in the case of RVF/LH stimuli, this has been a reflection of generalized deficit (see Table). Two studies have found RH abnormalities to be more significant than those pertaining to the LH. Pic'l et al., (1979) demonstrated poor RH performance on a dot enumeration experiment in non-paranoid schizophrenics, although LH performance on a verbal task was also poor. The unusually brief exposure time of 17 msec may have contributed to the RH inaccuracy (Sergent, 1983). Schweitzer (1982), using a complicated design which consisted of a single stimulus (shape or word) followed at differing intervals by an additional stimulus for matching, found that schizophrenics' RVF/LH accuracy approximated that of a normal control group whereas the patients' performance on shape matching was impaired.

Some authors (e.g. Gur, 1978; Connolly et al., 1983; Magaro & Page, 1983) have stressed the relatively preserved RH superiority for spatial tasks although it must be remembered that Gur (1978) showed the stimuli for a longer duration to schizophrenic subjects compared to controls and Connolly et al., (1983) subtracted 'response time' from 'processing time' which exaggerated the similarity between patients and controls.

A combination of right and left hemisphere dysfunction, the nature of which may differ qualitatively, forms the basis of an attractive theory explaining the typically schizophrenic features described by Bleuler (1911) including thought disorder and emotional disturbance (see Cutting, 1985; Gur, 1979). Neuropsychological evidence for this viewpoint from purely DVF studies is so far lacking.

Corpus Callosum Abnormality

Experimental designs which present visual stimuli to both VFs simultaneously and require the subject to make a same-different judgement depend on a degree of cooperation between the cerebral hemispheres and ipso facto communication between them (see Table). Beaumont and Dimond (1973) used this paradigm in their original study and found that the matching of shapes and letter was performed significantly more poorly across VFs than within them, though within VF matching was also defective. The mixed picture of less accurate matching within and across VFs was also found in other studies (Clooney & Murray, 1977; Eaton et al., 1979; Hillsberg, 1970; Magaro & Page, 1983). Merriam and Gardner (1987) modified the matching procedure by beginning with bilateral stimuli followed 2 seconds later by a single lateralized stimulus, with the subject asked to decide whether the latter matched the former in either the right or left VF. Matches where the single stimulus was the same as the one of the pair in the opposite VF were more difficult for all subjects and so the schizophrenics' impairment on this task could not have been due to a 'differential deficit'. In contrast, a colour matching task (David, 1987) revealed superior 'across' as opposed to 'within' VF matching (see Lieberman & Meehan, 1986) in affective and normal controls, compared to schizophrenics who found the 'across' matching more difficult. From the studies available, there appears to be a slight trend towards cross matching of non-verbal stimuli to be most impaired in schizophrenia (Eaton, et al., 1979; Hillsberg, 1979; David, 1987) with one study showing this tendency in paranoid schizophrenics only (Magaro & Page, 1983). These authors also found a cross matching deficit for verbal stimuli in nonparanoid schizophrenics which they attributed to poor LH verbal functioning rather than a CC abnormality.

Interhemispheric transmission time (IHTT) has been estimated by substracting manual reaction time (RT) obtained when stimulus and response involve different hemispheres (e.g. RVF/left hand) (crossed), from RT following stimulus and response in the same hemisphere (e.g. RVF/right hand) (uncrossed) (Bashore, 1981). Using this method, Connolly et al., (1983) failed to demonstrate increased IHTT in schizophrenics. As a group, they produced a faster RT for the hand ipsilateral to the VF of stimulation compared to the contralateral hand by approximately the same margin as controls (approximately 4 msec). However as individuals, this was not a consistent finding pointing to unreliability of the method and the confounding effect of (in this study) generally slow left hand responses. Shelton and Knight (1984) using a more simple visual stimulus did not show prolonged IHTT in their schizophrenic sample. Again this conclusion is suspect since the expected IHTT delay was not found in the normal group, and considerably slower right hand responses regardless of VF in the schizophrenics may have obliterated the IHTT component of the total RT.

A novel procedure was utilized to measure IHTT in schizophrenia by Schwartz et al., (1984) in which 2 dots were flashed in either one or both VFs with a small delay between them. The authors marshal previous work which suggests that the LH is responsible for temporal analysis and detection of successive stimuli. Therefore, information from the LVF/RH must be transfered via the CC to the LH for analysis. By delaying the RVF/LH stimulus until the subject reports apparent simultaneity, a measure of IHTT is obtained. The authors found that the LH advantage for temporal sequential analysis was present in both schizophrenics and normal controls, though the schizophrenics' response time was slower overall, but that IHTT was significantly longer (10 msec vs 4 msec) in the patient group. This is another example of a non-verbal stimulus revealing a putative CC defect.

Since speech is a predominantly LH function (Beaumont, 1982), any test which presents information to the LVF/RH and requires a spoken response is in part a test of CC function (see Bashore, 1981). By limiting the intrahemispheric processing requirement using simple color naming (David, 1987) there was a significant increase in the number of errors arising from LVF color naming compared to RVF in a proportion of schizophrenics, supporting an abnormality of the CC (see Geschwind & Fusillo, 1966). Other studies reviewed earlier employing a vocal response, found poorer performances in identifying RVF/LH compared to LVF/RH stimuli (Colbourn & Lishman, 1979; Connolly et al., 1979 though not Pic'l et al., 1979 for letters or Schweitzer 1982 for shapes) so that support for abnormal IHTT in these studies is virtually absent. It is possible as had been argued elsewhere (David, 1987) that the use of complex percepts requiring processing before transfer may cloud the effects of IHTT. More studies using simpler stimuli such as colors are required to clarify this issue.

New Directions

A more sophisticated approach to specifying the nature of information processing dysfunction in schizophrenia using DVF techniques has been attempted (Clooney & Murray, 1977; Pic'l et al., 1979; George & Neufeld, 1987). By increasing the size of an array of letters, Clooney and Murray, (1977) found that paranoid schizophrenics' RT increased (for 'same' judgements only). This was interpreted as reflecting a reliance on LH serial processing as opposed to RH parallel processing. Increasing the display size (number of dots) seemed to impair paranoid schizophrenics performance more than non-paranoids (as classified by the Maine Scale; Magaro et al., 1981) and this too was said to indicate an inappropriate reliance on serial processing by the paranoids. Since the non-paranoids performance was less influenced by the size of the array, the authors proposed that this indicated parallel processing. A more parsimonious explanation would be that the non-paranoids, who were the most impaired sub-group, were performing at ceiling even with low cognitive loads and hence their performance could hardly get worse. George and Neufeld (1987) increased the cognitive load by introducing 4 levels of complexity to each of their hemisphere-specific tasks. They found that the schizophrenics, especially non-paranoids, declined in their performance as the attentional demands increased but there was no obvious pattern with respect to the differential sensitivity of the hemispheres. Exceptions to this were that non-paranoids responded significantly more slowly than paranoids only at the fourth level for RVF stimuli and displayed a marked increase in response latency at the third load level for LVF stimuli.

Research of this kind has not so far been particularly rewarding but is more likely to yield useful data than more tests showing that schizophrenics are slow and make mistakes. Examining the effects of exposure time on hemisphere asymmetries is another strategy yet to be exploited. Longitudinal rather than cross-sectional data has led to interesting hypotheses from dichotic listening (Johnson & Crockett, 1982; Wexler, 1986) and non-lateralized visual information processing experiments (Nuechterlein & Dawson, 1984; Holzman, 1987) and there is no reason why these methods should not apply to DVF studies. Questions relating to whether the abnormalities detected are a consequence of a 'trait' or 'state' could be tackled by testing first degree relatives of schizophrenics as well as patients who have recovered.

CONCLUSIONS

A review of DVF studies in schizophrenia has revealed a bewildering mass of contradictory results. Many projects, none of which have exactly replicated their predecessors, each with their own methodological flaws, have contributed to an undifferentiated pool of knowledge. Nevertheless, despite formidable barriers to interpretation, certain consistencies emerge:

(1) Schizophrenics' performance is impaired in comparison to normal controls on tasks which present stimuli to the right or to the left visual fields.
(2) Cognitive tasks presented tachistoscopically to the RVF/LH have been performed less well more often than those involving the LVF/RH, but dysfunction in both has been recorded.
(3) Verbal tasks presented to the RVF/LH give rise to the largest performance decrement compared to non-verbal tasks, though both types are impaired.
(4) Experiments requiring integration of stimuli presented across the VFs, which presumably relies on an efficient CC, show impairment in schizophrenics, and this is especially so for non-verbal stimuli.

It remains to be determined whether these abnormalities relate to specific symptoms of schizophrenia or whether they are mere epiphenomena, whether they are stable over time and clinical course and whether they reflect a vulnerability to, or consequence of, the disorder. Furthermore, discovering the relationship between functional abnormalities and their presumed biochemical, physiological or structural substrate is still a distant but ever more tangible Holy Grail.

REFERENCES

Alpert, M. Rubenstein, & Kesselman, M. (1976). Asymmetry of information processing in hallucinators and nonhallucinators. Journal of Nervous and Mental Disease, 162, 258-265.

American Psychiatric Association (1980). Diagnostic and Statistical Manual of Mental Disorder (DSM-III) (3rd Edit.). Washington DC: APA.

Bashore, T.R. (1981). Vocal and manual reaction time estimates of inter-hemispheric transmission time. Psychological Bulletin, 89, 352-368.

Beaton, A. (1985). Left Side/Right Side. A Review of Laterality Research. London: Bratsford Academic & Educational.

Beaumont, J.G. (1982). Divided Visual Field Studies of Cerebral Organisation. London: Academic Press.

Beaumont, J.G. & Dimond, S. (1973). Brain disconnection and schizophrenia. British Journal of Psychiatry, 123, 661-662.

Bleuler, P.E. (1911). Dementia Praecox and the Group of Schizophrenias (translated, 1950). New York: International University Press.

Bradshaw, J.L. & Nettleton, N.C. (1981). The nature of hemispheric specialization in man. Behavioural and Brain Sciences, 4, 51-91.

Braff, D.L. & Saccuzzo, D.P. (1982). Effect of antipsychotic medication on speed of information processing in schizophrenic patients. American Journal of Psychiatry, 139, 661-662.

Chapman, L.J. & Chapman, J.P. (1973). Problems in the measurement of cognitive deficit. Psychological Bulletin, 79, 380-385.

Chapman, L.J. & Chapman, J.P. (1977). Selection of subjects in studies of schizophrenic cognition. Journal of Abnormal Psychology, 86, 10-15.

Clooney, J.L. & Murray, D.J. (1977), same-different judgements in paranoid and non-paranoid schizophrenic patients: a laterality study. Journal of Abnormal Psychology, 86, 655-658.

Colbourn, C.J. (1982). Divided visual field studies of psychiatric patients. in: J.G. Beaumont (ed.), Divided Visual Field Studies of Cerebral Organisation, London: Academic Press.

Colbourn, C.J. & Lishman, W.A. (1979). Lateralization of function and psychotic illness: a left hemisphere deficit? in: J.H. Gruzelier & P. Flor-Henry (eds.), Hemisphere Asymmetries of Function in Psychopathology, Amersterdam: Elsevier/North Holland Biomedical Press.

Connolly, J.F., Gruzelier, J.H., Kleinman, K.M. & Hirsch, S.R. (1979). Lateralised abnormalities in hemisphere-specific tachistoscopic task in psychiatric patients and controls. in: J.H. Gruzelier & P. Flor-Henry (eds.), Hemisphere Asymmetries of Function in Psychopathology, Amsterdam: Elsevier/North Holland Biomedical Press.

Connolly, J.F., Gruzelier, J.H. & Manchanda, R. (1983). Electrocortical and functional asymmetries in schizophrenia. in: P. Flor-Henry & J. Gruzelier (eds), Laterality and Psychopathology, Amersterdam: Elsevier/North Holland Biomedical Press.

Cutting, J.C. (1985). The Psychology of Schizophrenia. London: Churchill Livingstone.

David, A.S. (1987). Tachistoscopic tests of colour naming and matching in schizophrenia: evidence for posterior callosum dysfunction? Psychological Medicine, 17, 621-630.

David, A.S., Jeste, D.V., Folstein, M.F. & Folstein, S.E. (1987). Voluntary movement dysfunction in Huntington's disease and tardive dyskinesia. Acta Neurologica Scandinavica, 75, 130-139.

Eaton, E.M. (1979). Hemisphere-related visual information processing in acute schizophrenia. Before and after neuroleptic treatment. in: J.H. Gruzelier & P. Flor-Henry (eds.), Hemisphere Asymmetries of Function in Psychopathology, Amsterdam: Elsevier/North Holland Biomedical Press.

Eaton, E.M., Busk, J., Maloney, M.P., Sloane, R.B., Whipple, K. & White, K. (1979). Hemisphere dysfunction in schizophrenia: assessment by visual perception taks. Psychiatric Research, 1, 325-332.

Galin, D. (1974). Implications for psychiatry of left and right cerebral specialization. Archives of General Psychiatry, 31, 572-583.

Gazzaniga, M.S., Bogen, J.E. & Sperry, R.W. (1965). Observations on visual perception after disconnexion of the cerebral hemispheres in man. Brain, 88, 16-36.

George, L. & Neufeld, R.W.J. (1987). Attentional resources and hemispheric functional asymmetry in schizophrenia. British Journal of Clinical Psychology, 26, 35-45.

Geschwind, N. (1965). Disconnexion syndromes in animals and man. Brain, 88, 237-294 and 585-644.

Geschwind, N. & Fusillo, M. (1966). Color naming defects in association with alexia. Archives of Neurology, 15, 137-146.

Goldstein, G. (1986). The neuropsychology of schizophrenia. in: I.G. Grant & K.M. Adams (eds.), Neuropsychological Assessment in Neuropsychiatric Disorders, New York: Oxford University Press.

Gruzelier, J.H. (1981). Cerebral laterality and psychopathology: fact and fiction. Psychological Medicine, 11, 219-227.

Gruzelier, J.H. (1984). Hemispheric imbalances in schizophrenia. International Journal of Psychophysiology, 1, 227-240.

Gur, R.E. (1978). Left hemisphere dysfunction and left hemisphere overactivation in schizophrenia. Journal of Abnormal Psychology, 87, 226-238.

Gur, R.E. (1979). Cognitive concomitants of hemisphere dysfunction in schizophrenia. Archives of General Psychiatry, 36, 269-274.

Hammond, N.V. & Gruzelier, J.H. (1978). Laterality, attention and rate effects in the auditory temporal discrimination of chronic schizophrenics: the effect of treatment with chlorpromazine. Quarterly Journal of Experimental Psychology, 30, 91-103.

Hillsberg, B. (1979). A comparison of visual discrimination performance of the dominant and nondominant hemispheres in schizophrenia. in: J.H. Gruzelier & P. Flor-Henry (eds.), Hemisphere Asymmetries of Function in Psychopathology, Amsterdam: Elsevier/North Holland Biomedical press.

Holzman, P.S. (1987). Recent studies of psychophysiology in schizophrenia. Schizophrenia Bulletin, 13, 49-75.

Johnson, O. & Crockett, D. (1982). Changes in perceptual asymmetries with clinical improvement of depression. Journal of Abnormal Psychology, 91, 45-54.

Liddle, P.F. (1987). The symptoms of chronic schizophrenia: a reexamination of the positive-negative dichotomy. British Journal of Psychiatry, 151, 145-151.

Liederman, J. & Meehan, P. (1986). When is between-hemisphere division of labour advantageous? Neuropsychologia, 24, 863-874.

Lishman, W.A. (1971). Emotion, consciousness and will after brain bisection in man. Cortex, 7, 181-192.

Magaro, P., Abrams, L. & Cantrell, P. (1981). The Maine Scale of paranoid and non-paranoid schizophrenia: reliability and validity. Journal of Consultative Clinical Psychology, 49, 438-447.

Magaro, P.A. & Page, J. (1983). Brain disconnection, schizophrenia and paranoia. Journal of Nervous and Mental Disease, 171, 133-140.

Merriam, A.E. & Gardener, E.B. (1987). Corpus callosum function in schizophrenia: a neuropsychological assessment of interhemispheric information processing. Neuropsychologia, 25, 185-193.

Moscovitch, M. (1986). Afferent and efferent models of visual perceptual asymmetries: theoretical and empirical implications. Neuropsychologia, 24, 91-114.

Nelson, H.E. & O'Connell, A. (1978). Dementia: the estimation of premorbid intelligence levels using the new adult reading test. Cortex, 14, 234-244.

Neuchterlein, K.H. & Dawson, M.E. (1984). Information processing and attentional functioning in the developmental course of schizophrenic disorders. Schizophrenia Bulletin, 10, 160–203.

Newlin, D.B., Carpenter, B. & Golden, C.J. (1981). Hemispheric asymmetries in schizophrenia. Biological Psychiatry, 16, 561–582.

Pic'l, A.K., Magaro, P.A. & Wade, E.A. (1979). Hemispheric functioning in
paranoid and non-paranoid schizophrenia. Biological Psychiatry, 14,
891–903.

Robertson, G. & Taylor, P.J. (1987). Laterality and psychosis: neuropsychological evidence. British Medical Bulletin, 43, 634–650.

Robertson, R. & Bigelow, L.B. (1972). Quantitative brain measurements in
chronic schizophrenia. British Journal of Psychiatry, 121, 259–264.

Ross-Kossak, P. & Turkewitz, G. (1984). Relationship between changes in
hemispheric advantage during familiarization to faces and proficiency in facial recognition. Neuropsychologia, 22, 471–477.

Schweitzer, L. (1982). Evidence of right hemisphere dysfunction in
schizophrenic patients with left hemisphere overactivation. Biological Psychiatry, 17, 655–673.

Schwartz, B.D., Winstead, D.K. & Walker, W.G. (1984). A corpus callosal
deficit in sequential analysis by schizophrenics. Biological Psychiatry, 19, 1667–1676.

Sergent, J. (1983). The role of the input in visual hemispheric asymmetries. Psychological Bulletin, 93, 481–512.

Shelton, E.J. & R.G. Knight (1984). Inter-hemispheric transmission times
in schizophrenics. British Journal of Clinical Psychology, 24,
227–228.

Shenton, M.E., Solovay, M.R. & Holzman, P. (1987). Comparative studies of
thought disorder II: schizoaffective disorder. Archives of General
Psychiatry, 44, 21–30.

Sperry, R.W. (1968). Hemisphere deconnection and unity in conscious
awareness. American Psychologist, 23, 723–733.

Spitzer, R.L. & Endicott, J. & Robins, E. (1975). Research Diagnostic
Criteria. New York: New York State Psychiatric Institute.

Walker, E. & McGuire, M. (1982). Intra and inter-hemispheric information
processing in Schizophrenia. Psychological Bulletin, 92, 701–725.

Wexler, B.E. (1986). Alterations in cerebral laterality during acute
psychotic illness. British Journal of Psychiatry, 149, 202–209.

Wigan, A.L. (1844). The Duality of the Mind. London: Longman.

Wing, J.K. & Wing, L. (1982). Handbook of Psychiatry Vol 3. Psychoses of
Uncertain Origin. Cambridge: Cambridge University Press.

Young, A.W. (1982). Methodological and theoretical bases. in: J.G.
Beaumont (ed.), Divided Visual Field Studies of Cerebral Organisation, London: Academic Press.

LATE POSITIVE EVENT RELATED POTENTIALS IN SCHIZOPHRENIA

K P Ebmeier, A R MacKenzie, D D Potter and E A Salzen

WHAT IS P3?

As early as 1965 Sutton et al. described a late single positive component of the event related potentials (ERP) with a peak latency of about 300 ms which appeared to be related to stimulus uncertainty. This potential is 'endogenous' in that it does not reflect physical parameters of the eliciting stimuli and it can be elicited by stimuli of different sensory modalities or even by the absence of an expected stimulus. In this sense it can be said to reflect 'active cognitive processing of stimulus information on the part of the subject' (Pritchard, 1981). It is now clear that P3 is part of a late positive complex (LPC) rather than a unitary phenomenon. It consists of an early positive wave of 220 to 280 ms latency with fronto-central scalp distribution often termed P3a (Squires et al., 1975), a slightly later wave, called P3b, with a peak latency of 310-380 ms and maximal parietal distribution, and a slow wave (SW) overlapping with and following P3a and P3b and showing a parietal distribution similar to P3b but associated with increased negativity over the frontal leads. While the P3a is elicited by infrequent stimuli which were not attended to, a P3b occurs with the introduction of a discrimination task (e.g. counting target stimuli) involving infrequent stimuli (Squires et al., 1975). Apart from discriminative tasks, P3b can be elicited by stimuli which give feedback on the outcome of a prior task or stimuli which require a motor response. While SW and P3b covary in relation to many stimulus conditions, under certain conditions a dissociation can be observed (Ruchkin & Sutton, 1983).

P3b has been examined most extensively in its relation to various stimulus parameters. Its latency and amplitude can be experimentally manipulated independently from each other. P3b amplitude seems to be related to the subjective probability of the target stimulus, task and stimulus complexity, the reward gained for a correct response, stimulus equivocation, and task relevance of stimuli. These variables can act either independently, or additively and in some cases multiplicatively together (Johnson, 1986). P3 latency appears to be related to the difficulty the subject has in categorising the eliciting stimulus (Squires & Ollo, 1986), whether this is due to stimulus intensity (Papanicolaou et al., 1985), stimulus equivocation (Polich et al., 1985), stimulus complexity (Kutas et al., 1977), or task demands (Polich, 1986). Choice reaction time and P3 latency usually covary, particularly if the subject is instructed to make correct responses rather than fast responses (Kutas et al., 1977). P3 latency tends to increase with adult age (Pfefferbaum et al., 1984a), with smaller digit span in neurologically normal subjects (Polich et al., 1983), and with acute and some chronic organic psychiatric syndromes (Squires et al., 1979; Hansch et al., 1982; Goodin et al., 1983; Pfefferbaum et al., 1984b; St Clair et al., 1985).

The neural generators of P3a, P3b and SW are unknown; there are suggestions that P3a is generated within the frontal lobe (McCarthy et al., 1982), while P3b originates from medial temporal lobe structures (Halgren et al., 1980; Wood et al., 1984). However some author's have described a possible thalamic generator (Yingling & Hosobuchi, 1984), and there is some evidence from patients with temporal lobectomy (Stapleton et al., 1987) and from an experimental model of P3 (Paller et al., 1984) that normal P3 can be generated in subjects without temporal lobes.

IS P3 - AMPLITUDE REDUCED IN SCHIZOPHRENIA?

While researchers have used a variety of experimental paradigms and diagnostic criteria, reduced P3 amplitudes seem to be a robust character-istic of schizophrenic patients (Saletu et al., 1971; Levit et al., 1973; Roth et al., 1980; Baribeau-Braun, 1983; Pfefferbaum et al., 1984b; Barrett et al., 1986; Blackwood et al., 1987).

Apart from a genuine reduction of P3-amplitude several alternative explanations for a reduced peak voltage of P3 have to be considered. An increased 'inter-trial jitter' might produce a lower average peak voltage for single subjects. Similarly, an increased inter-subject variability of P3 latency can produce a reduction of 'P3' - peak voltage in the group's grand-average. Roth et al. (1980b) and Pfefferbaum et al. (1984b) exam-ined these possible causes of a reduction of P3 - amplitude by single trial analysis and correction for latency jitter and came to the con-clusion that although for schizophrenics both latency jitter and inter-subject variability of P3-latency was increased, the amplitude corrected for these factors was still smaller for schizophrenics than for controls.

Another possible reason for reduced P3 - voltage is a dispersal of late positive waves in schizophrenic patients. Saletu et al. (1971) des-cribed a single stimulus paradigm which produced more complex wave forms with 'N4' and 'P5' for schizophrenics with thought process disorder. In subsequent studies using P3-paradigms the variability of wave forms has been commented upon (eg. Blackwood et al., 1987) but never systematically examined.

In our own recent study of a group of DSM III diagnosed schizophren-ics (n=21) (American Psychiatric Association, 1980) and age-matched con-trols (n=16) we have also observed an increased variability in the ERP's of the schizophrenics. The subjects had to perform an auditory discrimin-ation task in which they counted randomly distributed target tones (1500 Hz) in a background of 90% non-target tones (1000 Hz). ERP's were recor-ded with a band-pass of 0.16-50 Hz and with linked earlobe reference. Averages, which excluded EOG artifacts greater than 45 microvolts, were computed off-line. Significantly more positive peaks were present in the evoked responses of the schizophrenics than amongst the controls at Cz and at Pz (see Fig.1) but not at lateral parietal sites (P3 and P4). Assuming that in schizophrenia there is a dispersal of peaks rather than an activation of additional generators, there would be an apparent reduc-tion of peak voltage for the commonly designated P3 (usually the maximum peak between 260 and 450 ms post-stimulus) for the patients compared with controls.

A further possible reason for reduction of P3-peak-voltage has been proposed by Barrett et al. (1986). These authors found not only a reduc-tion of P3 peak amplitude, but also of the mean amplitude between 275 and 425 ms post stimulus. This reduction only reached significance for fre-quent non-targets, but it led the authors to speculate that 'it is not really P3 per se which shows the marked amplitude difference between controls and schizophrenics but a considerably more protracted late positivity which overlaps P3' (Barrett et al., 1986).

Long-term medication is unlikely to play a major role in P3-amplitude reduction in schizophrenia (Baribeau-Braun et al., 1983; Strandburg et al., 1984; Blackwood et al., 1987), although some authors have reported a normalisation of amplitudes on clinical recovery (Levit et al., 1973; Matsubayashi et al., 1985). This raises the question of clinical correlates to amplitude reduction. While some authors have found no clinical correlates (Roth et al., 1972; Barrett et al., 1986), others have found small and moderate correlations with differing clinical characteristics. Saletu et al. (1971) found that schizophrenic patients with thought disorder had smaller P3 amplitudes. Blackwood et al. (1987) found negative correlations with total Hamilton Depression Score and certain items of the Brief Psychiatric Rating Scale, namely 'depressive mood' and 'motor retardation'. In contrast, we found significant correlations between P3-amplitude and certain positive and negative symptoms like 'distractable speech' (Kendall's tau=-0.55) and 'impersistence at work' (Kendall's tau=-0.45). The unavoidable (self-) selection of schizophrenics for electrophysiological studies makes it likely that spuriously significant correlations will appear which are likely to be different from study to study. In fact, some groups have found a persistence of amplitude reduction beyond clinical recovery (Barrett et al., 1986; Blackwood et al., 1987) which suggests that it might be a trait, rather han a state variable. This interpretation is supported by research conducted among relatives of schizophrenics (Friedman et al., 1982; Saitoh et al., 1984) or subjects with borderline or schizotypal personality disorder (Erwin et al., 1985; Blackwood et al., 1986; Kutcher et al., 1987), who all show a reduced P3 amplitude compared with controls.

In reaction time paradigms schizophrenics perform more slowly and less accurately so that the question arises whether reduced amplitude is simply a reflection of non-detection of targets. Baribeau-Braun (1983) examined accurate and fast responses to target stimuli separately and still found a smaller P3 amplitude in schizophrenics as compared with controls. They concluded that it was control and maintenance of a selective processing strategy rather than general slowness or absence of selectivity which accounted for the reduction in P3-amplitude in schizophrenics.

IS P3 - LATENCY INCREASED IN SCHIZOPHRENIA?

Many of the earlier studies and some recent studies (Roth & Cannon, 1972; Levit et al., 1973; Barrett et al., 1986) did not find abnormal P3-latencies in schizophrenics. Since Roth et al's first report of increased P3-latencies (1979) a few groups have replicated their findings (Pfefferbaum et al., 1984b; Blackwood et al., 1987; Romani et al., 1987). There are a number of possible reasons for those conflicting experimental findings. Pfefferbaum et al. (1984b) suggested that their increased P3-latencies in schizophrenics might be related to certain methodological improvements used in their study like the use of a 3-tone reaction time paradigm with single trial analysis of only the correct trials. It appears, however, that simple two tone experiments (Blackwood et al., 1987; Romani et al., 1987; Ebmeier et al., 1987) using stimulus synchronised averages can produce latency differences, while more complex reaction-time paradigms do not necessarily lead to latency differences (Barrett et al., 1986) (see Table 1).

TABLE 1

P3-Latency in Recent Studies and Possible Causes for Latency Increases

	Pfefferbaum et al, 1984	Barrett et al, 1986	Blackwood et al, 1987	Romani et al, 1987	Ebmeier et al, 1987
P3-latency increased	Yes	No	Yes	Yes	(Yes)
P3-paradigm	3 tone, RT	2x2 tone, RT	2 tone, count	2 tone, count	2 tone, count
Single trial analysis	+	-	-	-	-
P3-definition	Woody-filter	Max [275-425ms]	Tangents	[320-480ms]	a) Max [260-450ms] b) 1st>300ms
Slow wave (Low frequency filter)	? (3.5 Hz)	Mean voltage between 275-425ms significantly smaller (0.13 Hz)	? (1 Hz)	? (0.5 Hz)	no voltage diff. between groups > 360ms (0.16 Hz)
Stimulus intensity	70 dB above individual sensory threshold	90 dB	65 dB	70 dB	80 dB
Anti-cholinergic medication	?	?	?	no	b) Kendall's tau=0.48 at Pz
Cognitive deficit	on MMSE, correlated with P3-latency	?	?	on neuropsychological test battery, correlated with P3-latency	on WAIS, NART + WAIS correlated with P3-latency
Type of subjects	20 RDC schiz. 115 controls	20 RDC acute in/out-patients 20 controls	24 RDC in-patients 59 controls	20 DSM III in-patients > 5 yrs 20 controls	21 DSM III in- and out-patients 16 controls

More important seems to be the mode of definition of P3 for the purpose of latency - measurements. The presence of multiple peaks in the schizophrenic group necessitates the introduction of an arbitrary criterion for the definition of 'P3' and the determination of P3-latency. There appears to be no evidence that any one of the methods used is more valid than the others. Both Barrett et al. (1986) and the present authors could find no latency differences between schizophrenics and controls using as 'P3' the maximum peak between 275–425 ms and 260–450 ms, respectively. Blackwood et al. (1987) used the intersection of ascending and descending tangents when multiple peaks occurred in their patients and found latency differences. The present authors used a second definition for P3, i.e. the first maximum after 300 ms post - stimulus. This method leads to significantly increased P3-latencies for the schizophrenic group at Cz, but not at parietal positions (P2, P3, P4).

All of the studies which report consistent latency differences used low frequency filter settings which may have considerably reduced the contribution of slow wave activity to the evoked responses (see Table 1). Where this latency difference has not been found (Barrett et al., 1986; Ebmeier et al., 1987) the slow wave activity may have interacted with the P3 response, increasing the apparent P3 latency in the control group but not in the schizophrenics where slow wave activity is of reduced amplitude (Ebmeier et al., 1989).

Callaway (1984) described an increase in P300 latency after 1.2 mg of scopolamine, and we found significant correlations within the patient group between dose of anticholinergic medication and P3-latency (see Table 1). Apart from Blackwood et al. (1987) who examined non-medicated patients all other studies contained medicated patients, a subgroup of which would also have received anticholinergics.

In none of the described studies were patients and controls education-matched. Pfefferbaum et al. (1984b) found a moderately high correlation between MMSE-score and P3-latency in a group of schizophrenic and depressed patients tested with a visual P3 paradigm, but not with an auditory one. They argued that impairment of MMSE was 'consistent with the diagnosis of schizophrenia'. This finding begs the question whether schizophrenics have prolonged P3-latencies because they are cognitively impaired. Romani et al., (1987) examined a group of 20 chronic schizophrenics and controls with a neuropsychological test-battery and CT-scan

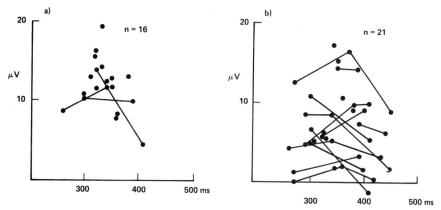

Figure 1. Maxima between 260 and 450 ms following target stimulus measured at Pz; if more than one maximum occurs in the same subject, these are linked.

in addition to an auditory oddball P3 paradigm. While for controls no significant correlations could be found between ERP's and neuropsychological measures, multiple determination coefficients (R squared) yielded significant associations in patients between the two main factors extracted from the test battery and the P3-latency. Ebmeier et al. (1987) examined a subgroup of their patients (n=14) with the National Adult Reading Test (Nelson, 1982) and the Wechsler Adult Intelligence Scale. NART - predicted IQs were significantly higher than actual WAIS - IQs (NART = 103.5 + 8.3, WAIS = 88.6+ 15.5). This difference was significantly greater for Performance IQ (NART = 104.6 + 6.5, WAIS = 84.7 + 13.9) than for Verbal IQ (NART = 101.9 + 9.1, WAIS = 92.9 + 17.1). While WAIS Performance IQ was not significantly correlated with P3-latency, there were significant correlations (P<0.01) with NART score, Full Scale IQ and Verbal IQ. These preliminary results suggest that, while P3-latency is related to cognitive function, it is more closely correlated with measures of pre-morbid function than with measures reflecting cognitive decline due to the schizophrenic illness.

While reaction times are more variable and increased in schizophrenics (Baribeau - Braun et al., 1983), this is not necessarily associated with a parallel change in P3-latency. Callaway and Naghdi (1982) argue that if stimulus evaluation time - and therefore P3-latency - is normal in schizophrenics the major reason for a slowing of reaction-time in schizophrenics must be an impairment of response selection.

Amongst clinical variables the duration and severity of the illness might play a role in the increase of P3-latency. Barrett et al. (1986) and the present authors used acute in-patients and out-patients while Romani et al. (1987), for example, used in-patients of more than 5 years standing. Matsubayashi et al. (1985) found an increase in P3-latencies in chronic, but not in acute schizophrenic patients. While in Blackwood et al.'s study (1987) P3-latency correlated positively with the total BPRS score and the subscore for 'emotional withdrawal and deficiency in relating to others', we found negative correlations with the sub-scores for 'anxiety', 'depression', 'guilt' and 'grandiosity'. This would support the notion that acute schizophrenics who often present with a substantial degree of affective symptoms (WHO, 1978) have a shorter P3-latency than chronic schizophrenics who present with emotional withdrawal and negative symptoms of schizophrenia. While P3-latency was not correlated with age in Blackwood et al.'s (1987) or our study, the fact that Romani et al.'s (1987) 'disorganised type' patients had an increased P3-latency and our 'paranoid type' patients did not, might simply be a result of their differing duration of illness (Tsuang et al., 1980). A long-term followup study would be required to decide the question whether we are dealing with two separate groups of patients, one with cognitive and neuropsychological impairment, emotional withdrawal and long P3-latencies and the other with no cognitive impairment but with affective symptoms and normal P3-latencies, or simply with patients at different stages of their illness.

ANATOMICAL AND PATHOPHYSIOLOGICAL CORRELATES OF ABNORMAL P3 IN SCHIZOPHRENICS

While the P3 has normally a concentric topographic development with its maximum in the centroparietal area, brain electrical activity mapping has shown that schizophrenic patients have a P3 maximum more anteriorly and shifted to the right with deficency of left temporal activity (Merstyn et al., 1983; Faux et al., 1987). This is compatible with pathological evidence showing left temporal lobe changes in schizophrenic brains (Brown et al., 1986). Romani et al. (1987) found abnormalities in

CT-scans of their patients, but these abnormalities were not correlated with P3-changes.

Smooth eye pursuit has been shown to be abnormal in many schizophrenic patients and their relatives, (Holzman et al., 1977; 1985). While we found no correlations between smooth eye pursuit errors in our patients and P3 abnormalities, St Clair et al. (1987) found P3 and smooth pursuit abnormalities to coincide in certain families with schizophrenic members. However, we did find that family history, apart from the diagnosis of schizophrenia, was the only significant independent factor to predict abnormal eye pursuit among our schizophrenic patients (n=23) and controls (n=18). The use of smooth eye pursuit disruption and, perhaps, P3 abnormalities might, therefore, lead to the identification of genetic markers for schizophrenia in certain families (St Clair et al., 1987).

CONCLUSION

The late positive complex, and particularly P3b, are relatively well defined by psychophysiological correlation studies in normals. Studies in schizophrenia have so far been mainly restricted to only a few simple paradigms, in particular 2- and 3-tone discrimination tasks with or without reaction time components. From a review of these studies some general conclusions can be drawn:

(1) The examined patient groups are hardly representative of 'schizophrenics', not least because delusional pre-occupation with electrical phenomena excludes a varying subgroup of patients who do not co-operate with the examination.
(2) Subjects have to be described, beyond a standardised diagnosis, in relation to their symptomatology, cognitive impairment and possible causes for impairment including alcohol consumption and anticholinergic medication. Pre-morbid estimations of intellectual performance like the NART should be used to match controls.
(3) The arbitrary definition of a 'P3' might be sufficient for clinical correlative studies or attempts to find markers for e.g. 'familial schizophrenia'. But the presence of multiple peaks and variable wave forms in schizophrenics is a challenge to psychophysiological research. The question whether multiple peaks represent a dispersal of waves like P3a, P3b and SW, which normally coincide, but which have a different functional significance, awaits exploration.

ACKNOWLEDGEMENTS

The authors wish to thank H McAllister for programming the smooth eye pursuit paradigm, as well as A Flett, K Hird, K Kleppang and S McLeod for their help with the experimental work and with preparing the script.

REFERENCES

American Psychiatric Association (1980). Diagnostic and Statistical Manual (3rd Edit.). Washington: American Psychiatric Association.
Baribeau-Braun Picton, T.E. & Gosselin, J.K. (1983). Schizophrenia: A neurophysiological evaluation of abnormal processing. Science, 219, 874-876.
Barrett, K., McCallum, W.C. & Poccock, P.V. (1986). Brain indicators of altered attention and information processing in schizophrenic patients. British Journal of Psychiatry, 148, 414-420.
Blackwood, D.H.R, Whalley, L.J., Christie, J.E., Blackman, I.M., St

Clair, D.M. & McInnes, A. (1987). Changes in auditory P300 event related potentials in schizophrenia and depression. British Journal of Psychiatry, 150, 154-160.

Brown, R., Coltler, N., Nicholas-Corsellis, J., Crow, T., Frith, C., Jagoe, R., Johnstone, E., & Marsh, L. (1986). Post mortem evidence of structural brain change in schizophrenia: difference in brain weight, temporal horn area, and parahippocampal gyrus compared with affective disorder. Archives of General Psychiatry, 43, 36-42.

Callaway, E. (1984). Human information processing: some effects of methylphenidate, age and scopolamine. Biological Psychiatry, 19, 649-662.

Callaway, E. & Naghdi, S. (1982). An information processing model for schizophrenia. Archives of General Psychiatry, 39, 339-347.

Ebmeier, K.P., Mackenzie, A.R., Potter, D., Crawford, J.R., Besson, J.A.O. & Salzen, E. (1987). Late event related potentials in schizophrenia. British Journal of Clinical and Social Psychiatry, 5, 124-125.

Ebmeier, K.P., Potter, D.D., Cochrane, R.H.B. and Salzen, E.A. (1989). Lower-bandpass filter-frequency in P3-experiments: a possible cause for divergent results in schizophrenic research. Biological Psychiatry, in press.

Faux, S.F., Torello, M.W., McCarthy, R.W., Shenton, M.E., Duffy, E.M. (1987). P300 topographic alterations in schizophrenia: a replication study. in: R. Johnson, J.W. Rohrbaugh & P. Parasuraman (eds.). Current Tends in ERP-Research, Suppl.40 to EEG + Clinical Neurophysiology. Amsterdam: Elsevier.

Goodin, D.S., Starr, A., Chippendale, T. & Squires, K.S. (1983). Sequential changes in the P3 component of the auditory evoked potential in confusional states and dementing illness. Neurology, 33, 1215-1218.

Halgren, E., Squires, N.K., Rohrbaugh, J.W., Babb, T.L. & Crandall, P.H. (1980). Endogenous potentials generated in the human hippcampal formation and amygdala by infrequent events. Science, 210, 803-805.

Hansch, E.C., Syndulko, K., Cohen, S., Goldberg, Z., Potvin, A. & Tourellotte, W.W. (1982). Cognition in Parkinson's disease: an event-related potential perspective. Annals of Neurology, 11, 599-607.

Holzman, P.S. (1985). Eye movement dysfunctions and psychosis. International Review of Neurobiology, 27, 179-205, London: Academic Press.

Holzman P.S., Kringlen, E., Levy, D.L., Procter, L.R., Haberman, S. & Yasillo, N.J. (1977). Abnormal pursuit eye movements in schizophrenia. Evidence for a genetic indicator. Archives of General Psychiatry, 34, 802-805.

Johnson, R. (1986). A triarchic model of P300 amplitude. Psychophysiology, 23, 367-384.

Kutas, M., McCarthy, G. & Donchin, E. (1977). Augmenting mental chronometry: The p300 as a measure of stimulus evaluation time. Science, 197, 792-795.

Kutcher, S.P., Blackwood, D.H.R., St Clair, D., Gaskell, D.F. & Muir, W.J. (1987). Auditory P300 in borderline personality disorder and schizophrenia. Archives of General Psychiatry, 44, 645-650.

Levit, R.A., Sutton, S. & Zubin, J. (1973). Evoked potential correlates of information processing in psychotic patients. Psychological Medicine, 3, 487-494.

Matsubayashi, M., Omura, F., Kobayashi, T., Miyasato, Y. & Ogura, C. (1985). Event-related potentials and cognitive function in schizophrenia. Electroencephalography and clinical Neurophysiology, 61, S33.

McCarthy, G., Wood, C.C., Allison, T., Goff, W.R., Williamson, P.D. & Spencer, D.D. (1982). Intracranial recordings of event related potentials in humans engaged in cognitive tests. Neuroscience Abstracts, 8, 976.

Morstyn, R., Duffy, F.H. & McCarley, R.W. (1983). Altered P300 topography in schizophrenia. Archives of General Psychiatry, 40, 729-734.

Nelson, H.E. (1982). National Adult Reading Test (NART): Test Manual. Windsor: NFER Nelson.

Paller, K.A., Zola-Morgan, S., Squire, L.R. & Hillyard, S.A. (1984). Monkeys with lesions of hippocampus and amygdala exhibit event-related brain potentials that resemble the human P300 wave. Neuroscience Abstracts, 10, 849.

Papanicolaou, A.C., Loring, D.W., Raz, N. & Eisenberg, H.M. (1985). Relationship between stimulus intensity and the P300. Psychophysiology, 22, 326-329.

Pfefferbaum, A., Ford, J.M., Wenegrat, B.G., Roth, W.T. & Kopell, B.S. (1984a). Clinical applications of P3.1. normal aging. Electroencephalography and Clinical Neurophysiology, 59, 85-103.

Pfefferbaum, A., Wenegrat, B.G., Ford, J.M., Roth, W.T. & Kopell B.S. (1984b). Clinical application of the P3 component of event-related potentials. II. dementia, depression and schizophrenia. Electroencephalography and Clinical Neurophysiology, 59, 104-124.

Polich, J. (1986). Attention, probability, and task demands as determinants of P300 latency from auditory stimuli. Electroencephalography and Clinical Neurophysiology, 63, 251-259.

Polich, J., Howard, L. & Starr, A. (1985). Stimulus frequency and masking as determinants of P300 latency in event-related potentials from auditory stimuli. Biological Psychiatry, 21, 309-18.

Polich, J., Howard, L. & Starr, A. (1983). P300 latency correlates with digit span. Psychophysiology, 20, 665-669.

Pritchard, W.S. (1981). Psychophysiology of P300. Psychological Bulletin, 89, 506-540.

Romani, A., Merello, S., Gozzoli, L., Zerbi, F., Grassi, M. & Cosi, V. (1987). P300 and CT-Scan inpatients with chronic schizophrenia. British Journal of Psychiatry, 151, 506-513.

Roth, W.T. & Cannon, E.H. (1972). Some features of auditory evoked responses in schizophrenics. Archives of General Psychiatry, 27, 466-471.

Roth, W.T., Horvath, T.B., Pfefferbaum, A., Tinklenberg, J.R. & Mezzich, J. (1979). Late event-related potentials and schizophrenia. in: H. Begleiter (ed.). Evoked Brain Potentials and Behaviour: Downstate Series of Research in Psychiatry and Psychology. New York: Plenum Press.

Roth, W.T., Pfefferbaum, A., Horvath, T.B., Berger, P.A. & Kopell, B.S. (1980). P3 reduction in auditory evoked potentials of schizophrenics. Electroencephalography and Clinical Neurophysiology, 49, 497-505.

Ruchkin, D.S. & Sutton, S (1983). Positive slow wave and P300 - association and dissociation. in: A.W.K. Gaillard & W. Ritter (eds.). Tutorials in ERP-research: Endogenous Components. Groningen: North Holland Publishing Company.

Saletu, B., Itil, T.M. & Saletu, M (1971). Auditory evoked response, EEG and thought process in schizophrenia. American Journal of Psychiatry, 128, 336-344.

Squires, N.K. & Ollo, C. (1986). Human EP-techniques: Possible applications to neuropsychology. in: H.J. Hannay (ed.). Experimental Techniques in Human Neuropsychology. New York: Oxford University Press.

Squires, N.K., Squires, K.C. & Hillyard, S.A. (1975). Two varieties of long-latency positive waves evoked by unpredictable auditory stimuli in man. Electroencephelography and Clinical Neurophysiology, 38, 387-401.

Squires, N., Galbraith, G., & Aine, C. (1979). Event-related potential assessment of sensory and cognitive deficits in the mentally retarded. in: D. Lehmann & E. Callaway (eds.). Human Evoked Potentials: Applications and Problems. New York: Plenum Press.

Stapleton, J.M., Halgren, E. & Moreno, K.A. (1987). Endogenous potentials after anterior temporal lobectomy. Neuropsychologia, 25, 549–557.

St Clair, D.M., Blackwood, D.H.R. & Christie, J.E. (1985). P3 and other long latency auditory evoked potentials in presenile dementia Alzheimer type and alcoholic Korsakoff syndrome. British Journal of Psychiatry, 147, 702–706.

St Clair, D.M., Muir, W.M. & Blackwood, D.M.R. (1987). Auditory P3 and smooth pursuit eye tracking in schizophrenic patients and their relatives. Abstracts of the 3rd Scottish Meeting of the Psychophysiological Society, 3rd October 1987.

Strandburg, R.J., Marsh, J.T., Brown, W.S., Asarnow, R.F. & Guthrie, D. (1984). Event-related potential concomitants of information processing dysfunction in schizophrenic children. Electroencephalography and Clinical Neurophysiology, 57, 236–253.

Sutton, S., Braren, M., Zubin, J. & John, E.R. (1965). Evoked potential correlates of stimulus uncertainty. Science, 150, 1187–1188.

Tsuang, M.T., Winokur, G. & Crower (1980). Morbidity risks of schizophrenia and affective disorders among first degree relatives of patients with schizophrenia, mania, depression and surgical conditions. British Journal of Psychiatry, 137, 497–504.

Wood, C.C., McCarthy, G., Squires, N.K., Vaughan, H.G., Words, D.L. & McCallum, W.C. (1984). Anatomical and physiological substrates of event related potentials: two case studies. in: J. Cohen, R. Karrer & P. Tueting (eds.). Annals of the New York Academy of Sciences, 425, 681–721.

World Health Organisation (1978). Report of the International Pilot Study of Schizophrenia, Vol 1. Geneva: World Health Organisation.

Yingling, C.D. & Hosobuchi, Y. (1984). A subcortical correlate of P300 in man. Electroencephalography and clinical Neurophysiology, 59, 72–76.

ELECTROPHYSIOLOGICAL CORRELATES OF FACIAL IDENTITY

AND EXPRESSION PROCESSING

D D Potter and D M Parker

INTRODUCTION

The recent growth of research into face recognition has resulted in increasingly refined models of this process based on evidence from behavioural, neuropsychological and neurophysiological studies (Bruce & Young 1986, Rhodes, 1985). The aim of this chapter is to illustrate some of the ways that the study of EEG and event related potentials (ERPs) can provide useful additional information about the timing and distribution of neural events associated with the processing of faces. Studies of scalp recordings of brain electrical activity during the processing of facial information have, in the main, concentrated on the following four issues. What special roles do the right and left hemispheres of the brain have in face processing? To what extent do unique mechanisms exist in the brain for the processing of facial information? Does familiarity affect matching processes in ways similar or different from that associated with words or objects? To what extent are the processing of facial expression and identity separable? The review is split up in to four main sections corresponding roughly to the four questions above but there is some overlap of ideas in these different sections. Not all of the issues relating to each question have been considered and additional information relating to some of these issues can be found in the chapters by Peng and Campbell and by Ellis in this volume.

HEMISPHERIC ASYMMETRIES

Much of the psychological research on hemispheric asymmetry in normal individuals has employed the divided visual field (DVF) technique. Early research suggested a left visual field (right hemisphere) advantage for the processing of face identity information but conflicting results indicating either no advantage, or a right visual field (left hemisphere) advantage also appeared. Sergent and Bindra (1981), in a review of this literature, suggested that visual-field advantage is to a large extent dependent on the type of information which must be extracted from the pattern for efficient performance of the task. For example in tasks such as deciding the sex of a face or deciding whether a pattern containing facial features is of the correct configuration, low spatial frequency information is sufficient and results in a left visual field (LVF) advantage in DVF studies. In tasks involving more complex discriminations such as classifying familiar individuals according to their occupations or deciding whether specific features of a face are correct is dependent on high spatial frequency information and results in right visual field (RVF) advantage (Sergent, 1986). In the case of expression processing the majority of studies show a right hemisphere advantage (Ley & Strauss,

1986). It seems though, that perhaps less attention has been paid to stimulus and task factors in these DVF studies. The brief presentation in peripheral vision of small sets of highly discriminable faces in tasks of low complexity may favour a holistic processing strategy resulting in a left visual field advantage which has nothing to do with any specific specialisation for the processing of facial expression.

Initially it appeared that the majority of patients suffering from prosopagnosia, the inability to recognise familiar faces, had unilateral lesions in the right inferior occipito-temporal region (Meadows, 1974). More recently it has been argued on the basis of post-mortem evidence that bilateral lesions are necessary (Damasio, 1986), though there is still considerable debate on this issue (De Renzi, 1986, Landis et al., 1986). In the case of expression processing, right hemisphere damage generally results in significant deficits in both naming and judging similarity of facial expressions. Left hemisphere damage can also produce a deficit in expression processing which is somewhere in between that seen in normal and right hemisphere damaged individuals and it has been suggested that this may be due to a dissociation between the the perceptual analysis of an expression and the derivation of the context dependent meaning of the expression (Feyereisen, 1986). Right frontal damage has also been implicated as a source of impairment in expression processing (Kolb et al., 1983). It should also be noted that left fronto-temporal damage can result in tendencies towards depressive symptoms whereas right fronto-temporal damage can result in euphoric symptoms (Campbell, 1982). This may be a confounding factor in studies of emotion perception by producing biases in individuals responses to particular expressions.

EEG STUDIES

One method of assessing the contribution of different regions to a task is by measuring cortical activation. This is accomplished by sampling ongoing EEG activity and analysing the frequency content of the signal. A decrease in power of alpha activity (a frequency of approximately 10 cycles/second) is interpreted as an increase in cortical activation. EEG studies of face processing have tended to concentrate on the posterior region of the head. One of the earliest studies (Dumas & Morgan, 1975) involved forming subjective impressions about the character, friendliness, and distinctiveness of a varying number of faces and then recalling this information 15 seconds later. An increase in alpha suppression was observed over the right hemisphere in the right-handed male subjects that they studied. Evidence of increased cortical activation over the right hemisphere associated with face processing was also observed in a study by Ornstein et al. (1980) in which 10 male and 10 female subjects identified target words or faces or abstract shapes in a questionnaire booklet. Synonym and mental rotation tasks produced left hemisphere alpha suppression while face recognition and gestalt picture completion tasks resulted in right hemisphere alpha suppression. Evidence of sex differences began to emerge when Rapzynski and Ehrlichman (1979), using a go/no-go continuous recognition task involving either words or faces, observed increased alpha suppression over the left hemisphere in all tasks in a group of 24 women. Face and word tasks did dissociate to the extent that alpha suppression over the left hemisphere was less for faces than words. Further evidence of the influence of sex and handedness has been reported by Glass et al. (1984). Right-handed males and females with or without left-handed relatives were used as subjects. Alpha power distribution was monitored during the performance of either an arithmetic task or a continuous recognition paradigm using face stimuli. In the arithmetic task there was more evidence of left hemisphere activation in both males and females without left-handed relatives but, in the case of the face task, males with left handed relatives tended to show greater right hemisphere activation and females without left handed relatives greater left hemisphere activation. All other groups showed no lateralisation. Over-all these studies suggest that there may be sex differences in hemispheric lateralisation and indeed that familial handedness may influence the patterns of asymmetry observed.

There are however considerable difficulties in making inferences about functional asymmetries in a particular individuals' brain based on the handedness of close relatives. There are also problems with some of the tasks used in these experiments in that they may have encouraged the use of linguistic skills in their performance (see Bruyer, 1988 for a critical review of many of the early electrophysiological studies of face processing). One study which looked at frontal and parietal regions (Ahern & Schwartz, 1985) was concerned with the effect on EEG activity of viewing faces showing expressions of positive and negative affect. The investigators reported that positive emotional expressions resulted in decreased alpha over left frontal sites and that expressions of negative affect caused decreased alpha at the right frontal sites. No corresponding changes were observed at parietal sites. These results above have an interesting correlate in a study of frontal EEG in human infants tasting sweet or sour liquids. The alpha activity was again modulated in a way that suggested that pleasant stimuli produced increased cortical activation at left frontal sites and unpleasant stimuli at right frontal sites (Fox & Davidson,1986).

A limitation of current EEG techniques is that fast changes in dynamic activity cannot be clearly detected. This is because estimates of the frequency content of the EEG signal are typically derived from data collected over a time period of from two to eight seconds whereas changes in frequency content associated with specific cognitive events may be occurring in tens to hundreds of milliseconds. One therefore gets a somewhat limited estimate of the interactions between different areas that are monitored. ERP studies provide one approach which has this temporal resolution.

EVENT RELATED POTENTIAL STUDIES

Before discussing findings from studies of the averaged visual evoked responses to briefly presented images of faces it is perhaps useful to look at typical responses observed to such stimuli (Figure 1, a and b). Only those features which will be discussed in the subsequent sections of this review have been highlighted. Figure 1a illustrates the response observed to the first face stimulus in an experiment where the subjects' task is to judge whether two successively presented faces are of the same identity or not. The first peak one observes, at a latency of approximately 120 msec (depending on average luminance and pattern contrast of the stimulus), is observed predominantly at posterior sites and will be referred to as the P120. This is followed by a fronto-centrally distributed peak at a latency of approximately 200 msec which will be described as the P200. There then follows a peak, or more accurately a cluster of peaks, with latencies in the range 270-350 msec which will be referred to as the P300. This positive going region is maximal at the parietal electrode sites and should not be confused with the 'P300' component that one observes to rare target stimuli in classical 'auditory oddball paradigms' (see chapter by Ebmeier et al., this volume). The visual modality equivalent to the auditory P300 occurs at a latency of approximately 500 msec (Simson et al., 1977). In the same latency range as this parietal positivity is a fronto-central negativity at a latency of

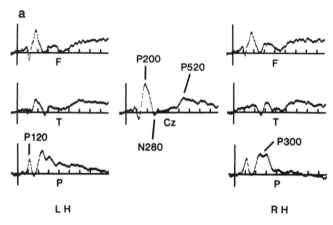

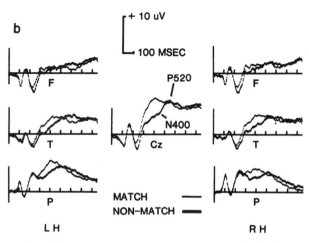

Figure 1. Grand averaged evoked responses (N=14) recorded to (a) the first and (b) second faces in an identity judgement task. See test for further description. (F = frontal, T = temporal, P = parietal).

approximately 280 msec (N280). Finally there is a positive going slow wave which is symmetrically distributed over the fronto-central region in the latency range 450–800 msec. There is, in the same latency range, a sustained increase in negativity in the parietal region which is asymmetrically distributed with greater negativity over the right hemisphere.

The responses illustrated in Figure 1b are those associated with a match or non-match decision in the same identity judgement task. The first feature to note is a component known as the N400, which occurs when the current stimulus does not match a previously primed target representation in memory. This phenomenon is also observed in number of different tasks using both word and picture stimuli (Kutas & Hillyard, 1984; Stuss et al., 1986). The visual equivalent of the auditory P300 is also highlighted (P520). This component is of the same amplitude in both conditions as the probability of a same or different decision is equal in this experiment. A number of different reference points have been used in the studies described below (linked-mastoids, nose, Fz, Cz, Pz and Laplacian). As a result the polarity, latency and amplitude of specific features of the ERP can be quite different from study to study. The labels which have been attached to specific features of the ERP are, to some extent arbitary and in some cases are a simplification of the situation. This has been done in an attempt to highlight what we believe are the recurrent trends that emerge in these different studies.

Small (1983) was one of the first to report evoked response hemispheric asymmetries, in the parieto-occipital region, to the brief presentation of face stimuli. Responses to familiar and unfamiliar faces were compared to those produced by other complex geometric stimuli or checkerboard pattern reversal in a group of right handed subjects. No task was involved other than fixating on the stimuli. The main findings of this study were that the amplitude of response was greater at right hemisphere sites at a latency of 300 msec only in the case of the face stimuli and that the latencies of both P120 and P300 were shorter in the case of geometric designs and pattern reversal. This latter effect is probably due to the higher contrast in the geometric and pattern reversal stimuli. In a subsequent study (Small, 1986) the responses from a group of right and left handers were compared, using the same stimuli as the previous experiment, except the familiar and unfamiliar faces were also presented inverted. The main findings of this study were that there was a significant P300 asymmetry to all stimuli in the right-handed group but that this was greater for faces than other stimuli. Left handed subjects showed no significant P300 right hemisphere asymmetries. In this study it was noted that there was a non-significant trend in all groups for larger P120 amplitudes over the right hemisphere. In her most recent study (Small, 1988) these data were compared to the responses observed in a prosopagnosic patient with C.T. scan evidence of lesions in the right posterior parietal region and above the left lateral ventrical. The main difference between the controls and the patient were that the latency of the P120 was significantly slower than the normal population particularly at right hemisphere sites and this was interpreted as evidence that in this particular case of prosopagnosia the problem was at a perceptual rather than a cognitive level of processing.

Srebro (1985) studied the evoked responses to briefly presented images of faces and other simple meaningful geometric shapes which had been degraded by varying degrees of random noise. The task was to detect whether a face or geometric pattern was present in the image. The Laplacian technique was used to sample the ERP data from the scalp. In this technique activity at a site of interest is compared to the activity occurring in a group of electrodes surrounding it and only that activity unique to the target electrode is recorded. Using this approach, Srebro was able to demonstrate that a response occurring at the latency of the P200 was primarily located in the temporal lobe region and that this response is asymmetrically distributed with more activation observed over the right hemisphere than the left both for faces and simple meaningful geometrical shapes. There was some evidence of differences in the distribution of activity in the temporal lobe associated with the face or pattern responses which, Srebro tentatively suggested, may have indicated a mapping for shape in the temporal cortex in the same way that there is a mapping for location in primary visual areas. Only a limited number of stimuli were used on a limited number of subjects and so this suggestion remains highly speculative. Sobotka et al. (1984) combined the DVF technique with the recording of visual ERPs in a study in which subjects were required to decide whether the identity of two sequentially presented faces matched or not. Whereas asymmetry of the P120 response was shown to be dependent on the field of presentation, the P300 response was always larger over the right parietal region. A sustained increase in negativity was also observed over the right parietal region in the latency range 400–1000 msec after every stimulus. A similar sustained increase in negativity has also been observed by Deeke et al. (1986) in a task involving decisions about the occupations of famous faces. In perhaps the first study which made a direct comparison between word and face processing in which subjects had to decide whether two sequentially presented stimuli were same or different, Butler and Glass (1981) investigated the hemispheric distribution of the contingent negative variation (CNV) which occurs in the interstimulus interval. A significant CNV asymmetry was observed over the left hemisphere in the case of word stimuli but no significant increase in CNV over the right hemisphere was observed in the case of the face stimuli. In a study using a similar design but recording from occipital and posterior temporal sites Sobotka (1986) reported that responses were larger over the right hemisphere for faces and over the left hemisphere for words at a latency of 240 msec though it is not clear which specific feature of the ERP was being measured.

In summary then, a number of studies indicate a greater role for the right hemisphere in face recognition in right-handed individuals. This has to be qualified by the observation that all of these studies use briefly presented stimuli which may favour a right hemisphere processing strategy (Sergent & Bindra, 1981). Right hemisphere asymmetries are also observed in response to meaningful patterns other than faces (Srebro, 1985).

Specificity of Face Processing

We now turn to the question of whether or not there are specific systems for processing face information. There are a number of lines of evidence which are used to support this notion. Studies of human infants suggest some level of innate predisposition to attend to face-like configurations (Goren et al., 1975, Dzurawiec & Ellis, 1989). Neurophysiological studies of neurones in monkey temporal cortex indicate the presence of clusters of cells which are selectively responsive to face stimuli (Perrett et al., 1985a) and electrical stimulation in discrete areas of human parietal and temporal cortex have been shown to disrupt face recognition (Fried et al., 1982).

A recent ERP study bearing on this issue (Jeffreys & Musselwhite, 1987) was concerned with the location of a P200 type component which occured with maximum amplitude to briefly presented high contrast drawings and photographic images of faces. The distribution of this response, which was sampled using an array of electrodes at the midline running from ear to ear over the vertex, suggests bilateral generators in temporal cortex responding at a latency of approximately 180 msec. The location and latency of this response is very similar to that observed in studies of single cells which are selectively responsive to face stimuli in the temporal cortex of monkeys (Perrett et al., 1985a). They were further able to demonstrate that manipulating stimulus parameters, such as the orientation, degree of detail, amount of visual noise or degree of completeness of the image, influenced the latency and amplitude of the response to these differing stimuli in ways which mirrored changes observed in neuronal responses in monkeys. Boetzel and Gruesser (1988), using simple line drawings of a face, chair and tree, observed a similar centrally distributed P200 type response with largest amplitude and shortest latency in the case of the face stimulus. In a second experiment a series of faces, vases and shoes, chosen for their symmetry and individuality, were used as the stimuli. In this case the P200 response was very similar in all cases but the N280 component was largest in the case of the face stimuli.

It is possible that the P200 response is similar to neuronal responses observed in primate neurophysiological studies indicating a major
role for the temporal lobe region in high level pattern representations.
The problem with using this as evidence for specificity is that neurones
in this region of cortex are selectively responsive to a range of of biologically meaningful stimuli (Perrett et al., 1985b; 1985c), and it has
not been conclusively proven that these different populations of cells
exist as functionally distinct processing systems in temporal cortex or
that transformations, such as inversion or using photographic negatives,
which affect both the P200 and cell responses to faces, may also affect
the processing of other stimuli.

From a neuropsychological point of view interest in face familiarity
stemmed from the observation of specific face recognition deficits (Meadows, 1974; Damasio, 1982). Some prosopagnosics can discriminate between
faces but appear not to know whether the face is familiar or not. In some
cases it has been possible to demonstrate that even though a prosopagnosic is unable to behaviourally discriminate familiar and unfamiliar
faces their galvanic skin response shows a clear dissociation between
familiar and unfamiliar faces. This 'covert' recognition of familiarity
has been interpreted as evidence of two independent pathways of face
information (Bauer, 1986). Behavioural studies of familiarity have concentrated, for example, on the relative importance of internal and external features of a face (Ellis et al., 1979) or changes in hemispheric
advantage, in DVF studies, with increasing familiarity (Ross-Kossak &
Turkewitz, 1986). In electrophysiological studies face familiarity has
become of interest primarily because faces are examples of complex meaningful non-verbal visual stimuli. This allows the comparison of ERPs to
faces with those observed in similar tasks using linguistic stimuli
(Kutas & Hillyard, 1984) and allows the dissociation of stimulus specific
cortical activity from activity associated with more general cognitive
mechanisms.

Two recent experiments looking at the effects of familiarity on
identity required subjects to make match/non-match decisions about the
identity of sequentially presented pairs of faces. ERPs were recorded
from frontal, temporal, parietal and central sites. In one study familiarity was manipulated by using pictures of individuals known personally
to the subjects and pictures of unfamiliar faces (Potter et al., 1987)
and in the other study famous faces and unfamiliar faces were used (Barrett et al., 1988). The main findings of these two experiments were that
the evoked responses to unfamiliar faces showed a sustained and widespread relative increase in negativity in the latency range 300-600 msec,
particularly after the first stimulus. There was also a significant relative increase in negativity in the same latency range at the right parietal sites after both the first and second stimuli. The ERP to the second stimulus on non-match trials showed a wide-spread increase in negativity in the latency range 350-450 msec (N400) and this difference was
larger in the case of familiar faces than in the case of unfamiliar
faces. It is also of interest to note that, in the study by Barrett et
al., the ERPs associated with match and non-match responses dissociated
significantly in the latency range 120-160 msec particularly for familiar
faces (Barrett et al., 1988). A related study involved the presentation
of of a continuous sequence of face stimuli in a go-no-go task in which
subjects had to respond to a previously memorised set of target stimuli
(Smith & Halgren, 1988). ERPs to faces which did not match the target set
were characterised by the presence of an N400 type component distributed
maximally over the parieto-occipital region, in contrast to the centrally
distributed P520 observed to the target faces. There was again evidence
of a sustained increase of negativity over the right posterior region of
the head. The increased negativity in the latency range 350-500 msec is

generally distributed over the head and is very similar to the N400 negativity seen in tasks in which judgements about words are made (Kutas & Hillyard, 1984; Rugg, 1984).

IDENTITY AND EXPRESSION PROCESSING

Current theoretical models of face recognition assume a functional dissociation of identity and expression processing (Bruce & Young, 1986). There are a number of neuropsychological studies which indicate a double dissociation between impairments of recognition of identity and expressions (Etcoff, 1985, see also Peng & Campbell, this volume). A recent study of normal individuals which supports this notion is that of Young et al. (1986), in which they report that although familiarity affected the speed and accuracy of judgements of identity it had no effect on judgements of expression.

Our recent research has been concerned with the comparison of the behavioural and electrophysiological responses observed in tasks involving similarity judgements of facial identity or expression. Only two particular aspects of this work will be discussed here. The changes in ERPs which are associated with match and non-match decisions in identity and expression judgements will be compared and in a second experiment, with equivalent procedures and an equivalent matching task, the effect of removing the external features of the face will be considered.

The experimental design can be briefly summarised as follows. The stimuli consisted of Black and White photographs of the faces of 6 different males each posing 6 different expressions (fear, surprise, happiness, sadness, anger and disgust). The 36 stimuli were used to generate four continuous sequences of 72 slides which were presented at a rate of one slide every 4.5 seconds. A response was required from the subject after every slide except the first slide in the sequence. In the identity judgement task the subject had to decide whether the currently presented slide displayed an individual who had the same identity as the individual shown in the previously presented slide. In the expression judgement task subjects decided whether the current slide displayed the same expression as the preceding slide. In other words each slide had to be compared with the previous slide and also remembered for the next comparison. During identity judgements, the expression always changed from one slide to the next and during the expression judgement task, the identity always changed from one slide to the next. Separate blocks of identity and expression judgements were performed by each subject. The sequence of stimuli were ordered such that there was an equal number of match and non-match decisions within each block of trials. The index finger of each hand was used for match and non-match responses and the hand used for match responses was balanced. Twelve right-handed subjects took part in each experiment.

Behavioural data consisting of median reaction times and percentage errors were assessed using Anova and Tukey tests for post-hoc comparisons. ERPs were analysed by using Anova on mean voltage measurements from specific regions of the waveforms and Geisser-Greenhaus corrections were made where appropriate.

Reaction times were significantly faster and error rates lower in the case of decisions about the identity of a face (Fig.2). Non-match decisions took significantly longer only in the case of expression judgements and more errors were made on same judgements only in the case of expression judgements. Removal of the external features of the face resulted in a significant increase in reaction time for identity judgements

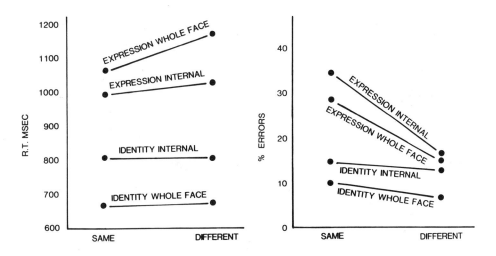

Figure 2. Reaction time and error rates observed in judgements of identity and expression. Removal of external features significantly affected identity judgements but not expression judgements.

but not for expression judgements.

In the case of identity judgements on whole faces the ERPs for match and non-match decisions (for correct trials only) show a very typical pattern of differentiation (Figure 3a). The responses associated with non-match decisions are more negative in the latency range 310-430 msec than the evoked response associated with match decisions. This difference is observable at all sites, though onset is approximately 100 msec earlier at frontal and temporal sites than at parietal sites. This difference between match and non-match trial ERPs is symmetrically distributed across the two hemispheres. The pattern of results is quite different in the case of expression judgements (Figure 3b). Match and Non-match decision responses only differentiate significantly at the right parietal site in the latency range 490-540 msec.

Removal of the external features of the face had two major effects. The fronto-centrally distributed N280 component (Figure 3a and 3b) was greatly reduced in amplitude for both identity and expression (Figure 3c and 3d), and this was associated at parietal sites with a sustained increase in negativity. The second effect was that in the case of identity judgements (Figure 3c), the N400 response in non-match trials was no longer observable but the match/non-match differences observed in expression judgements (Figure 3d) were unaffected.

The distribution of activity associated with match/non-match differences is clearly different when decisions about identity or expression are being made. This is associated with a considerable increase in reaction time when processing expression information and one is bound to ask how similar the cognitive demands are in these two tasks. Removal of the external features, though not affecting late cognitive ERPs in expression judgements, had a profound effect on behavioural performance in identity judgements which was mirrored in the ERP by the virtual abolition of the N400 type component, highlighting the importance of the external features in identity processing.

We started this review by asking in what way studies of ERPs might influence current views on face processing and a number of points have emerged. The first feature which emerges repeatedly in these studies is that asymmetries are observed at all latencies of the ERP in the form of greater response amplitudes over the right posterior region of the head, even during interstimulus intervals. In the case of the centrally distributed P200 response, evidence of asymmetry is less apparent in the literature. The observation of this asymmetry is perhaps not surprising given the fact that almost all these studies were carried out on right-handed subjects, especially as those studies which used left-handed subjects do not report evidence of asymmetry. Given that studies using other

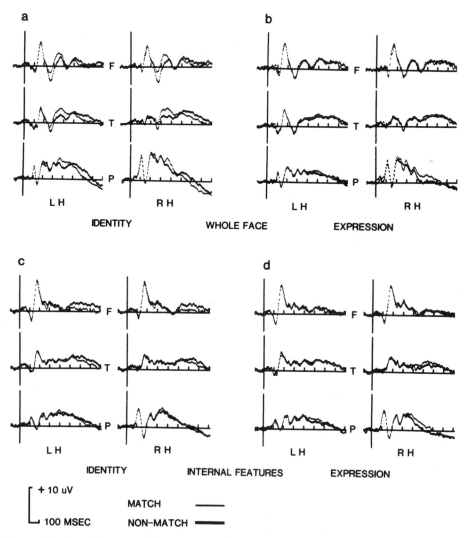

Figure 3. Grand averaged responses from two groups of subjects. The main effects to note are as follows. Removal of the external features of the face in identity judgement (c) results in disappearance of N400 component observed in (a). Expression judgements (b and d) are characterised by an asymmetrically distributed N400 type component. (F = frontal, T = temporal, P = parietal).

other meaningful non-verbal visual stimuli (Srebro, 1985; Barrett & Rugg, personal communication) also indicate a greater involvement of the right hemisphere, then this suggests a basic functional asymmetry rather than something specific to faces.

Much of the evidence in support of the notion of specificity has centred around the P200 response which appears to have an origin in the temporal lobe regions. These findings are clearly of importance in that they highlight the role of this region of cortex in the high level representation of complex meaningful non-verbal visual patterns. Until studies using a range of meaningful patterns are carried out in the same subjects and on adequate samples of individuals then the issue remains an open question.

Studies of the effects of face familiarity on the ERP indicate that unfamiliarity produces a widespread increase in cortical activation, though onset is earlier and more sustained at frontal and temporal sites than at parietal sites. These studies have also highlighted the double dissociation between the right hemisphere processing negativity observed when subjects are maintaining representations of meaningful non-verbal stimuli and the left hemisphere processing negativity observed when subjects are maintaining representations of linguistic stimuli. These studies further emphasise the generality of the increased negativity (N400) observed when the current stimulus does not match a previously primed representation.

Finally, there is some evidence of a shift of cortical activation when processing the identity or expression of a face. The fact that these differences emerge relatively late in the ERP might suggest a shift in cognitive strategy rather than evidence of independent processing of identity and expression information. In normal day to day interactions much of the information about emotion is derived from dynamic changes in facial features whereas identity is much more dependent on the static features of the face. Unequivocal demonstration of independence of identity and expression processing will probably require the use of dynamic stimuli.

ACKNOWLEDGEMENT

D.D. Potter was supported by the E.S.R.C. U.K..

REFERENCES

Ahern, G.L. & Scwartz, G.E., (1985), Differential lateralisation for positive and negative emotion in the human brain: EEG spectral analysis. Neuropsychologia, 23, 745-755.

Barrett, S.E., Rugg, M.D. & Perrett, D.I. (1988). Event-related potentials and the matching of familiar and unfamiliar faces. Neuropsychologia, 26, 105-117.

Bauer, R.M. (1986). The cognitive psychophysiology of prosopagnosia. in: H.D. Ellis, M.A. Jeeves, F. Newcombe, & A. Young, (eds.), Aspects of Face Processing. Dordrecht: Martinus Nijhoff.

Boetzel, K. & Grusser, O.-J. (1988). Electrical brain potentials evoked by pictures of faces and non-faces. A search for 'face specific' EEG-potentials. Submitted for publication.

Bruce, V. & Young, A. (1986). Understanding face recognition. British Journal of Psychology, 77, 305-327.

Bruyer, R. (1988). Brain asymmetries in face processing: a critical review of electrophysiological studies from a psychological point of view. Submitted for publication.

Butler, S.R., Glass, A. & Heffner, R. (1981). Asymmetries of the contingent negative variation (CNV) and its' after positive wave (APW) related to differential hemispheric involvement in verbal and non-verbal tasks. Biological Psychology, 13, 157-171.

Campbell, R. (1982). The lateralisation of emotion. International Journal of Psychology, 17, 211-229.

Campbell, R., Landis, T. & Regard, M.. (1986). Face recognition and lip-reading: a neurological dissociation. Brain, 109, 509-521.

Damasio, A.R., Damasio, H. & Van Hoesen, G.W. (1982). Prosopagnosia: anatomical basis and behavioural mechanisms. Neurology, 32, 331-341.

Damasio, R., Damasio, H. & Tranel, D. (1986). Prosopagnosia: anatomical and physiological aspects. in: H.D. Ellis, M.A. Jeeves, F.Newcombe, & A.Young (eds.). Aspects of Face Processing. Dordrecht: Martinus Nijhoff.

De Renzi, E. (1986). Prosopagnosia in two patients with C.T. scan evidence of damage confined to the right hemisphere. Neuropsychologia, 24, 385-389.

Deeke, L., Uhl, F., Spieth. F., Lang, W. & Lang, M. (1987). Cerebral potentials preceding and accompanying verbal and spatial tasks. in: R. Johnson, J.W. Rohrbaugh & R. Parasuraman (eds.). Current Trends in Event-related Potential Research (EEG Suppl. 40). New York: Elsevier.

Dumas, R. & Morgan, A. (1975). EEG asymmetry as a function of occupation, task, and task difficulty. Neuropsychologia, 13, 219-228.

Dziurawiec, S. & Ellis, H.D. (1988). Neonates attention to face-like stimuli. Manuscript in Preparation.

Ellis, H.D., Shepherd, J.W. & Davies, G.M. (1979). Identification of familiar and unfamiliar faces from internal and external features: some implications for theories of face recognition. Perception, 8, 431-439.

Etcoff, N.L. (1985). The Neuropsychology of emotional expression. in: G. Goldstein & R.E. Tarter (eds.). Advances in Clinical Neuropsychology Vol. 3. New York: Plenum.

Feyereisen, P. (1986). Production and comprehension of emotional facial expressions in brain-damaged subjects. in: R. Bruyer (ed.). The Neuropsychology of Face Perception and Facial Expression. Hillsdale N.J.: Lawrence Erlbaum Associates.

Fox, N.A. & Davidson, R.J. (1986). Taste-elicited changes in facial signs of emotion and the asymmetry of brain electrical activity in human newborns. Neuropsychologia, 24, 417-422.

Freid, I., Mateer, C., Ojemann, G., Wohns, R. & Fedio, P. (1982). Organisation of visuospatial functions in human cortex: evidence from electrical stimulation. Brain, 105, 349-371.

Glass, A., Butler, S.R. & Carter, J.C. (1984). Hemispheric asymmetry of EEG alpha activation: effects of gender and familial handedness. Biological Psychology, 19, 169-187.

Goren, C.G., Sarty, M. & Wu, R.W.K. (1975). Visual following and pattern discrimination of face-like stimuli by newborn infants. Pediatrics, 56, 544-559.

Jeffreys, D.A. & Musselwhite, M.J. (1987). A face responsive visual evoked potential in man. Journal of Physiology, 390, 26.

Kolb, B., Milner, B. & Taylor, L. (1983). Perception of faces, facial expression and emotion by patients with localised cortical excisions. Canadian Journal of Psychology, 37, 8-18.

Kutas, M. & Hillyard, S.A. (1984). Brain potentials during reading reflect word expectancy and semantic association. Nature, 307, 161-163.

Landis, T., Cummings, J.L., Christen, L., Bogen, J.E. & Imhof, H-G. (1986). Are unilateral right posterior cerebral lesions sufficient to cause prosopagnosia? clinical and radiological findings in six additional patients. Cortex, 22, 243-252.

Ley, R.G. & Strauss, E. (1986). Hemispheric asymmetries in the perception of facial expression by normals. in: R. Bruyer (ed.). The Neuropsychology of Face Perception and Facial Expression. Hillsdale N.J.: Lawrence Erlbaum Associates.

Meadows, J.C. (1974). The anatomical basis of prosopagnosia. Journal of Neurology, Neurosurgery and Psychiatry, 37, 489-501.

Ornstein, R., Johnstone, J., Herron, J. & Swencionis, C. (1980). Differential right hemisphere engagement in visuospatial tasks. Neuropsychologia, 18, 49-64.

Perrett, D.I., Smith, P.A.J., Potter, D.D., Mistlin, A.J., Head, A.S., Milner, A.D. & Jeeves, M.A. (1985a). Visual cells in the temporal cortex sensitive to face view and gaze direction. Proceedings of the Royal Society of London, 223, 293-317.

Perrett, D.I., Smith, P.A.J., Mistlin, A.J., Chitty, A.J., Head, A.S., Potter, D.D., Broennimann, R., Milner, A.D. & Jeeves, M.A. (1985b). Visual analysis of body movements by neurones in the temporal cortex of the macaque monkey: a preliminary report. Behavioural Brain Research, 16, 153-170.

Perrett, D.I., Chitty, A.J., Mistlin, A.J. & Potter, D.D. (1986). Visual cells in the temporal cortex selectively responsive to the sight of hands manipulating objects. Behavioural Brain Research, 20, 31.

Potter, D.D., Parker, D.M. & Ellis, H.D. (1987). Processing of familiar and unfamiliar faces: an event-related potential and reaction time study. Journal of Psychophysiology, 1, 187.

Rapackzynski, W. & Ehrlichman, H. (1979). EEG asymmetries in recognition of faces: comparison with tachistoscopic technique. Biological Psychology, 9, 163-170.

Rhodes, G. (1985). Lateralised processes in face recognition. British Journal of Psychology, 76, 249-271.

Ross-Kossak, P. & Turkewitz, G. (1986). A micro and macrodevelopmental view of the nature of changes in complex information processing: a consideration of changes in hemispheric advantage during familiarisation. in: R. Bruyer (ed.). The Neuropsychology of Face Perception and Facial Expression. Hillsdale N.J.: Lawrence Erlbaum Associates.

Rugg, M.D. (1984). Event-related potentials in phonological matching tasks. Brain and Language, 23, 225-240.

Sergent, J. & Bindra, D. (1981). Differential hemispheric processing of faces: methodological considerations and reinterpretation. Psychological Bulletin, 89, 541-554.

Sergent, J. (1986). Microgenesis of face perception. in: H.D. Ellis, M.A. Jeeves, F. Newcombe & A. Young (eds.). Aspects of Face Processing. Dordrecht: Martinus Nijhoff.

Simson, R., Vaughan, H.G. & Ritter, W. (1977). The scalp topography of potentials in auditory and visual descrimination tasks. Electroencephalography and Clinical Neurophysiology, 42, 528-535.

Small, M. (1983). Asymmetrical evoked potentials in response to face stimuli. Cortex, 19, 441-450.

Small, M. (1986). Hemispheric differences in the evoked potential to face stimuli. in: H.D. Ellis, M.A. Jeeves, F. Newcombe & A. Young (eds.). Aspects of Face Processing. Dordrecht: Martinus Nijhoff.

Small, M. (1988). Visual evoked potentials in a patient with prosopagnosia. Electroencephalography and Clinical Neurophysiology, 71, 10-16.

Smith, M.E. & Halgren, E. (1987). Event-related potentials elicited by familiar and unfamiliar faces. in: R. Johnson, J.W. Rohrbaugh & R. Parasuraman (eds.). Current Trends in Event-related Potential Research (EEG Suppl. 40). New York: Elsevier.

Sobotka, S., Pizlo, Z. & Budohska, W. (1984). Hemispheric differences in evoked potentials to pictures of faces in the left and right visual fields. Electroencephalography and Clinical Neurophysiology, 58, 441-453.

Sobotka, S. (1986). Opposite superiorities of the right and left cerebral hemispheres in visually evoked potentials to physiognomic and alphabetic material. Behavioural Brain Research, 23, (EBBS Abstract).

Srebro, R. (1985). Localisation of cortical activity associated with visual recognition in humans. Journal of Physiology, 360, 247-259.

Stuss, R., Picton, T.W. & Cerri, A.M. (1986). Searching for the names of pictures: an event related potential study. Psychophysiology, 23, 215-223.

Young, A.W., McWeeny, K.H., Hay, D.C. & Ellis, A.W. (1986). Matching of familiar and unfamiliar faces on identity and expression. Psychological Research, 48, 63-68.

PAST AND RECENT STUDIES OF PROSOPAGNOSIA

Hadyn D Ellis

INTRODUCTION

Prosopagnosia is usually characterised by a sudden loss in ability to recognise faces of familiar people. Sufferers typically have then to rely on voices or dress for identifying spouse, family, friends or famous individuals; and, not infrequently, do not even recognise themselves in the mirror. Before discussing prosopagnosia in more detail, I should like to give an outline account of some of the historical landmarks in its identification and investigation. In doing so I shall not attempt to give a comprehensive review of the literature: instead the more signifi-cant papers will be briefly mentioned.

Probably the earliest clinical record of a case where face memory was impaired was given in 1844 by Wigan (Isler & Regard, 1985), who believed it to be caused by unilateral brain damage. Twenty eight years later Hughlings Jackson described a man who, after right hemisphere damage, lost his ability to recognise both people and places (Harrington, 1985). Following a similar case in 1876, Jackson labelled the inability to recognise objects, people and places 'imperception' which he classi-fied as being in many ways comparable to aphasia (Harrington, 1985).

Very detailed accounts of prosopagnosic patients were later given by Charcot (1888) and Wilbrand (1892). Charcot described a man who also failed to recognise places as well as faces and who also could not draw them. His other intellectual faculties were intact. Fraulein G., describ-ed by Wilbrand (1892), was even more interesting because she not only displayed reasonably preserved verbal processes, but she was also able to discuss her own condition with some insight. 'Going by my state', she said to Wilbrand, 'we see more with the brain than with the eye. The eye is only the means of seeing, because I see everything quite clearly but I don't recognise it and often don't know what it is I see .... If I look in the mirror I can't understand that that's me ...'.

Fraulein G., however, was not a straightforward case of prosopag-nosia, she reported more problems in recognising newly encountered people than old friends, which is atypical; and on at least two occasions, she made the bizarre error of confusing a person with an inanimate object. The only other case where the latter kind of error appears to have been reported was so noteworthy, that it gave the title to Sachs' (1985) coll-ection of neurological essays, 'The Man who Mistook his Wife for a Hat'. The eponymous Dr. G. also sometimes saw faces that weren't: for example, patting the tops of fire hydrants and parking meters believing them to be the heads of children. The fact that Fraulein G. and Dr. P. were prone to such errors may support Ellis's (1983) suggestion that the first stage in face recognition is the classification of an object as a face rather than some other category. Both Fraulein G. and Dr. G. had reasonable visual acuity so any failure at this early stage of processing cannot be attributed simply to sensory impairment: instead it may imply that perceptual classification may be disrupted and consequently the global information somehow misdirected. Great caution must be exercised before this particular hobby horse is ridden too far: until patients with similar symptoms to Fraulein G. and Dr. G. have been studied under rigorous experimental conditions and found to suffer reliably from misclassification errors it is futile to make theoretical inferences.

The reporting of patients with prosopagnosia was not widespread until Bodamer in 1947 discussed three new cases. He coined the term 'prosopagnosia' (Greek, not knowing faces) and gradually throughout the 1950's and 1960, reports of more and more cases were published, including some landmark studies. For example, Hecaen and Angelergues (1962), analysing 22 cases, came to the conclusion that prosopagnosia resulted from posterior right hemisphere damage. As we shall see this conclusion in turn has been challenged, denied and recently resurrected - but there is no immediate resolution in sight. Bornstein's (1963) paper contained a number of interesting points, among which is that arising from the case of an ornithologist who, upon becoming prosopagnosic, also lost the ability to discriminate different species of birds - which sharply calls into question the absolute specificity implied in the name 'prosopagnosia' which will be briefly examined later.

The classical distinction between apperceptive and associative agnosias (Lissauer, 1890) was revived by Hecaen (1981) when he distinguished two kinds of prosopagnosias: that resulting from distortions arising from faulty input mechanisms; and that caused by an inability to connect veridical input to stored representations. Some prosopagnosics complain of quite gross perceptual distortions when looking at faces. In these cases the term metamorphosia seems appropriate. Others, who seem to have perceptual problems that are more or less confined to faces, report that they are cartoon-like (Shuttleworth, Syring & Allen, 1982) or all look identical (Bodamer, 1947) or are all Asiatic looking (Tiberghien & Clerc, 1986) or grey and expressionless (Pallis, 1955). The associative prosopagnosics were labelled 'mnestic' by Hecaen (1981). These patients do not report that faces look in any way odd: they simply do not evoke any sense of familiarity (e.g. Bruyer et al., 1983). It is possible to categorise prosopagnosic patients into more than two groups using a classification scheme based upon contemporary information-processing models of face recognition, such as the one described later, but, given the rarity of the disorder, it has to be admitted that this exercise is of limited clinical value (Ellis, 1986a).

One distinction that may be made between perceptual and mnestic prosopagnosics is that the former could have a preserved ability to image or revisualise a face whereas the latter may not be able to do so. This paradox arises if it is assumed that imagery relies upon preserved internal representations of faces. Mnestic prosopagnosics have either had these representations destroyed or have lost access to them; perceptual prosopagnosics should have them preserved but, because of perturbation at one of the input stages, the representations are not accessed by external stimuli but may be used to generate images. There are, of course, a lot of unsupported assumptions here concerning the nature of recognition and imagery but, even more worrying, is the finding that one cannot necessarily assume that patients who have claimed to be able to image a face were, in fact, able to do so. Indeed when Levine, Warach and Farah, (1985) did ask a prosopagnosic patient, who had reported some facial imagery, to describe the face of Abraham Lincoln they received a description of someone with a beard but with a short round face. He could not

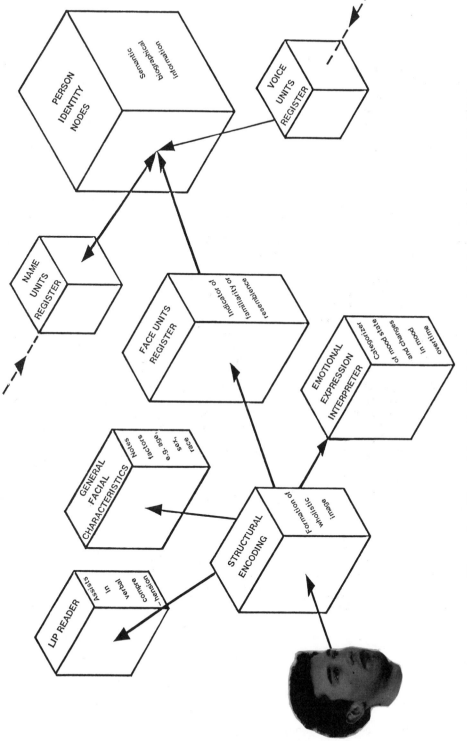

Figure 1. The modules thought to be associated in normal face recognition.

153

even begin to describe John Kennedy or Winston Churchill. Furthermore, his descriptions of animals from image were even more bizarre. For example, an elephant was described as having 'Long legs, a neck that is long enough to bend down to the ground and pick things up...'(p.1011).

This finding must make suspect any self-reported facial imagery by prosopagnosics that is not checked by a test such as that used by Levine, Warach and Farah (1985). Regrettably, this means that in every other published case where good imagery is reported particular results must remain questionable and so the notion that 'perceptual' prosopagnosics may be distinguished from 'mnestic' prosopagnosics must remain an interesting theoretical speculation with potential clinical applications until better data become available.

MODEL OF FACE RECOGNITION

While at present the significance of prosopagnosia with and without facial imagery remains non-proven, other observations made on prosopagnosics have proved quite useful to those wishing to model normal recognition processes (Ellis, 1981; Hay & Young, 1982; Bruce & Young, 1986; Ellis, 1986b). Figure 1 illustrates the general principles.

Recognition is depicted as a three-stage process: a module for the formation of a structural description; a module where an analysis for familiarity via face recognition units takes place; and a module for semantic processing, in which biographical and episodic information about the person is accessed. Other processing of primary facial information is thought to be carried out by parallel, independent satellite modules that are devoted variously to analysing emotional expressions in the face; lip reading; and extraction of general categorical information concerning sex, age and race of the person. The possible existence of the first two satellite modules is supported by observations of double dissociations whereby patients with difficulties in recognising emotional expressions, Kurucz and Feldmar (1979), or in lip reading, Campbell, Landis and Regard (1986), have been contrasted with other patients who have profound prosopagnosia yet can recognise expressions or read lips. The third is a little problematical because no patients without prosopagnosia have yet been found who exhibit difficulties in categorising a face as male or female, black or white, young or old (Ellis, 1986b). Bruce et al. (in press), however, when examining this issue by reaction time (RT) techniques found that varying the difficulty of sex discrimination (using male faces that were either very masculine or rather feminine) did not influence RTs to decide whether the face was familiar. This would not have been the case if sex information were carried out prior to the extraction of familiarity information via the face recognition units. If sex were established after that stage, however, RT would not be affected; but because RTs to make sex judgments are faster than those for familiarity judgments (Sergent, 1986) it seems unlikely that the decision of sex would follow that for familiarity in any hierarchical perceptual process. For this reason alone the module dealing with global facial characteristics is illustrated in Figure 1 as an independent process from the primary recognition route.

NEUROPHYSIOLOGICAL EVIDENCE

Parallel work on the neurophysiology of face recognition has emerged from a number of laboratories. Perrett and his colleagues, for example, have found a variety of cells in the superior temporal sulcus of macaque monkeys that variously respond to any face, to specific facial features, or to particular faces (see Perrett, et al., 1986). No-one has yet satisfactorily mapped these neurophysiological findings on to the kind of model shown in Figure 1, but this will surely be systematically attempted in the near future. At the same time 'artificial' primate prosopagnosia studies may also be made.

As an aside, I cannot forbear to mention some very recent work on sheep who appear to show very similar temporal cells maximally responsive either to sheep in general, or to specific breed, or to familiar sheep or to human and dog faces (Kendrick & Baldwin, 1987). These observations extend the study of face recognition beyond primates to include other 'social' mammals.

One aspect of the neurophysiological research in relation to prosopagnosia is worthwhile mentioning at this point and that refers to the absence of a theoretically possible deficit in recognising faces that does not seem to happen. Perrett and his associates, while observing cells that respond to particular facial features, have not reported cells that fire only to a feature from a specific, familiar individual. Doubtless they have not so far actually looked for such cells. Interest here centres on the fact that prosopagnosics do not ever say 'That face is familiar but I don't recognise the eyes'. In other words, the failure to identify a face is absolute: there is no suggestion that some parts may be identifiable and others not.

SPECIFICITY

The fact that face-specific cells are found in the brains of monkeys and sheep may suggest that, for social animals, the evolution of a highly-specific centre for processing faces may confer biological advantages. But this begs the wider question of specificity, viz. is the system for recognising faces unique insofar as it is carried out separately from other object recognition systems and by a different kind of process? This question has been fully debated elsewhere (Ellis & Young, in press); but, briefly, there is not a great deal of evidence to support such an extreme position. Instead, a weaker version of specificity seems more attractive. This view was expressed most clearly by Konorski (1967) who argued that structures that he termed 'gnostic units' exist within the brain which are specialised to handle particular classes of input: faces are just one of a number of such classes within the visual domain and similar classes exist within other domains.

The only area where faces appear to reveal unique properties is that concerned with the possibility that they may be innately attractive stimuli. Goren, Sarty and Wu (1975) discovered that neonates attended to a face-like pattern significantly more than they did to scrambled face features or to a blank head shape. Though methodologically flawed this study has proved replicable (Dziurawiec & Ellis, in preparation). The fact that babies may arrive into the world already equipped to be attracted by a pattern with face-like configuration, however, does not rule out the possibility that other patterns may also be attractive. It has been found, for example, that very young babies not only imitate facial expressions, but also imitate finger gestures (Melzoff & Moore, 1977). Perhaps breasts may prove equally attractive to neonates.

Following on Bornstein's (1963) observation, Damasio et al. (1982) have argued very strongly that prosopagnosia is not confined to problems of face recognition. Instead, it is usually accompanied by difficulties in recognising individual examples of other object categories. These include foods (Pallis, 1955), cars (Bruyer et al., 1983), and animals

(Macrae & Trolle, 1956). This view has been recently reiterated and cogently defended (Damasio, in press). However, two things make me reluctant to accept Damasio's position. One is the fact that prosopagnosics seem to display such a variety of accompanying agnosias, suggesting that these could arise from damage to neighbouring cerebral structures. This explanation allows for the likelihood that individual cases of prosopagnosia involve slightly different areas of brain damage, thereby producing different accompanying function disorders. The second reason for doubting Damasio's argument is that at least one apparently pure case of prosopagnosia has been reported. De Renzi (1986a) described the case of a 73 year old notary who became prosopagnosic following a stroke. This patient's ability to select his own personal items from among a range of similar items appears to undermine Damasio's theoretical position. It must be allowed, of course, that in addition to his inability to recognise previously familiar faces, he may have had other recognition difficulties that had not been uncovered during clinical assessment, but in the absence of such evidence, it seems reasonable to conclude that De Renzi's patient had suffered damage only to those visual structures supporting facial recognition.

ANATOMY OF PROSOPAGNOSIA

Prosopagnosia usually involves bilateral damage to the occipito-temporal areas involving the inferior longitudinal fasciculus and/or neighbouring gyri (Meadows, 1974; Damasio et al., 1982). At least that is the prevailing received wisdom. Recently, however, some have questioned the need for bilateral lesions for prosopagnosia to occur. De Renzi (1986b), for example, has presented evidence on two patients with prosopagnosia who, on CT scan evidence, had damage confined to the right hemisphere. One of these cases was the notary described above. His damage involved the areas served by the right posterior cerebral artery, encompassing the parahippocampal gyrus, the lingual and fusiform gyri, both lips of the calcarine fissure, the cuneus and the splenium, but no abnormality was evident in the left hemisphere. The second case, a 66 year old man, also with a right hemisphere infarct, involved almost identical damage.

It may be argued that CT scan data, or at least negative evidence from this brain imaging technique, is not unquestionably correct. Landis (personal communication), however, has reported that he and colleagues have post-mortem evidence from a patient who died shortly after becoming prosopagnosic and who had recently sustained right hemisphere lesions. Unfortunately for their argument, however, this patient had also incurred older left hemisphere damage which leaves open the possibility (however remote) that it was the old plus the new lesions that, in combination, produced prosopagnosia.

De Renzi (in press) has discussed the fact that laterality phenomena are not always consistent. A significant proportion of normal subjects, for example, do not have a clear left visual field advantage for linguistic material and a right hemisphere advantage for visuo-spatial stimuli. In the same vein, Milner (1985) had earlier pointed out that up to half the population may not conform exactly to these text-book dominance patterns. Male brains may be generally more asymmetrically organised (McGlone, 1978) and Mazzucchi and Biber (1983), have calculated that there are roughly four male prosopagnosics for every female one - a finding not easily accounted for by any corresponding imbalance in occurrence of precipitating factors (strokes, tumours etc.)

After my rather lengthy review of older issues in the study of prosopagnosia, I shall now turn to a discussion of three relatively new lines of research that either introduce novel and potentially interesting theoretical themes or provide some much needed practical observations on rehabilitation of prosopagnosic patients.

COVERT RECOGNITION

Bauer (1984) described L.F. a 39 year old victim of a motorcycle accident that caused bilateral posterior damage. L.F. like so many patients, was found to achieve a normal score on the Benton Face Matching Test, where unknown target faces while in view, have to be picked out from an array of faces. Because this test only scores for accuracy, however, it is insensitive to the abnormal, feature-by-feature strategies frequently observed when prosopagnosics attempt the task.

L.F. however, cannot recognise previously familiar faces but Bauer was reluctant to accept that, though prosopagnosic, he was entirely unable to respond differentially to 'familiar' as opposed to unfamiliar faces. In order to examine this hunch, Bauer employed the Guilty Knowledge Test devised for lie detection. He presented pictures of L.F.'s family as well as famous faces and measured the patient's autononomic responses principally using the skin conductance (SC) index as a measure of autonomic arousal. As each face appeared five different names were read out, only one of which was the correct one. While L.F. couldn't spontaneously name any of the faces, for more than 60% he showed the highest SC response to the correct name. In other words, his autonomic system made a differential response usually to the correct name – rather as a guilty suspect might respond maximally to some detail of a crime that innocent people would not know about.

Bauer (1986) also described similar results using the same methodology with P.K., a 59 year old stroke victim who was prosopagnosic yet revealed covert recognition. Tranel and Damasio (1985) employed a more straightforward technique in which they presented a mixture of known and unknown faces in a series. They found in two prosopagnosic patients greater electrodermal activity for known faces compared with unknown faces, confirming Bauer's observations.

There are other clues to suggest that prosopagnosics, though entirely unconscious of being able to discriminate facial familiarity, may respond differentially. Bruyer et al. (1983), for example, observed that their patient, a relatively "pure" case of prosopagnosia, could learn previous face-name combinations more easily than novel ones. The concept of covert recognition has been most comprehensively explored, however, in a series of experiments by De Haan, Young and Newcombe (in press). De Haan et al. discovered that P.H., a 19 year old who became prosopagnosic following a motorcycle accident, displayed covert recognition in a variety of situations. I shall only summarise some of their experiments.

(i) Pairs of faces, half of which were of two famous and half of two unfamiliar faces were shown to P.H. and he was required on each trial to decide if they were different views of the same individual or if they were photographs of two different individuals. Normal subjects make faster decision to pairs of familiar faces and P.H's reaction times revealed the same pattern.

(ii) Internal or external features of pairs of faces were masked and displayed as in (i). Normal subjects find famous faces easier to identify from internal compared with external features (Ellis, Shepherd & Davies, 1979) and they also match pairs of familiar faces faster when internal

157

features are shown (Young, et al., 1985). P.H. showed the same pattern of results: despite not recognising the faces his matching decisions were obviously influenced by their familiarity.

(iii) <u>Interference effects</u> occur for normal subjects asked to categorize names of famous people as either pop-star or politician when alongside the name is a photograph of someone from another category, e.g. Neil Kinnock's name is categorized as 'politician' more slowly if it occurs alongside Mick Jagger's face (Young, et al., 1986). In two experiments, involving pop-stars/politicians and politicians/TV personalities, P.H's name classifications were similarly interfered with when a famous face from the other category accompanied it - but not when same category faces occurred.

(iv) <u>Learning</u> true name-occupation pairings and true name-face pairings were learned more quickly than untrue pairings.

When De Haan et al. (in press) asked PH how he was able to produce results such as those given above, he stated that his responses were pure guesses. But clearly at some level below conscious awareness a face recognition system is operating. Where could this be?

Bauer (1984, 1986) has suggested one plausible, but as yet unproven, hypothesis. He argues that, in addition to the principal recognition route from the visual cortex through the inferior temporal lobes to the limbic system (the ventral route), there is a dorsal route between visual cortex and limbic structures (see Figure 2). In prosopagnosia, whereas the ventral route is damaged, the dorsal route may be intact and give rise to "autonomic recognition". Now this suggestion does not necessarily explain the results of De Haan et al. (in press), but doubtless, it could be made to do so. An alternative idea is that there are numerous routes to recognition operating at different levels of consciousness and that if any of these remain intact covert recognition may occur.

CAPGRAS' SYNDROME

Strictly speaking the following should not be regarded as constituting recent work in prosopagnosia but it does give me an opportunity to

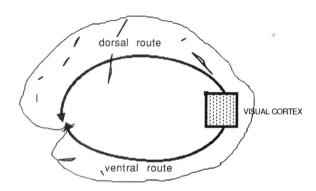

Figure 2. Bauer's (1984) dual face recognition routes.

amplify a proposed link between prosopagnosia and a psychiatric syndrome that may prove ultimately to be theoretically useful (Young & Ellis, in press a).

Capgras' Syndrome is one of the delusional misidentification syndromes (Tzavaras et al., 1986). It was first described by Capgras and Rebel-Lachaux (1923). They observed a female patient who asserted that her husband, children and numerous acquaintances had been replaced by doubles who were impersonating them. They first termed this 'l'illusion des sosies' before the term Capgras' Syndrome was generally adopted. Todd, Dewhurst and Wallis (1981) described two other typical cases. One was a 56 year old man who, upon recovering from neurosurgery believed his wife was an imposter - not quite a perfect one, being older and greyer. Another example was of a 68 year old woman who first believed her psychiatrist was an imposter; then her daughter was accused similarly of being a dissembler. Finally she developed the idea that there were 4 'Dr. Ts', the voice being the same in all cases but 3 were wearing masks. Frontal lobe lesions were suspected from EEG data which was confirmed by CAT scans.

In many other cases of Capgras' Syndrome signs of brain damage have been found to be present (e.g. Hayman & Abrams, 1977; Joseph, 1986; De Pauw & Szulecka, in press). So that, although normally classified as a functional disorder of a paranoid nature, there is a growing suspicion that it may have organic bases. This view has been recently reiterated and extended to the field of prosopagnosia by Lewis (1987). He presented details of a 19 year old epileptic who, when given an increased dose of phenytoin, developed Capgras' Syndrome: she failed to recognise her sister, claiming instead that she was her long-dead aunt. Then she became convinced that her mother, father and sisters had been replaced by 'dummies'. Further reduplicative paramnesias occurred as she asserted that even the house and cat were not originals. Nuclear Magnetic Resonance imaging revealed bilateral occipito-temporal lesions coupled with smaller bilateral frontal lesions. Lewis (1987) in noting the similar pathologies in Capgras' Syndrome and prosopagnosia suggests there may be a connection. One possibility which has yet to be explored systematically is that Capgras' Syndrome is the mirror image of prosopagnosia. Figure 3A

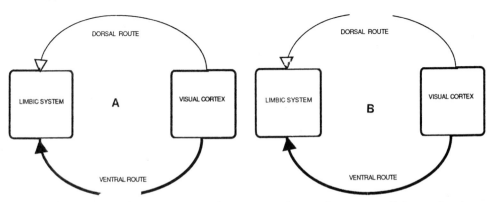

Figure 3A. Schematic representation of Bauer's (1984) dual routes to face recognition.

Figure 3B. A possible mechanism for producing Capgras' Syndrome (See Figure 3A).

shows Bauer's (1984) model of prosopagnosia in schematic form. In figure 3B the reverse state that may produce Capgras' Syndrome is shown.

In prosopagnosia the principal route to face recognition is blocked but some sort of 'emotional' recognition may be possible. In Capgras' Syndrome it may be that the 'emotional' route is interrupted but that the main route remains intact. Phenomenalogically this would mean that faces are recognised but something about them is missing: there is not the usual emotional response that accompanies recognition of any familiar faces - particularly those of people very close. Patients may resolve this dilemma by proclaiming the person to be a double, dummy or robot. Mishkin and Appenzeller (1987) have summarised much of their own work that indicates one of the roles of the amygdala is to integrate familiar stimuli with their corresponding emotional associations and this line of evidence may provide a useful lead for any further work attempting to link prosopagnosia and Capgras' Syndrome.

TRAINING

Prosopagnosia is a rare neurological condition usually afflicting elderly people. In most reported cases voice recognition serves as an alternative means of identifying familiar people - albeit a much poorer route to recognition than the face. It is not surprising, therefore, that, until recently, no-one has reported any attempt to train prosopagnosics to recognise faces. Wilson (1987) however, has published an account of successful training in the use of mnemonics enabling a prosopagnosic patient to learn a small set of face-name associations.   It   is difficult to know if he learned to spot specific facial features or whether he developed a more global knowledge of the faces he learned to name. But the mnemonic technique is undeniably helpful not only for prosopagnosics but for other brain-damaged individuals as well (Wilson, 1987).

A few years ago, Andy Young and I began what turned out to be a lengthy study of a rather unusual prosopagnosic (Young & Ellis, in press, b). K.D. is the only reported case of prosopagnosia acquired during childhood. She was 9 years old when we began studying her, by which time she had been prosopagnosic for about 6 years. It developed after meningitis and numerous operations to reduce hydrocephaly had left her with not only mild left hemiparesis and impaired vision but also with profound prosopagnosia. Full details of the clinical assessment of K.D. are given elsewhere (Young & Ellis, in press). Here I shall give a brief resume.

When we began to study her, K.D. was a lively child attending a special unit for the visually handicapped. Her IQ and reading were approximately normal, despite having reduced contrast sensitivity across the full range of spacial frequencies. Her object recognition, visually and stereognostically was good but, with increasing representational abstractness (photograph, line drawing) her performance became poorer. She scored in the normal range on the Benton Face Matching Test, although like other prosopagnosics she took a long time to arrive at decisions, and seemed to employ a feature-by-feature scan. She could even score creditably on a two-alternative forced-choice face memory test, provided the retention interval was no more than a few seconds. Once the interval was increased beyond that her accuracy fell to chance level. More strikingly, K.D. could not identify faces of familiar people, or their photographs, though she was reasonably able to recognise their voices. She could also interpret emotional expressions on faces.

Over an 18 month period Young and I administered K.D. a series of

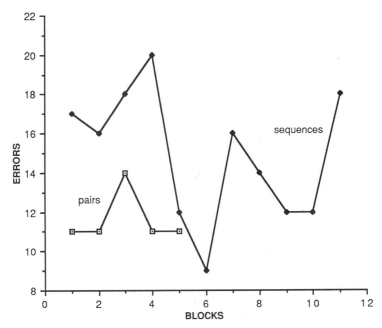

Figure 4. K.D's. performance on discriminating pairs of schematic faces. Each block represents 50 trials.

four training programmes designed to make use of repetition together with feedback on performance during which we continually monitored her accuracy. Full details of these programmes and the results are given elsewhere (Ellis and Young, in preparation); so I shall confine myself to a very brief description of each.

(i) <u>Matching familiar and unfamiliar pairs of faces</u>. K.D. was presented with two faces that could be two of 36 different views of the same child or of different children. On half the trials the faces were of the 5 children in the visually-handicapped unit, including K.D., and 5 were children unknown to her.

Over a series of trials K.D. showed rather poor accuracy in deciding whether each pair comprised same or different faces. Moreover, she displayed no signs of improving with experience of the set of faces and being given immediate feedback after every trial.

(ii) <u>Schematic faces</u>. For this programme stimuli were pairs of simple cartoon 'faces' that differed on 0, 1, 2, 3 or 4 features. The stimuli were presented on a monochrome monitor via a BBC B microcomputer which K.D. had recently learned to use. The pairs of faces were programmed to occur in blocks of 10, either simultaneously or sequentially separated by 2 secs. Audio feedback followed every response. Figure 4 illustrates K.D's. accuracy in deciding 'Same' or 'Different' over trials. She was clearly operating at better than chance level but did not improve with practice. G.M., who has similar visual difficulties to K.D., was also given a block of trials in each condition.

(iii) <u>Digitized faces</u>. In order to establish whether or not K.D. was

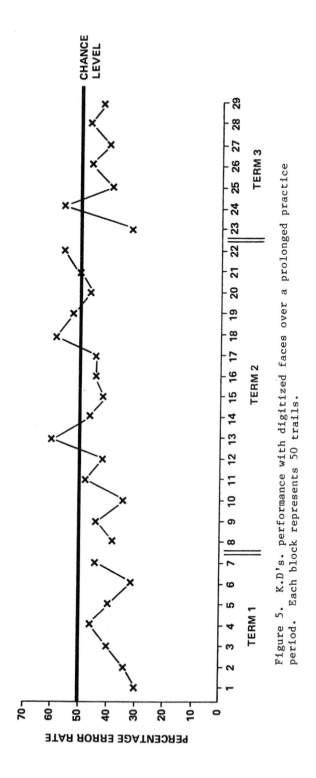

Figure 5. K.D's. performance with digitized faces over a prolonged practice
period. Each block represents 50 trails.

handicapped by the use of schematic faces a similar test was designed in which the faces were 128 x 128 pixel portraits of 19 men. On any trial two faces were generated by the computer that were randomly and equi- probably either identical or of two different men. However, as with sche- matic faces, K.D's. ability to determine whether the pairs were same or different did not improve over successive blocks of trials. Moreover, when the exercise was repeated, using sequential pairs of faces only, on a daily basis over 3 school terms there was still no improvement (Figure 5).

(iv) Name-face learning. Finally, K.D. was tested on her ability to learn 8 simple names to 8 faces. Again, stimuli were generated using a computer program that showed each face as a 128 x 128 pixel portrait to- gether with a name. When all 8 face-name combinations had been displayed a block of 10 trials was given on each of which a face was randomly sel- ected and alongisde it the 8 names were shown. All K.D. had to do was key in the number alongside the chosen name. Audio feedback was then supplied to indicate a correct or incorrect choice. Figure 6 shows that she was unable to learn the names. Compared with R.S. another classmate with similar visual difficulties K.D's. performance was very poor indeed.

I am conscious that I have dwelled rather at length on what are essentially negative data. That K.D. did not evince any ability to learn facial discrimination tests does not, of course, necessarily mean that all prosopagnosics will be equally unable to benefit from similar train- ing schedules, but it is probably unlikely that they would do so. Since we completed our study of K.D., Young and I have learned of Wilson's (1987) limited success in teaching a stroke victim face-name combinations using a vivid imagery mnemonic scheme. Perhaps a similar programme may work with K.D. when she is a little older and it is one we shall attempt in due course, though not with any great optimism since Wilson (personal communication, 1988) did not find that her training led to particularly reliable recognition by her patient.

REFERENCES

Bauer, R.M. (1984). Autonomic recognition of names and faces: a neuro- psychological application of the Guilty Knowledge Test. Neuropsycho- logia, 22, 457-469.
Bauer, R.M. (1986). The cognitive psychophysiology of prosopagnosia. in: H. Ellis, M. Jeeves, F. Newcombe & A. Young (eds.). Aspects of Face Processing. Dordrecht: Martinus Nijhoff.
Bodamer, J. (1947). Die Prosopagnosie. Archiv fur Psychiatrie und Nerven- krankheiten, 139, 949-964.
Bornstein, B. (1963). Prosopagnosia. in: L. Halpern (ed.). Problems of Dynamic Neurology. Jerusalem: Hadassah Medical Organization.
Bruce, V. & Young, A.W. (1986). Understanding face recognition. British Journal of Psychology, 77, 305-327.
Bruce, V., Ellis, H.D., Gibling, F. & Young, A.W. Parallel processing of the sex and familiarity of faces. Canadian Journal of Psychology, in press.
Bruyer, R., Latterre, C., Seron, X., Feyereisen, P., Strypstein, E., Pierrand, E. & Rectem, D. (1983). A case of prosopagnosia with some preserved covert remembrance of familiar faces. Brain and Cognition, 2, 257-284.
Campbell, R., Landis, T. & Regard, M. (1986). Face recognition and lip reading: a neurological dissociation. Brain, 109, 509-521.
Capgrass, J. & Rebel-Lachaux, J. (1923). Illusion des sosies dans un delire systematise chronique. Bulletin de la Society Clinique de Medecine Mentale, 2, 6-16.

Charcot, J.M. (1888). Un cas de suppression brusque et isole de la vision mentale des signes et objets (formes et couleurs). Progres Medecine, 11, 568.

Damasio, A.R. (1989). Mechanisms of face recognition. in: A. Young & H. Ellis (eds.). Handbook of Research on Face Processing. Amsterdam: North-Holland.

Damasio, A.R., Damasio, H. & Van Hoesen, G.W. (1982). Prosopagnosia: anatomical basis and behavioural mechanisms. Neurology, 32, 331-341.

De Pauw, K.W. & Szulecka, T.K. Dangerous delusions: Violence and the misidentification syndromes. British Journal of Psychiatry, in press.

De Haan, E., Young, A. & Newcombe, F. (1987). Face recognition without awareness. Cognitive Neuropsychology, 4, 385-415.

De Renzi, E. (1986a). Current issues in prosopagnosia. in: H. Ellis, M. Jeeves, F. Newcombe, A. Young (eds.). Aspects of Face Processing. Dordrecht: Martinus Nijhoff.

De Renzi, E. (1986b). Prosopagnosia in two patients with CT scan evidence of damage confined to the right hemisphere. Neuropsychologia, 24, 385-389.

De Renzi, E. (1989). Prosopagnosia: A multi-stage specific disorder? in: A. Young & H. Ellis (eds.). Handbook of Research on Face Processing. Amsterdam: North-Holland.

Dziurawiec, S. and Ellis, H.D. Neonates' attention to face-like stimuli. Manuscript in preparation.

Ellis, H.D. (1981). Theoretical aspects of face recognition. in: G. Davies, H. Ellis & J. Shepherd (eds.). Perceiving and Remembering Faces. London: Academic Press.

Ellis, H.D. (1983). The role of the right hemisphere in face perception. in: A. Young (ed.). Functions of the Right Cerebral Hemisphere. London: Academic Press.

Ellis, H.D. (1986a). Disorders of face recognition. in: K. Poek, H. Freund & H. Ganshirt (eds.). Neurology. Berlin: Springer-Verlag.

Ellis, H.D. (1986b). Introduction: Processes underlying face recognition. in: R. Bruyer (ed.). The Neuropsychology of Face Perception and Facial Expression. Hillsdale, N.J.: Lawrence Erlbaum Associates.

Ellis, H.D. & Young, A.W. (1989). Are faces special? in: A. Young and H. Ellis (eds.). Handbook of Research on Face Processing. Amsterdam: North-Holland.

Ellis, H.D. and Young, A.W. Training in face processing skills for a child with acquired prosopagnosia. Manuscript in preparation.

Ellis, H.D., Shepherd, J.W. & Davies, G.M. (1979). Identification of familiar and unfamiliar faces from internal and external features: some implications for theories of face recognition. Perception, 8, 431-439.

Goren, C.G., Sarty, M. & Wu, R.W.K. (1975). Visual following and pattern discrimination of face-like stimuli by newborn infants. Pediatrics, 56, 544-559.

Harrington, A. (1958). Nineteenth-century ideas on hemisphere differences and 'duality of mind'. The Behavioural and Brain Sciences, 8, 617-660.

Hay, D.C. & Young, A.W. (1982). The human face. in: A. Ellis (ed.). Normality and Pathology in Cognitive Functions. New York: Academic Press.

Hayman, M.A. & Abrams, R. (1977). Capgras' syndrome and cerebral dysfunction. British Journal of Psychiatry, 130, 68-71.

Hecaen, H. (1981). The neuropsychology of face recognition. in: G. Davies, H. Ellis & J. Shepherd (eds.). Perceiving and Remembering Faces. London: Academic Press.

Hecaen, H. & Angelergues, R. (1962). Agnosia for faces. Archives of Neurology, 7, 92-100.

Isler, H. & Regard, M. (1985). The case for applied history of medicine, and the place of Wigan. The Behavioural and Brain Sciences, 8, 640-641.

Joseph, A.B. (1986). Focal central nervous system abnormalities in patients with misidentification syndromes. Bibliotheca Psychiatrica, 164, 68–79.

Kendrick, K.M. and Baldwin, B.A. (1987). Cells in the temporal cortex of conscious sheep can respond preferentially to the sight of faces. Science, 236, 448–450.

Konorski, J. (1967). Integrative Action of the Nervous System. Chicago: University of Chicago Press.

Kurucz, J. and Feldmar, G. (1979). Proso-affective agnosia as a symptom of cerebral organic disease. Journal of the American Geriatrics Society, 27, 225–230.

Levine, D.N., Warach, J. & Farah, M. (1985). Two visual systems in mental imagery. Neurology, 35, 1010–1018.

Lewis, S.W. (1987). Brain imaging in a case of Capgras' Syndrome. British Journal of Psychiatry, 150, 117–121.

Lissauer, H. (1890). Ein Fall von Seelenblindheit nebst einem Beitrage zur Theorie derselben. Archiv fur Psychiatrie und Nervenkrankheit, 21, 222–270.

Macrae, D. & Trolle, E. (1956). The defect of function in visual agnosia. Brain, 79, 94–110.

McGlone, J. (1978). Sex differences in functional brain asymmetry. Cortex, 14, 122–128.

Mazzuchi, A. & Bibner, C. (1983). Is prosopagnosia more frequent in males than females? Cortex, 19, 509–516.

Meadows, J.C. (1974). The anatomic basis of prosopagnosia. Journal of Neurology, Neurosurgery and Psychiatry, 37, 489–501.

Melzoff, A.N. & Moore, M.K. (1977). Imitation of facial and manual gestures by human neonates. Science, 198, 75–78.

Milner, A.D. (1985). Two hemispheres do not make a dichotomy. The Behavioural and Brain Sciences, 8, 643–644.

Mishkin, M. & Appenzeller, T. (1987). The Anatomy of memory. Scientific American, 256, 80–89.

Pallis, C.A.C. (1955). Impaired, identification of faces and places with agnosia for colours: report of a case due to cerebral embolism. Journal of Neurology, Neurosurgery and Psychiatry, 18, 218–244.

Perrett, D.I., Mistlin, A.J., Potter, D.D., Smith, P.A.J., Head, A., Chitty, A.J., Broennimann, R., Milner, A.D., Jeeves, M.A.J. Functional organization of visual neurones processing face identity. in: H. Ellis, M. Jeeves, F. Newcombe, A. Young (eds.). Aspects of Face Processing. Dordrecht: Martinus Nijhoff.

Sachs, O. (1985). The Man Who Mistook His Wife for a Hat. London: Duckworth.

Sergent, J. (1986). Methodological constraints on neuropsychological studies of face perception in normals. in: R. Bruyer (ed.). The Neuropsychology of Face Perception and Facial Expression. Hillsdale, N.J.: Laurence Erlbaum Associates.

Shuttleworth, E.C., Syring, V. & Allen, N. (1982). Further observations on the nature of prosopagnosia. Brain and Cognition, 1, 307–322.

Tiberghien, G., and Clerc, I. (1986). Familiarity, context and prosopagnosia. in: R. Bruyer (ed.). The Neuropsychology of Face Perception and Facial Expression. Hillsdale, N.J.: Lawrence Erlbaum Associates.

Todd, J., Dewhurst, K. & Wallis, D. (1981). The syndrome of Capgras. British Journal of Psychiatry, 139, 319–327.

Tranel, D. & Damasio, A.R. (1985). Knowledge without awareness: an autonomic index of facial recognition by prosopagnosics. Science, 228, 1453–1454.

Tzavaras, A. Luaute, J. & Bidault, E. (1986). Face recognition dysfunction and delusional misidentification syndromes. (D.M.S.) in: H. Ellis, M. Jeeves, F. Newcombe, A. Young (eds.). Aspects of Face Processing. Dordrecht: Martinus Nijhoff.

Wilbrank, H. (1892). Ein Fall von Seelenblindheit and Hemianopsie mit Sectionsbefund. Deutsche Zeitschrift fur Nervenheilkunde, 2, 361387.

Wilson, B. (1987). Rehabilitation of Memory. London: The Guilford Press.

Young, A.W. & Ellis, H.D. (1989). Semantic processing. in: A. Young & H. Ellis (eds.). Handbook of Research on Face Processing. Amsterdam: North-Holland.

Young, A.W. & Ellis, H.D. Childhood prosopagnosia. Brain and Cognition, in press.

Young, A.W., McWeeny, K.H., Ellis, A.W. & Hay, D.C. (1986). Naming and categorizing faces and written names. Quarterly Journal of Experimental Psychology, 38A, 297-318.

Young, A.W., Hay, D.M., McWeeny, K., Flude, B. & Ellis, A.W. (1987). Matching familiar and unfamiliar faces on internal and external features. Perception, 14, 737-746.

DIFFERENT FORMS OF FACE-KNOWLEDGE IMPAIRMENT

Catherine Yee-Yuen Peng and Ruth Campbell

PROSOPAGNOSIA AS A FAILURE TO RECOGNISE FACES

Clinical Definition of Prosopagnosia

Bodamer (1947) invented the term Prosopagnosia to describe the isolated inability to recognise people by their face. Patients are usually able to judge a face to be a face, and some of them may even be able to discriminate and match face photographs normally (Benton & Van Allen, 1968). The major symptom is the failure to recognise familiar faces in real life and in reproduction (photographs, television etc.). In some cases, patients may not even recognise their own face (Bauer & Rubens, 1985). Prosopagnosic patients may be able to identify people despite this disability. They can learn to rely on paraphernalia such as clothing, gait, hair style, height and distinguishing birthmarks and on identification cues from other modalities, like voice and perfume.

Prosopagnosia is often associated with other deficits; in particular the following problems have been reported: cerebral achromatopsia, constructional disability, topographic amnesia, dressing apraxia, left hemianopia and various types of agnosia for objects (Hecaen & Angelergues, 1962; Bauer & Rubens, 1985; Damasio, 1985; De Renzi, 1986a). While prosopagnosia may co-exist with one or more of those symptoms, it is not consistently accompanied by any one or more of them.

Other Face Recognition Disorders

Other fairly specific problems in recognising individuals by their face have been reported. One is the Capgras syndrome. Patients believe that familiar persons have been replaced by imposters. The underlying ability to recognise a familiar face is, however, intact (Christodoulou, 1977; Synodinou et al., 1978).

Prosopagnosia may sometimes be misdiagnosed as a global amnesia. Patients may report that they 'forget who other people are.' It is important to find out whether patients have problems in retrieving people's names in all situations or if they only have problems when they are asked to put names to faces. That said, global amnesia can, obviously, include prosopagnosia (Corkin, 1984). The patient's difficulties then encompass both the recall of previously familiar names and the overt recognition of previously familiar faces.

Dementing disorders can also give rise to fairly specific face processing problems at some stages of the disease (Kurucz & Feldmar, 1979; Crawford et al., 1986). Indeed, there may be misdiagnosis of prosopagnosia following CVA as 'confusion' or 'dementia' if there is a paucity of indications to the contrary. Prosopagnosia will not usually be followed by further indications of cognitive disorder. If its onset is due to a CVA, it tends to be a sustained disorder, typically maintained over months or years, although transient face processing disorders have been reported, too.

The correct diagnosis of prosopagnosia, rather than a more general amnesia, a dementing disease or a psycho-neurological disorder, is of importance for rehabilitation. It is not impossible for such patients to function relatively normally. Employment prospects are improved when the diagnosis is circumscribed and neurological.

Testing for Prosopagnosia

A widely used test for face-processing impairment is Benton & Van Allen's Face Recognition task (1968). This uses photographs of unfamiliar individuals which must be matched by the patient to other photographs of the same individual under different conditions of lighting or viewpoint. Thus it is a test of face-matching skill. It can also be used to test memory for new faces by presenting the target individual followed after a delay, by the test set.

Tests for familiar face recognition should be constructed by clinicians. In our studies, we used photographs of patients' relatives, friends and colleagues (i.e. formerly familiar faces) as well as photographs of staff of the rehabilitation centre who frequently worked with the patients (i.e. faces that should be familiar following the accident). These were presented to the patient with all extraneous cues to identity (hairline, hair colour, jewellery etc.) masked out. Famous Face photographs can also be used, but demographic variables, such as age of subject and their interests are crucial and test requirements must be carefully tailored to the individual's pre-morbid interests. When the patient was an avid TV watcher, then a test of famous TV personalities is in order, but it cannot be relied on if these faces were not in the patients' identification repertoire before a brain lesion intervened. Both the cases reported below were avid watchers of TV soap-operas and were tested with faces of stars of soap series. But the class of Famous Faces that can be reliably identified across different cultures and ages is remarkably small and changes swiftly with the passage of fame.

Anatomical and Physiological Considerations

Damasio et al. (1982) analysed 11 cases of prosopagnosia at autopsy, and found that the lesions were all bilateral and mostly symmetrical. All were in the occipito-temporal areas. The picture is the same when the same investigators used neuro-imaging techniques on new patients (Damasio et al., 1985). On this evidence Damasio reaffirms the opinion of Meadows (1974) that prosopagnosia is produced by bilateral lesions, and extends this earlier conclusion by pinpointing the specific loci as occipito-temporal on both sides (Meadows had suggested that only the RH damage had to be specific to this locus; any posterior LH damage of sufficient extent, contributed to the prosopagnosic pattern). However, the question of laterality is not closed. Both De Renzi (1986b) and Landis et al. (1986) report unilateral (RH cases). Landis et al.'s evidence is based on CT scans on 6 patients and autopsy findings are not yet available. Limitations of CT scanning are discussed at length in this volume: we would point out only that firm localisation based on CT alone may not always be reliable.

Neurophysiological Considerations

Perrett and his colleagues (e.g. see Perrett & Rolls, 1983) report that a substantial number of neurons in the superior temporal sulcus (STS) of the macaque monkey respond selectively to visually presented faces of monkeys and of relevant human caretakers. These cells are found in both hemispheres. The area corresponding histologically to the STS in humans would include much of the lateral surface of the temporal lobe to the occipital junction. Mateer has conducted studies on human patients undergoing cortical surgery. Following Penfield's pioneering technique, she examines the effects of local cortical electrical stimulation on cognitive performance. She reports that RH stimulation (LH reports are not given) of the posterior and middle temporal gyri disrupts face identification (Mateer, 1983). These findings are consistent with the anatomical findings from primates.

Theories and Findings in Clinical Neuropsychology

Theories and models attempting to explain prosopagnosia are cast in two ways: one tends to describe prosopagnosia as a specific impairment to face processing, and the other sees prosopagnosia as a component of a more general impairment. Both are information theoretic accounts, for in both approaches it is understood that the recognition of familiar faces involves a series of stages of processing, from perception through to action.

The first view is expounded by some experimental psychologists. Using evidence from experiments with normal subjects they have shown many ways in which the perception and memory of faces is 'special' compared with that for words and objects. Thus they often postulate an independent, modular system for the processing of information specific to faces (Fodor, 1983; Bruce & Young, 1986). On this view, prosopagnosia results from damage to this system (see also H. Ellis, this volume).

The second view is more widely held by clinical neuropsychologists and clinical neurologists. Warrington appears to have been the first investigator in current times to investigate specific face processing difficulties in this way (Warrington & James, 1967; Whitely & Warrington, 1977). She characterises face-processing deficits in terms of a defective component of either perception or category-specific memory. In this account face recognition is particularly sensitive to impairment because faces are differentiated by small form or feature differences (a high perceptual load), hundreds of whom are typically known by any one adult (high associative memory load for individuals within this class). Thus a 'perceptual' and a 'mnestic' type of prosopagnosia can be distinguished (De Renzi, 1986a). Damasio et al. (1985) indicate four possible stages of information processing where damage will result in prosopagnosia. These are (1) a perceptual stage, concerned with the abstraction of perceptual detail or form; (2) a matching stage, where a template-type description, stored in long-term memory, is matched to the outputs from the perceptual analysers; (3) a stage concerned with the activation of this internal template – a memory stage and finally (4) overt recognition – presumably a readout stage from the memory description. This fourfold description can clarify some reported dissociated disorders within prosopagnosia (see e.g. Malone et al., 1982; De Renzi, 1986a; Tiberghien, 1986). It suggests that associated disorders should be expected to correspond with the presumed site of impairment; – a deficit at stage (1), for instance, should be anticipated to impair the processing of unfamiliar and familiar faces alike, and to cause problems in within-category discrimination for other classes of object whose members are visually similar (flowers, vehicles, dogs, cattle etc.). Patients with a deficit at stage (4) may show covert signs of recognition in the absence of overt recognition ability (Bruyer et al., 1983; Bauer & Rubens, 1985; De Haan et al., 1987). The 'general deficit' view should predict that this dissociation might be observed for other object classes than faces, too. As far as we know covert recognition of objects other than faces has not been tested in these patients.

It is certainly true that prosopagnosic patients have impairments other than face recognition; no 'pure' prosopagnosic, in this sense, has yet been reported. But is this likely? Human lesions are likely to affect independent as well as associated functional systems. 'When God lesions, he does not localise' (Passingham, 1986). Furthermore, there is evidence (Baylis et al., 1985) that a single neuron in the macaque STS can perform multiple functions, by virtue of its contribution to a small ensemble of multiply interconnected neurons; the ensemble of neurons may deal with faces, but its distributed architecture allows different face processing functions, as well as different identities, to be signalled by the firing of a single cell. That Mateer finds a range of different problems when small cortical regions in the corresponding human area are stimulated can be taken to support this multiple distributed processing view of the organisation of some face-sensitive cortical regions. It seems that, even when Man interferes selectively in brain areas (including single cells), multiple symptoms may arise.

We would suggest that the clinical and the experimental psychological views indicated earlier may reflect different interpretations of 'functional specificity'. Processing specificity and functional independence are not synonymous. It is quite possible for functional specificity to arise in the context of general processing stages and functions. This can be important in the interpretation of dissociations; double dissociations in particular. Teuber (1955) highlighted the importance of the concept of dissociation. The argument is simple: when a lesion in brain area X affects function A but not B, and a lesion in brain area Y affects function B but not A, brain areas X and Y are functionally dissociable, and functions A and B are anatomically dissociable. This need not exclude the possibility that A and B are dependent on more general functions, nor that brain areas X and Y may be responsible for other functions.

When clinical evidence is viewed in the light of double-dissociation, prosopagnosia can be described as a functionally and anatomically specific impairment. Although prosopagnosic patients have a variety of symptoms apart from impairments of face processing, all of these associated symptoms can be observed in non-prosopagnosic patients with lesions in other brain areas (Kertesz, 1983). No prosopagnosic patient has been reported with all these associated symptoms. This is already a convincing dissociation, allowing the inference that prosopagnosia, while it may reflect multi-stage impairments <u>within</u> the overall label, is nevertheless a specific impairment in face processing contrasting with other cognitive deficits.

In the next section we contrast the present, quite well formulated view of face processing disorder with a different aspect of face knowledge impairment in order to show that double dissociations exist between two processing systems for the abstraction of information from faces.

PROSOPAGNOSIA AS A FAILURE TO PROCESS FACE MEANINGS

Bodamer's paper on Prosopagnosia had the title 'Die Prosop-agnosie (Die Agnosie des Physiognomieerkennens)'. 'Kennen' means knowing by previous experience. This is the word Bodamer used to describe prosopagnosia as an impairment of face recognition. But 'Wissen' means 'knowing' by knowledge not necessarily obtained by direct experience; that is, semantic/conceptual, rather than associative or episodic knowledge. We ask - could there be 'Die Prosop-agnosie (Die Agnosie des Physiognomieer-wissens')? Are there patients who fail to understand the meaning of faces or facial actions? Would such a disorder doubly dissociate from an 'Agno-sie des Physiognomieerkennens'?

There are roughly three classes of meaning that can be derived from faces; one can know something about the social/personal aspects of the person from the face; one can read emotional expression from faces and faces are important in processes involved in verbal communication. So, in the first category, age and sex can be inferred from face characteris-tics. In the second category, emotional expressions and non-verbal com-municative gestures can be identified, while in the third category - which comprises what we call 'face-to-face communication', gaze reg-ulation and gestural regulation of conversation are informative (Argyle, 1987; Kendon, 1986). These phenomena are relatively under-investigated within neuropsychology.

With respect to face-to-face interaction, Campbell et al. (1986) report a double dissociation between lipreading skill and face-emotion and face-recognition skills. A patient with a slight alexia was unable to lipread but had perfect face recognition. A patient with impaired face recognition and impaired facial expression processing was unimpaired in matching faces on the basis of the sounds they were speaking.

With regard to the processes of person description, some prosopag-nosic patients have been tested in judging the age and sex of an individ-ual from a photograph and are as impaired at that as in the recognition of a familiar face (see, for example, Bornstein, 1963; Cole & Perez-Cruet, 1964; Shuttleworth et al., 1982). It is not yet clear whether this impairment is associated particularly with the loss of high spatial frequency information processing, nor is it clear how far this impairment is dissociable from prosopagnosia (Ellis, 1986).

Impairment of the interpretation of facial expression has been observed in prosopagnosic patients. One of Bodamer's cases could not recognise facial expression nor identity (and see Campbell, Landis & Regard, 1986; Bruyer et al., 1983). But impairment of facial expression identification may be associated with deficits other than face recog-nition. Ross (1983) reports a patient with deficits in interpreting facial expression and expression in tone of voice, and face-expression impairment can dissociate from face recognition impairment. A number of studies have shown facial expression classification to be sensitive to right hemisphere lesions in non-prosopagnosic patients (see Feyereisen, 1986 for review).

Ellis (1986) suggests face expression analysis is a process distinct from face identification and, up to a point, the dissociations observed in the clinical literature support that view. Nevertheless, the common co-occurrence of prosopagnosia with emotion identification disorder is intriguing. Further investigations of face identity and emotion process-ing in neurological patients seem to us to be worth pursuing. We are still far from understanding the necessary and sufficient conditions under which face recognition and the categorisation of facial expression can be observed to dissociate. Nor do we know whether all types of face-meaning analysis are functionally related, or whether dissociations might occur between its different aspects. And we believe that it is particu-larly important, in the light of the discussion above on functional bases for face recognition impairment, to try to distinguish some possible general processing impairments that might contribute to face-meaning problems in contrast with specific face-identification (i.e. recognition) impairments.

We are fortunate to have encountered two patients who provide some evidence on these questions. One could not recognise familiar faces, the other could not recognise facial expressions. They were tested by the same investigator with identical materials. Results of our investigation are summarised and discussed in the next section.

FACE RECOGNITION AND FACE EXPRESSION JUDGEMENT IN TWO PATIENTS

Patient MJS

This man aged 36 was a radar operator in the Canadian airforce, educated to eleventh-grade level. He had a motor vehicle accident in 1979 resulting in traumatic brain injury. During the investigation, he was working as a carpenter in the Lethbridge Rehabilitation Centre, Montreal, Canada. He was married with two children. MJS sustained bilateral middle temporal damage following his accident. Two subdural haematomas were removed from the left and right middle temporal cortical area on 24 September 1979. Following his accident, MJS also suffered from bilateral complex partial epileptic seizures. EEG measured in December 1980 showed diffused slow waves 5-6 cycle/second in areas T3 and T4. This EEG abnormality was consistent with the localisation of the surgical lesions. On testing prior to the reported sessions, MJS had an overall IQ of 90 (Verbal 93, Performance 86) with particular difficulties in Object Assembly and Block Design. His M.Q. was 56.5 with particularly low performance on Digit Span, Paired Associate and Visual Reproduction subtests.

Patient MBM

This man aged 26 was a car mechanic, educated to eleventh grade. He had a motor vehicle accident in 1983 resulting in traumatic brain injury. During the investigation, he was undergoing rehabilitation in the Lethbridge Rehabilitation Centre, Montreal, Canada. He was divorced prior to his injury. MBM's injury was bilateral to the orbito-frontal areas, including a right cerebral contusion extending 5x1x1mm along the orbital surface to the anterior pole. Two bilateral subdural haematomas were removed. MBM's overall IQ was tested before the reported sessions. His overall score was 76 (Verbal 77, Performance 75) with particular difficulties in paired associate learning, logical reasoning, concept formation and general knowledge. MQ was 34.5 with particularly impaired performance on Paired Associate, Information, Logical Memory and Mental Control subtests.

Both patients were given the Boston Aphasia Examination, Token Test and the Boston Naming Test. These revealed no impairment. Language, including naming skill, and immediate verbal memory processes are intact in these patients, and testing was done verbally, in English.

Description of Tests

i) Tests of face recognition. Patients were shown photographs of their family members, relatives, friends and colleagues as well as faces of 10 famous politicians and 15 famous TV soap-opera stars to test their face recognition ability (they both had watched TV a great deal before and since injury). They were also given the Benton Test to assess their ability to match and memorise unknown faces.

ii) Tests of facial expression classification. Patients were shown Ekman & Friesen's (1976) photographs of 7 actors portraying seven different facial expressions. They were asked to categorise them by performing the following tasks: naming the expression portrayed on each photograph, sorting the photographs into piles according to expression category; distinguishing different individuals within the same expression category and matching photographed expressions to videotapes of the same expression projected by a different encoder.

iii) Apperception test: the identification of visually similar individual exemplars within a single category. Pictures of different animals, buildings, cars and common Canadian flowers were shown. The subject was asked to name each individual object (e.g. 'that flower is a trillium, that car is a Ford Mustang of the 1960s.'); to discriminate between similar objects having the same name (e.g. 'those are both types of cattle, but I don't know the name...they are different types, though...') and to recognise the same object from a different viewpoint. This assesses the ability to make within-category decisions based on complex visual analysis and on knowledge of the characteristic attributes of those objects. It is a test of apperceptive skill (Leibniz, Herbert: - see Reber, 1985).

Both patients had worked with cars either professionally or as a hobby, prior to their accident; it is very likely indeed that this category was extremely well known and well differentiated by them premorbidly.

iv) Conceptual test: identification of object classes and categories. Using the picture set indicated in the above test, subjects were asked which species each animal belonged to, what function the buildings had, the approximate price of the cars and the likely categorical organisation of pictures of roses (for which neither patient had any botanical knowledge). We reasoned that this test taps the ability to search in a directed way through semantic knowledge in order to categorise and conceptualise (naturally, performance on this task might be impaired for perceptual reasons, but if perceptual ability - say in simultaneous matching - is good, it should not be expected to be compromised in this task).

v) Delayed match to sample. The subject is shown a single photograph and asked to memorise it. After a fixed delay (10 seconds in the present task), a set of photographs is presented from which the subject is asked to choose the one that was shown before. A correct match comprises the selection of a different picture of the same object. In this test, once again, the same picture set as was used for the apperceptive and conceptual tests (see above) were used. In this way the patients' ability to match for (1) face identity (across different expressions); (2) for face expression (across different identities) and (3) for the same object (across different viewpoints) was tested.

vi) Visual imagery. Patients were instructed to visualise objects, animals and persons. Then they were asked questions about the images and their responses, including eye-movements, were recorded.

vii) Verbal categorisation. A modification of Hampson's (1985) test of category asymmetry was used to tap the subjects' skill in the uses of verbal categorisation. The modifications were to include some questions about emotion. Thus, subjects are asked to choose "which is the better sentence 'to smile is a way of being happy' or 'being happy is a way of smiling'?" and to explain their choices. A second test investigated the patients' 'emotional lexicon' (see Tiller, unpublished). They were asked to generate and then to classify emotion-related words (like 'calm', 'distressed', 'happy' etc. etc.). The generation task was to an emotional category label (e.g. 'words to do with sadness...'), the sorting task was undirected. These tasks were designed to test conceptual, verbal aspects of emotion processing.

viii) <u>Voice, gaze and touch and cross-modal matching</u>. Patients who have problems in interpreting voice tone, in perceiving direction of gaze of an interactant and in sensitivity to the location and quality of touched parts of the body are likely to have problems in the analysis of information relevant to social interaction. These sensory-specific characteristics were tested by asking the patients to distinguish between different voice qualities, including loudness, sex of the speaker and emotional tone; to point to direction of gaze and to locate and describe which parts of the subjects' body were touched by the experimenter. It should be noted that neither patient had any central or peripheral sensory deficit that was likely to impede these processes.

The categorisation of emotional voice-tone was also tested. Patients were asked both to name the emotion of the tone of voice and to match it to an Ekman face-emotion picture, thus testing emotion matching cross-modally.

ix) <u>Social cognition</u>. Patients were asked to describe themselves and other people in terms of their personal and social attributes and identities. They were asked to assess their own and others' social situations. They were asked to generate information from given social stereotypes. They were asked to provide descriptions of social situations associated with emotional states and their public display. Both autobiographical and hypothetical ('what would you do if....') situations were used to elicit these test responses. These were designed to test the patients' abilities to perform covert elaborations of social processes, including emotional ones. In addition, for rehabilitation purposes, Trower, Argyle and Bryant's (1977) Social Situation Difficulties Measurement Test was administered as a diagnostic test of possible ongoing social adjustment difficulties.

These patients were compared with 2 control subjects. The controls were carefully chosen from relatives and friends to match the patients as closely as possible on sex, age, demographic variables including social class, education level, general interests and pre-morbid intelligence.

RESULTS

Dissociated Deficits

As table 1 shows, MJS was impaired at facial recognition. He could not even recognise pictures of himself. However he could name and categorise facial expressions of emotion, discriminate between expressions having the same name, match photographed expressions to video-taped ones, and match facial expression to tone of voice correctly.

MBM was not impaired in face recognition. However, he was unable to perform <u>any</u> of the matching tasks on facial expression, within or across modalities.

Neither patient was impaired in complex visual analysis and perceptual matching of the Benton faces. Nor were they impaired in perceptual discrimination of nonverbal signals (Gaze, Voice, Touch). These dissociated impairments do not reflect central sensory disorders. Both patients reported severe and profound social problems in adjusting to life after their accident.

Deficits Associated with MJS's Impairment

MJS was severely impaired on <u>all</u> delayed match-to-sample tasks. If

174

TABLE 1

PERFORMANCE OF MJS AND MBM COMPARED WITH CONTROLS

key: - = no impairment, + = impaired performance

	MJS	CONTROL	MBM	CONTROL
i). FACE RECOGNITION				
Benton	-	-	-	-
Family, etc	0/15	15/15	15/15	15/15
TV	0/15	12/15	15/15	11/15
Famous	1/10	9/10	8/10	8/10
ii). FACIAL EXPRESSION CLASSIFICATION				
Naming	50/51	48/51	12/51	47/51
Sorting	33/33	31/33	3/33	30/33
Identity/Expression	12/12	12/12	12/12	12/12
Photo-video	20/24	18/24	2/24	18/24
iii). APPERCEPTIVE: COMPLEX VISUAL ANALYSIS				
Car	14/14	14/14	14/14	14/14
Animal	58/58	58/58	58/58	58/58
Building	11/12	11/12	11/12	11/12
Flower	8/8	8/8	8/8	8/8
iv). CONCEPTUAL: COMPLEX VISUAL ANALYSIS				
Car	12/14	11/14	0/14	11/14
Animal	58/58	58/58	4/58	58/58
Building	12/12	12/12	1/12	12/12
Flower	8/8	8/8	0/8	8/8
v.) APPERCEPTIVE: DELAYED MATCH TO SAMPLE				
Car	3/14	12/14	14/14	12/14
Animal	18/58	50/58	56/58	52/58
Building	2/12	12/12	12/12	11/12
Flower	0/8	8/8	8/8	7/8
vi). CONCEPTUAL: VERBAL CATEGORISATION				
Hampson	14/15	14/15	7/15	14/15
Tiller	30/30	30/30	7/30	30/30
vii). VISUAL IMAGERY				
Eye movement	-	-	-	-
Verbal report				
of detail	+	-	-	-
viii). VOICE, GAZE, TOUCH & CROSS-MODAL MATCHING				
Voice	12/12	12/12	12/12	12/12
Gaze	24/23	24/24	24/24	24/24
Touch	12/12	12/12	12/12	12/12
Cross-modal	12/12	12/12	1/12	12/12
ix). SOCIAL COGNITION				
Social Identity	-	-	+	-
Soc. situation	-	-	+	-
Prototype	-	-	+	-
Stereotype	-	-	+	-
Display-rule recall	-	-	+	-
Display-rule				
hypothetical	-	-	+	-
SOCIAL DIFFICULTIES (TROWER et al., 1978)				
	+	-	+	-

we were to follow earlier neurological classifications we would categorise him in accordance with Warrington's suggestions as one of De
Renzi's mnestic prosopagnosics with an associated within-category memory
deficit associated with his prosopagnosia.

It is interesting to note that MJS had great problems with visual
imagery. He was able to produce images, but he reported a failure to
visualise details of objects, animals or particular people or expressions
within an imagined frame. While some eye-movement was observed it was not
consistent and appeared only when he was directed to quite distant parts
of the image (e.g., when imagining a dog his eyes moved when asked to
describe the dog's tail). Within Damasio's framework this might mean his
problems arise at stage 3, where the representation of detailed knowledge
about a particular individual's face is activated.

Apart from face recognition, delayed match to sample and visual
imagery, MJS was not impaired in any other tested task.

MBM's associated impairments

Unlike MJS, MBM was not impaired in delayed match-to-sample, nor in
visual imagery. As we say above, he was also unimpaired in recognising
faces. He was, however, severely impaired in tasks which MJS performed
normally. So, as well as being impaired in classifying emotion pictures,
MJS could not perform tasks (iv), (vii) and (ix). He was quite unable to
provide rich conceptual classifications of the world.

It is important, however, to note that this was not a simple manifestation of 'frontal cognitive disorder' as described, for example by
Milner (1982), nor is it well captured by Shallice's (1982) planning-
deficit conceptualisation nor Duncan's (1986) characterisation of frontal
dysfunction in terms of goal-directed control of cognitive action (though
this may be involved). Thus, MJS' errors were not perseverative, and in
face recognition, which was quite intact, he was able to identify correctly by name, as well as match by identity, thus indicating intact semantic associations up to this level of processing and a controlled ability to extract the relevant information. Rather, his descriptions and
behaviours in the classification tasks indicate to us a grossly impaired
ability to use stored representations of individuals and events in order
to make conceptual distinctions and comparisons beyond the level of identification.

DISCUSSION

These patients demonstrate that the two German meanings of 'knowledge' can dissociate with brain lesions. MJS cannot recognise faces
(Agnosie des Physiognomieerkennens) and MBM cannot process face meanings
(Agnosie des Physiognomieerwissens). These two functions are therefore
doubly dissociable. Precisely the same tests were used on both patients.
This double dissociation has not been clearly pinpointed in precisely
this way before. It is equally important to note that neither patient had
been diagnosed as deficient in face processing, though both reported
severe social problems following their accidents.

But it is clear that more general impairments underly these dissociated deficits in these patients. MJS was impaired in all within-
category identification tasks that involved a delay between presentation
and test, while his ability to handle tests of conceptual categorisation
and evaluation, including social/emotional aspects, was intact. MBM was
impaired in the conceptual analysis of information, as shown by his per-

formance on tasks of categorisation, evaluation, and functional description. These patients' face recognition and face-expression matching abilities are, we suggest, indicative of an underlying dissociation between apperceptive skills that are important for recognising identity of individual objects, persons or events on the one hand, and, on the other, conceptual skills that appear to be vital for effective categorisation - including the classification of facial expression and in particular for the ability to assess one's social setting effectively.

This conclusion is reinforced by MBM's particularly poor ability to make judgements about real and hypothesised social situations, despite intact face recognition skills. We could, on this basis, label this as yet another dissociation: one between social and non-social information processing. In terms of social management within the Rehabilitation Unit, it was MBM who caused the most severe problems, for his behaviour, while not particularly impetuous, was certainly inappropriate.

Our final suggestion is that this dissociation between apperceptive and conceptual processes may not only have consequences for the distinction between social and non-social behaviour, but also have distinct anatomical and neurophysiological bases. The localisation of injuries for both patients is far from sufficient to suggest a model. However, they suggest a special role for the temporal lobes for processing apperceptive information in contrast to a special role played by the orbito-frontal areas in processes involved in stable categorisation. Two distinct anatomical pathways are responsible for the two suggested dissociable functional systems. The temporal pathway receives multimodal sensory input from the superior temporal gyrus and projects to the amygdala and hippocampus via the parahippocampal gyrus. Poeck's (1985) description of syndromes associated with deficits in this pathway can, we believe, be classified as apperceptive. The orbito-frontal pathway also receives multimodal sensory information from the superior temporal gyrus and projects eventually to the amygdala and hippocampus, but it is connected with the hypothalamus via the magnocellular layer in the dorsomedial thalamic nucleus and with the cingulate gyrus prior to its entry to the hippocampus. This pathway is a likely candidate for the processing of conceptual information involved in emotional and social behaviour, particularly when one considers some of the possible functions suggested for the hypothalamus, the dorsomedial thalamus, and the cingulate gyrus (Stuss & Benson 1986, Damasio & Van Hoesen 1983, Cambier & Graveleau 1985). These pathways are also neurochemically distinct. It should be noted that the central amygdaloid nucleus, which is involved in the orbito-frontal pathway, is part of the mesolimbic dopamine pathway.

These anatomical and neurochemical considerations are, at present, only suggestive. We have shown a distinct difference in processing faces as a function of whether that processing is essentially apperceptive or conceptual; face recognition is apperceptive, but face expression categorisation cannot be performed on this basis. We suggest possible anatomical sites associated with this functional distinction. Whether these distinctions emerge in a clearer fashion for faces when only the right hemisphere is damaged is a question for further research. So, too, is the implication of our inference that frontal lobe damage may cause neither a specific impairment of the classification of emotion nor an obvious problem in 'control of action', but rather, that a profound conceptual impairment underlies flawed performance in frontal patients. Because face identification does not tap this but expression identification does, the observed dissociation occurs. This makes problematic some studies (e.g. Jackson & Moffat, 1987) indicating specific face expression processing difficulties which are tested without tests of other conceptual skills or knowledge of site of brain injury. In our opinion, deficits in face-expression processing might often (though not always) indicate other conceptual problems.

MBS knows <u>who</u> and <u>what</u> but not <u>how</u> and <u>why</u>. MJS knows <u>how</u> and <u>why</u> but cannot reliably remember <u>who</u> or <u>what</u>.

CONCLUSIONS

This paper started with a brief review of the current opinions concerning prosopagnosia - the impairment of the ability to recognise familiar people by their face. We then pointed out that 'knowledge' of faces extends to other aspects than identification, and reveal a double dissociation between 'Physiognomieer<u>kennens</u>' and 'Physiognomieer<u>wissens</u>'; that is, between the ability to identify known individual 'instances' of faces and the quite separate ability to classify and judge on the basis of such knowledge.

This dissociation, in two particular patients, was not specific to faces; but faces - which provided the same stimulus conditions for these tasks - showed themselves to be sensitive to it. We suggest, then, that two major cognitive processing systems can be functionally and anatomically distinguished in the human brain; an apperceptive system, which learns identities and their perceptual correlates on the basis of experiences, and a conceptual system which may or may not use outputs from the identification process to perform classification functions - including the processing of human emotion from faces.

These studies also confirm that one cerebral function, that of processing socially important information, may not be paid due <u>neuropsychological</u> attention despite patients' own reports of social problems. Social behaviour is particularly vulnerable to the disruption of the classification, rather than the identification, processing system. We believe this to be an important area for further research.

ACKNOWLEDGEMENTS

We are grateful to J. Baribeau and M. Ethier of the Human Neuropsychology Laboratory, Concordia University, Montreal, Quebec, Canada and to C. Braun of the Human Neuropsychology Laboratory, University of Quebec in Montreal, Canada, for their cooperation and for organising access to these patients. We thank the staff of the Lethbridge Rehabilitation Centre, Quebec, Canada for their help and encouragement in testing these patients. C. Peng is supported by an ESRC (UK) grant and this study was supported by a travel grant from Wolfson College, Oxford. R. Campbell is supported by an Oxford University Pump-priming Grant.

REFERENCES

Argyll, J.M., <u>Bodily Communication</u>. London: Methuen, in press.
Bauer, R.M. & Rubens, A.B. (1985) Agnosia. <u>in</u>: K.M. Heilman, & E. Valenstein, (eds.). <u>Clinical Neuropsychology.</u> New York: Oxford University Press.
Baylis, G., Rolls, E.T. & Leonard, M. (1985). Selectivity between faces in the response of a population of neurons in the cortex in the superior temporal sulcus of the monkey. <u>Brain Research, 342</u>, 92-102.
Benton, A.L. & Van Allen, M.W. (1968). Impairment in facial recognition in patients with cerebral disease. <u>Cortex, 4</u>, 344-358.
Bodamer, J. (1947). Die Prosop-Agnosie (Die agnosie des Physiognomieerk-

ennens). Archives fur Psychiatrie und Zeitschrift fur Neurologie, 179, 6-53.

Bornstein, B. (1963). Prosopagnosia. in: L. Halpern (ed.). Problems of Dynamic Neurology Jerusalem: Haddessah Medical Organisation.

Bruce, V. & Young, A. (1986). Understanding Face Recognition. British Journal of Psychology, 77, 305-327.

Bruyer, R., Laterre, C., Seron, X., Feyereisen, P., Strypstein, E., Pierrard, E., & Rectem, D. (1983). A case of prosopagnosia with some preserved covert recognition of familiar faces. Brain & Cognition, 2, 257-284.

Cambier, J. & Graveleau, Ph. (1985), Thalamic syndromes. in: J.A.M. Frederiks (ed.). Handbook of Clinical Neurology vol. 45, Amsterdam: Elsevier.

Campbell, R., Landis, T. & Regard, M. (1986). Face recognition and lip-reading. Brain 109, 509-521.

Cole, M. & Perez-Cruet, J. (1964). Prosopagnosia. Neuropsychologia 2, 237-246.

Corkin, S. (1984). Lasting consequences of bilateral medial temporal lobectomy: clinical course and experimental findings in HM. Seminars in Neurology 4, 249-259.

Crawford, J.R., Besson, J.A.O., Ellis, H.D., Parker, D.M., Salzen, E.A., Gemmell, H.G., Sharp, P.F., Beavan, D.J. & Smith, F.W. (1986). Facial Processing in the Dementias. in: H.D. Ellis, M.A. Jeeves, F. Newcombe & A. Young (eds.) Aspects of Face Processing. Dordrecht: Martinus Nijhoff.

Christodoulou, G.N. (1977). The Syndrome of Capgras. British Journal of Psychiatry, 130, 556-564.

Damasio, A.R. (1985). Disorders of complex visual processing: agnosia, achromatopsia, Balint syndrome and related difficulties of orientation and construction. in: M.M. Mesulam (ed.). Principles of Behavioural Neurology. Philadelphia: F.A. Davis.

Damasio, A.R., Eslinger, P.J., Damasio, H., Van Hoesen, G.W., & Cornell, S. (1985). Multimodal amnesic syndrome following bilateral temporal and basal forebrain damage: the case of patient DRB. Archives of Neurology, 32, 331-341.

Damasio, A.R., Damasio, H. & Van Hoesen, G.W. (1982). Prosopagnosia: anatomical basis and behavioural mechanisms. Neurology, 32, 331-351.

Damasio, A.R. & Van Hoesen, G.W. (1983). Emotional disturbances association with focal lesions of the limbic frontal lobe. in: K.M. Heilman & P. Satz. (eds.) Neuropsychology of Human Emotion. New York: Guilford.

De Haan, E.H.F., Young, A. & Newcombe, F. (1987). Face recognition without awareness. Cognitive Neuropsychology,4, 385-415.

De Renzi, E. (1986a). Current issues on prosopagnosia. in: R. Bruyer (ed.). The Neuropsychology of Face Perception and Facial Expression. Hillsdale, New Jersey: Lawrence Erlbaum Associates.

De Renzi, E. (1986b). Prosopagnosia in two patients with CT scan evidence of damage confined to the right hemisphere. Neuropsychologia, 24, 385-391.

Duncan, J. (1986). Disorganisation of behaviour after frontal lobe damage Cognitive Neuropsychology, 3, 271-290.

Ekman, P. & Friesen, W. (1976) Pictures of Facial Affect. California: Consulting Psychologist Press.

Ellis, H.D. (1986). Introduction: processes underlying face recognition. in: R. Bruyer (ed.). The Neuropsychology of Face Perception and Facial Expression. Hillsdale, New Jersey: Lawrence Erlbaum Associates.

Feyereisen, P. (1986). Production and comprehension of emotional facial expressions in brain-damaged subjects. in: R. Bruyer (ed.). The Neuropsychology of Face Perception and Facial Expression. Hillsdale, New Jersey: Lawrence Erlbaum Associates.

Fodor, J. (1983). The Modularity of Mind. Cambridge, Mass: MIT Press.

Hampson, S. (1985). Personality traits as cognitive categories. in: A. Angleiter, G.L.M. Van Heck & A.F. Furnham (eds.) Personality Psychology in Europe vol 2. Lisse: Swets & Zeitlinger.

Hecaen, H. & Angelergues, R. (1962). Agnosia for faces (prosopagnosia). Archives of Neurology, 7, 92–100.

Jackson, H. & Moffat, N.J. (1987). Impaired emotional recognition following severe head injury. Cortex, 23, 293–300.

Kendon, A. (1986). Current issues in the study of gesture. in: J.L. Nespoulas, P. Perron & A.R. Lecours (eds.). The Biological Foundations of Gesture: Motor and Semiotic Aspects. Hillsdale, New Jersey: Lawrence Erlbaum Associates.

Kertesz, A. (1983). Localisation in Neuropsychology. London: Academic Press.

Kurucz, J. & Feldmar, G. (1979). Prosopo-affective agnosia as a symptom of cerebral organic disease. Journal of the American Geriatric Society, 27, 225–230.

Landis, T., Cummings, J.L., Christen, L., Bogen, J.E. & Imhof, H-G. (1986). Are unilateral right posterior cerebral lesions sufficient to cause prosopagnosia? Cortex, 22, 243–252.

Malone, D.R., Morris, H.M., Kay, M.C., and Levin, H.S. (1982). Prosopagnosia: a double dissociation between the recognition of familiar and unfamiliar faces. Journal of Neurology, Neurosurgery and Psychiatry, 37, 489–501.

Mateer, C.A. (1983). Localisation of language and visual spatial functions by electrical stimulation. in: A. Kertesz. (ed.). Localisation in Neuropsychology. London: Academic Press.

Meadows, J.C. (1974). The anatomical basis of prosopagnosia. Journal of Neurology, Neurosurgery and Psychiatry, 37, 489–450.

Milner, B. (1982). Some cognitive effects of frontal lobe lesions in man. in: D.E. Broadbent & L. Weiskrantz (eds.). The Neuropsychology of Cognitive Function. London: The Royal Society.

Passingham, R. (1986). Unpublished lectures, University of Oxford.

Perrett, D.I. & Rolls, E.T. (1983). Neural mechanisms underlying the visual analysis of faces. in: J-P. Ewert, R.R. Capranica, & D.J. Ingle. (eds.). Advances in Vertebrate Neuroethology. New York: Plenum Press.

Poek, K. (1985). Temporal lobe syndromes. In J.A.M. Frederiks. (ed.). Handbook of Clinical Neurology vol 45. Amsterdam: Elsevier.

Reber, A.S. (1985). The Penguin Dictionary of Psychology. Harmondsworth Mddx: Penguin.

Ross, E. (1983). Right-hemisphere lesions in disorders of affective language. in: A. Kertesz (ed.). Localisation in Neuropsychology. London: Academic Press.

Shallice, T. (1982). Specific Impairments of planning. in: D.E. Broadbent & L. Weiskrantz (eds.) The Neuropsychology of Cognitive Function. London: The Royal Society.

Shuttleworth, E.E., Syrina, V., & Allen, N. (1982). Further Observations on the nature of prosopagnosia. Brain & Cognition, 1, 307–322.

Stuss, D.T. & Benson, D.F. (1986). The Frontal Lobes. New York: Raven Press.

Synodinou, C., Christodoulou, G.N. & Tzavaras, A. (1978). Capgras syndrome and prosopagnosia. British Journal of Psychiatry, 132, 413–414.

Teuber, H.L. (1955). Physiological psychology. Annual Review of Psychology, 6, 267–269.

Tiberghien, G. (1986). Context effects in recognition memory of faces: some theoretical problems. in: H.D. Ellis, M.A. Jeeves, F. Newcombe & A. Young. (eds.). Aspects of Face Processing. Dordrecht: Martinus Nijhoff.

Tiller, D. (unpublished). The Emotional Lexicon. D.Phil. thesis, University of Oxford.

Trower, P., Argyle, J.M. & Bryant, B. (1977). Social Skills and Mental Health. London: Tavistock.

Warrington, E.K. & James, M. (1967). An experimental investigation of facial recognition in patients with unilateral cerebral lesions. Cortex, 3, 317-326.

Whiteley, A.M. & Warrington, E.K. (1977). Prosopagnosia: a clinical, psychological and anatomical study of three patients. Journal of Neurology, Neurosurgery and Psychiatry, 40, 395-403.

HUMAN ORGANIC MEMORY DISORDERS: PROBLEMS AND INTERPRETATIONS

Andrew Mayes

INTRODUCTION

Whereas it is known that verbal abilities such as reading and writing break down in several different ways following brain lesions it is commonly believed that multiple specific disorders of memory have not yet been identified. This erroneous impression, which is partly based on the false equation of organic amnesia with all memory disorders, is also associated with the view that the neuropsychology of memory is in a more primitive state than that of language. Such a conclusion cannot be supported for two reasons. First, as will be described in this chapter, there are several kinds of memory disorder that are distinct from organic amnesia and even organic amnesia may comprise more than one kind of functional impairment. Second, there are reasons for thinking that memory disorders will not fractionate in the same way as those of, for example, language.

There is a widespread view in neuroscience that those brain regions responsible for processing particular kinds of information will also store that information. This view has been supported by studies of learning and memory in invertebrates like Aplysia and is also implicit in current thinking about parallel distributed memory systems (for example, see Allport, 1985). In a system of this kind complex information is processed and represented in a network of units with storage depending on altering the connection strengths between units. If the view is correct, there should be a strong expectation that lesions will not affect encoding, storage or retrieval of a given kind of information in isolation, but rather, will affect encoding, storage and retrieval together for that kind of information. In other words, there will be a strong expectation of finding only distinct material specific kinds of memory disorder rather than also finding different kinds of memory disorder for the same type of information.

Even if, as seems likely, it is true that information is processed and stored at the same neural sites, however, there may be exceptions to the strong expectation of finding memory disorders that differ only in terms of material specificity. Certain lesions may affect brain regions that modulate the consolidation and storage of information that is held in connected, but distinct neural structures. The affected brain regions might, for example, normally either maintain neural activity in the connected information processing and storing structures or release chemical agents, such as noradrenalin, vasopressin or other peptides, that facilitate storage in such structures without significantly affecting their processing abilities. Damage to the modulating regions should produce a storage deficit without affecting processing of the kind of information for which memory is poor. As yet there is no compelling

TABLE 1

Kinds of Human Organic Memory Disorders

Type	Critical Lesion	Comments
1. Short-term memory deficits.	Posterior association neocortex.	Several material-specific kinds; long-term memory probably also affected; processing deficits more likely than storage ones.
2. Deficits of previously well-established memory.	Posterior (and perhaps frontal) association neocortex.	Multiple material-specific partial dissociations; disconnections from or degradations of stores; may involve both semantic and episodic memory; can affect priming as well as explicit memory.
3. "Frontal lobe" memory disorders.	Frontal association neocortex.	Multiple deficits, most of which are secondary to a planning disorder; recency/frequency judgement deficit may have separate explanation.
4. Organic amnesics.	Limbic-diencephalic structures and perhaps cholinergic basal forebrain.	Often associated with frontal lobe lesions; may comprise several deficits; implicit memory relatively preserved, very poor explicit memory for context.
5. Disorders of skill memory and conditioning (habits)	Primarily basal ganglia and cerebellum, but other regions probably involved.	Poorly researched. Need to explore effect of lesions on different kinds of skill and conditioning.

evidence that specific memory deficits of this kind exist, but if there are no exceptions to the strong expectation one is left with a serious puzzle, if processing and storage of information are inseparable, then it might seem there should be no specific organic memory deficits. This seems contrary to the available evidence, but the puzzle may be resolved by considering what is meant by the concept of a specific memory disorder. The concept is typically used to refer to deficits in which processing of a particular kind of information is basically intact although memory for it is very poor despite the apparently intact ability to express the relevant knowledge if it was there (the problem can apply to past learnt memories or ones that must be created de novo). Thus, if a striate cortex lesion causes cortical blindness, then it would be fatuous to say that the lesion had caused a specific impairment in visual memory although no new visual memories could be acquired. To characterize an impairment as a specific memory deficit one needs to be satisfied that some basic processing abilities for the affected kind of information have been left intact. For example, in organic amnesia, lesions affect memory for semantic and episodic information but leave intelligence intact. Most kinds of information processing must therefore be preserved and many workers argue that the impairment is caused by an encoding, storage and retrieval deficit of only a small component of episodic and semantic information, retrieval of which is essential if the complex information as a whole is to be remembered (see Mayes et al., 1985). Nevertheless, as information processing is basically intact in amnesia it is reasonable to regard it as a specific memory deficit even though most researchers do not believe it is caused by a selective storage failure.

This chapter will review the main groups of putatively specific memory disorders, which are outlined in Table 1, in order to characterize the functional deficits that underlie them. In doing so the points discussed above will be borne in mind. In particular, very strong evidence will be required before it is accepted that a deficit is caused by a specific impairment of storage, encoding or retrieval although such possibilities will not be excluded. Finally, the provisional analysis of the underlying functional deficits will be used to illuminate how the healthy brain mediates memory activities. The five main groups of memory disorders shown in Table 1 can each be subdivided into several similar, but distinct kinds of deficit (although this is polemical in the case of organic amnesia). The kinds of deficit seen in many patients will be compounds of these possibly elementary memory disorders. For example, patients even in the early stages of Alzheimer's disease may show amnesia, short-term memory deficits, recall, recognition and priming failures with previously well-established memories and deficient performance on memory tests sensitive to frontal lobe lesions. It needs to be determined therefore whether a deficit is subdivisible or truly elementary. Each of the five groups comprises disorders in which there is bad performance on selected memory tests, but not evidence of major types of processing failure. Five groups are provisionally used because (with the exception of the ragbag group 5, which will need to be subdivided in the future) the disorders comprising each group are caused by lesions to the same brain area and the deficits underlying them seem to be functionally similar.

SHORT-TERM MEMORY DISORDERS

Problems with short-term memory are primarily caused by lesions to the posterior association cortex although performance on certain short-term memory taks, such as the Brown-Peterson test, may be affected by frontal association cortex lesions. These disorders are of interest because of their relevance to the questions of whether there are short-term stores distinct from long-term ones, how many there are, what their functions are and what the relationship between short- and long-term storage actually is. The occurrence of such disorders only provides evidence for distinct short-term stores if it can be shown that (1) they are caused by selective storage failures of short-term memory and (2) long-term memory disorders exist for the same kind of information (as well probably as other kinds) in the face of normal short-term memory. It will be argued that these desiderata have not yet been met. If they had been for the types of short-term memory disorder so far described, then there would be neuropsychological evidence for the existence of several kinds of short-term store as implied by the working memory model of Baddeley and Hitch (1974). Thus, some patients have been described with poor auditory-verbal short-term memory (see Shallice & Warrington, 1979), some with poor visual verbal and non-verbal short-term memory (see Warrington & Rabin, 1971), some with selective reductions of visuospatial short-term memory (De Renzi & Nichelli, 1975) and one with selectively poor short-term memory for colour (Davidoff & Ostergaard, 1984). Other material specific kinds of short-term memory deficit may yet be found and some of the ones listed above may be further fractionated. By far the best studied of these disorders has been that involving auditory-verbal memory. Patients with this disorder usually show normal short-term memory for non-verbal auditory inputs and visual-verbal inputs so their deficit has been interpreted as one of phonological short-term memory. Furthermore, it has been argued by most workers, who have researched it, that the syndrome is one that affects short-term storage selectively and that it double dissociates with the long-term phonological (and other) memory failures found in organic amnesia. This issue will now be discussed.

Most patients with poor auditory-verbal short-term memory are conduction aphasics and hence show good comprehension of spoken language and fairly fluent speech output although some show paraphasias in spontaneous speech or when repeating spoken language. This indicates they have no gross processing or motor output problems with respect to phonology although it also suggests that patients may differ in important respects. Their poor short-term memory may have different causes. All these patients have reduced auditory immediate memory spans. For example, compared to the normal range of five to nine digits, some patients can only repeat back one or two digits. In those patients who have been tested it has also been found that they show reduced recency effects and that they are deficient on the Brown-Peterson task even when only required to remember one spoken item (see Shallice & Warrington, 1979; Vallar & Baddeley, 1984). When tested, recognition has also been impaired so the failure does not result from a crude output problem. Three main accounts of these specific deficits have been advanced. The first is that a subtle deficit in the processing of phonemes underlies the short-term memory failure (see Allport, 1985). The second is that a partial disconnection between the adequately analysed phonological input and some kind of articulatory output reduces both rehearsal and the rapid read-out of correctly analysed inputs so that memory for phonological structures seems to be lost abnormally quickly (a view derivable from Kinsbourne, 1972). The third is that patients are suffering from a selective short-term storage deficit specific to phonological inputs. As the patients so far studied have not all been the same it is, of course, possible that all three of these accounts may be correct but for different patients. The storage account should, however, only be adopted when the other two explanations have been convincingly eliminated because of its a priori improbability.

Allport (1985) has found some support for the processing deficit account in a patient previously believed to have a selective storage failure. When he required her to make 'same-different' judgements about normally spoken syllables she performed poorly even though the task did not exceed the bounds of her reduced memory span. Vallar's patient P.V. has, however, been shown to perform normally on a task of this kind. Although P.V. might make more errors on the subtler 'same-different' judgements that would be needed when factors like voice onset time are varied in synthetic speech it is unclear whether such minor processing inaccuracies could produce the short-term memory deficits seen in this patient. On the other hand, P.V. and all other patients with poor phonological memory could be abnormally slow at making 'same-different' judgements that may be as accurate as those of normals. If this reflects slowed processing, a processing impairment would have been identified that is capable of causing very poor immediate memory for phonology. The issue needs to be properly tested, but Starr and Barrett (1987) have found that patients show longer latencies in an auditory digit probe identification task even with a digit series of one. These workers also found that patients showed a reduced amplitude late positive component in their evoked potentials to digits even when only reaction times matched to controls were averaged, which suggests the presence of a further processing deficit. Their task could be modified so as to probe identification with phonologically similar items in patients and controls, testing up to the limits of subjects' spans to ensure that slowed judgements do not simply reflect the fact that with single item repetition patients are nearer than controls to their memory limit.

Slowness is also the key to the disconnectionist explanation of the syndrome although the account given of it is different. An adequately analysed phonological input is held to be poorly connected to a covert or overt articulatory output so that the output will be slow and probably inaccurate. This disconnection will have two main effects. First, it will prevent or reduce rehearsal. It is known that without rehearsal auditory digit span is reduced and failure to rehearse covertly probably also impairs performance on the Brown-Peterson task even with single items. Second, the disconnection will slow output and hence allow more time for forgetting even with immediate memory phenomena that do not depend on rehearsal such as the recency effect. The hypothesis has not been systematically tested, but some evidence supports it. Thus, the patient P.V. fails to show a word length effect in serial recall of auditorily presented words, which suggests that she does not rehearse (Vallar & Baddeley, 1984). This failure to rehearse could, however, be a strategic choice because she remembers too little to make rehearsal worthwhile rather than reflect a primary rehearsal deficit. Evidence for the latter possibility comes from the Starr and Barrett (1987) study, already mentioned, showing that patients make slower judgements even about single spoken digits and from a study by Friedrich et al. (1984). It has been argued that in normal people repetition rehearsal is a privileged route because verbatim repetition of single words does not interfere with, nor is disrupted by, the simultaneous execution of a matching task with visually presented letters. Friedrich et al., found that repetition rehearsal was not privileged in this way with a conduction aphasic E.A., who showed mutual interference between repetition and the visual task. This suggests that the patient had to rely on an effortful alternative rehearsal route from semantic representations back to phonology. The finding is interesting but not compelling because single item repetition is nearer to E.A.'s short-term memory capacity than to that of a normal person's and repetition close to one's span is likely to be more effortful. Performance on the dual task paradigm could be examined in young children with auditory spans matched to those of patients. Alternatively, it could be examined in normal adults with memory loads as close to span as those used with E.A. Evidence of an intact privileged route in these cases would support the disconnection view although its absence would not be a refutation.

The evidence that any conduction aphasic has a selective storage deficit is therefore unconvincing. Furthermore, their deficit should not be described as specific to short-term memory. Although patients can access the meaning of spoken inputs and, indeed, appear to show normal long-term memory for the gist of such inputs it has been shown recently that phonological long-term memory is drastically impaired (Baddeley, personal communication). P.V. (an Italian) was, unlike her controls, unable to learn a series of spoken Russian words with repeated present-ations. The deficit might therefore be caused by a subtle processing or disconnection impairment that affects a single short- and long-term memory phonological store. If so, it still has to be explained why amnesics show normal immediate memory for phonologically encoded inputs. One plausible possibility is that items can be recalled from immediate memory without retrieving their contextual markers because spatiotemporal context has not changed whereas such retrieval is critical for longer term recall at which amnesics are poor. Amnesics may have a specific problem with contextual retrieval.

At present, therefore, conduction aphasics do not provide proof of the existence of a short-term phonological store. There may be such distinct short-term stores for phonological and other kinds of inform-ation, but lesions may never selectively disrupt them in which case the evidence for their existence will have to be drawn from other sources. It is known, for example, that neurons in posterior association cortex can remain active for a few seconds after a stimulus is removed. This could be the basis of short-term storage as reflected in tasks like the digit span as continued neural activity might represent recently presented information.

DISORDERS OF PREVIOUSLY WELL-ESTABLISHED MEMORY

There has been a trend in recent years to interpret disorders of complex functions, such as aphasias, agnosias, apraxias and acalculias, as partially caused by disturbances in the ability to recall information that has previously been massively practised. For example, Warrington (1982) analysed the problems of an acalculic patient and concluded that his impairment at mental arithmetic largely resulted from a selective memory loss for previously well-known and greatly overlearnt facts, such as '3+2=5'. The lesions responsible for these impairments are typically of the posterior association cortex and this is compatible with the view that complex semantic information is predominantly stored in this region.

If there are truly selective disorders of previously well-established semantic memory, then identifying the nature and number of such disorders should reveal much about the structure of semantic memory. There is growing evidence for the existence of many such disorders, some of which are surprisingly specific. Thus, it has been claimed that there are memory disorders specific to the body image, previously familiar faces, arithmetic facts and for words and word meanings. In particular, some patients mainly have problems with concrete words whereas others have more difficulty with abstract words. Within the category of concrete words some patients have most difficulty with the names of animate objects whereas others have most difficulty with the names of inanimate objects. More extreme still, there seems to be some dissociation between problems with large and small animate objects and one patient has been described with an anomia specific for fruits and vegetables and another has been described with a problem specific to action words (see Mayes, 1987 for a review). Usually, however, the specificity of the impairment is not complete. For example, Warrington and Shallice described some post-encephalitic patients who were very bad at defining the spoken names of animate objects, but who were also probably not completely normal at defining the spoken names of inanimate objects either.

The above disorders should throw light on the problem of how the brain organizes the storage of semantic information. In order to determine their implications for this problem it is important, however, to try and answer three questions about these deficits. First, can any or all of them be explained as failures in processing sensory inputs or motor outputs? Second, if memory failures, are they caused by deficits in retrieval, storage or both, and are they accompanied by any kinds of encoding problem? This question clearly relates to the view, discussed in the introduction, that most lesions will disrupt processing and storage simultaneously. Third, are the materially specific semantic memory deficits invariably associated with corresponding episodic memory impairments?

The first question has been inadequately explored. There is evidence, however, that some prosopagnosics show good perceptual discrimination ability with faces and that some show implicit memory for previously familiar faces that they fail to recognize. Implicit memory is present when subjects behave so as to reveal that they have stored certain information even though they may fail to recall or recognize that information (explicitly remember it). Thus, patients have shown electrodermal responses that discriminate between correct and incorrect names of faces (Bauer, 1984) or between familiar and unfamiliar faces (Tranel & Damasio, 1985). In these cases it is hard to argue that perception is impaired because the patients are showing indirect evidence of identifying the faces that they fail to recognize. It is more plausible to argue that brain structures in the patients encode an adequate facial representation, but that this cannot be used to access further stored information, essential for recognition but not implicit memory, because the structures that store this information have either been destroyed or have been disconnected from the face encoding structures. Although similarly preserved implicit memory has been claimed with Wernicke aphasics most other putative semantic memory disorders have not been similarly examined so it remains possible that they are caused by a processing failure the result of which is an imperfect representation that is an inadequate cue for accessing a semantic memory that may be completely intact and normally accessible to adequate cues.

The intactness of processing should of course be assessed by direct tests of perceptual ability as well as of implicit memory. Implicit memory may be impaired, as it appears to be in Alzheimer patients, at least on some tests (Shimamura et al., 1987), without there being any other evidence of a relevant processing deficit. Indeed, Shallice (1986) has argued that the presence or absence of priming (a form of implicit memory characterized by altered or more efficient processing of previously presented items) is one of five criteria that distinguish selective storage from selective retrieval failures of formerly well-established memory. On his view, a storage failure causes (1) consistently good, indifferent or poor recall of particular items across occasions, (2) superordinate information to be more retrievable than subordinate information, (3) a failure to show priming to unrecalled or unrecognized items, (4) less disruption of more frequently encountered items, (5) a failure to show improved recall when more time is allowed for retrieval. Retrieval failures show a contrasting set of disturbances. Three comments should be made about these criteria. First, patients do differ on them and Shallice has even analysed preliminary data on eight semantic memory impaired patients and claims that they fall into two groups on the basis of the criteria. Second, despite this very provisional data, the rationale underlying the criteria is shaky and each could be given an opposite interpretation depending on one's model of how memory works. For example, if the store is partially degraded, then item retrieval could be inconsistent across occasions because available cues will vary as will their likelihood of matching features in the fragmented memory. Patients may fall into groups as Shallice's data suggests but such clustering may not identify patients with selective storage or retrieval deficits. The third point is the more basic one, raised in the introduction of whether one should expect to see specific storage and retrieval deficits.

The third point may be clarified by considering the prosopagnosics who show implicit memory for unrecognized faces. The interpretation offered for these cases was that patients either have a retrieval failure that disconnects adequately encoded 'face' cues from certain kinds of semantic information or a storage failure for those kinds of semantic information. In the former case, other cues should access the semantic information normally whereas they will not in the latter. But will the encoding of new facial information be normal? If the failure is caused by disconnection, facial features will be normally encoded but not linked to the semantic features vital for explicit memory so familiarity will not develop for new faces because relevant semantic information will neither be encoded or stored. If the failure is one of storage, then it should be impossible to encode, store or retrieve the kind of semantic information relevant to recognizing faces as familiar whatever the input route. These predictions need to be tested. All semantic memory impairments whether caused by disconnection or direct destruction of storage sites should, on this interpretation, be associated with particular kinds of encoding and retrieval failure. If this is found not to be so, then a new interpretation must be found.

The claimed existence of semantic memory deficits has been treated as evidence that semantic and episodic memory are subserved by different brain regions and are functionally independent. Such a view could be false because no-one has shown that patients do not also have associated deficits of similar previously well-established episodic memories. For example, if a patient cannot remember animate concepts, then his episodic memories related to animate things should also be grossly defective. This possibility remains untested but if fulfilled could either mean that episodic and semantic memory are identical and are mediated by identical brain structures or that episodic memory involves semantic information and other information that is processed and stored in other brain regions.

This brief overview indicates that most important questions about disorders of previously well-established memory remain unanswered. We need more evidence that they are primary memory failures rather than secondary to processing deficits and more needs to be done to identify at which kinds of processing patients are impaired. For example, if storage degradation causes a patient to have selectively poor memory for concepts of animate objects, then the equation of storage sites with processing sites, advanced in the introduction would suggest that some processing deficits should also be present. Precisely which ones should be present depends on the account of semantic memory organization that is offered. For example, on Allport's (1985) view, according to which stored concepts about animate objects might comprise an interconnected neural network of elements that represent the sensory components that constitute the living things in question, partial degradation of the store would have to be accompanied by inadequate processing of those sensory components affected by the lesion because the full representation of such components should be impossible. Failure to find processing failures of these kinds would refute Allport's view, but not the general equation of storage with processing sites. Finally, the degree to which disorders are specific must be examined more critically and systematically.

FRONTAL LOBE MEMORY DISORDERS

The effects on memory of frontal lobe lesions are still poorly understood. As the region is probably functionally heterogeneous one would expect lesions of it to produce more than one kind of impairment. At present, most memory deficits induced by lesions to the region can be explained as secondary to reduced ability to plan elaborate encoding and retrieval operations. Although such deficits may be dissociable because they are caused by distinct lesions, they are nevertheless closely functionally related. There is, however, also evidence that frontal lobe lesions can cause impairments in memory for event recency and frequency and it has been argued by Hasher and Zacks (1979) that these kinds of contextual information are automatically encoded with minimal attentional effort. If their view is correct, then frontal lobe lesions may cause two radically different kinds of memory disorder, one secondary to deficits in effortful processing and one independent of such deficits.

The memory disorders that can be interpreted as secondary to fail-ures of elaborative processing have been reviewed elsewhere (see Mayes, 1987) so will only be outlined here. It has usually been found that frontal lobe lesions either fail to impair recognition or minimally disrupt it whereas they cause a much more serious disruption of free recall (for example, see Milner et al., 1985; Hirst, 1985). Whereas recognition is little helped by elaborative encoding recall may be greatly improved. There is also direct evidence that patients with frontal lobe lesions do not spontaneously show normal semantic cate-gorization of complex verbal or pictorial stimuli and that the extent of this failing correlates with their recall deficit for such material. The recall deficit can also be reduced or abolished if patients are given an encoding plan by the experimenter. Thus, a deficit in learning unrelated word pairs is largely abolished when patients are shown how to form mediating images between the words (see Signoret & Lhermitte, 1976).

Consistent with having memory deficits secondary to planning and judgemental failures, patients show impairments with metamemory (see Hirst, 1985). For example, unlike normal people, patients with frontal lobe lesions often say that it is a good idea to pour themselves a glass of water between hearing a 'phone number and telephoning rather than calling immediately. Clearly, judgemental failures like this will impair the ability to plan memory processing operations. They may also help explain the association between frontal lobe lesions and a group of dramatic retrieval disorders. There is a good evidence that frontal lobe lesions cause confabulation, that is the recall of incorrect, and some-times bizarre information in response to standard questions (see Stuss & Benson, 1984). For example, in answer to the question of what he is doing in hospital, instead of saying he does not know, a patient will give a detailed and fantastical story, bearing little relationship to reality. This disorder is compatible with poor metamemory. Frontal lobe pathology has also been linked to reduplicative paramnesia, in which a patient claims that two or more places exist with nearly identical properties when, in fact, only one exists, and Capgras syndrome, in which the reduplicative disorder applies to familiar people rather than places (see Stuss & Benson, 1984). Both these disorders probably involve a slightly disturbed perception of familiar places or people, which is then comp-ounded with a judgemental distortion caused by frontal lobe damage.

There is also some evidence that frontal lobe lesions cause poor

recall of pretraumatically acquired memories, and that their retrograde
amnesias differ from those shown by organic amnesics in being characterized by no relative sparing of older memories (see Albert, Butters &
Brandt, 1981; Stuss & Benson, 1984). But the evidence about retrograde
amnesia after frontal lobe lesions is still very weak and based on observations of Huntington's choreics and leucotomized schizophrenics. There
needs to be a systematic study of patients with selective frontal lobe
lesions on tests of retrograde amnesia. If they have a problem in organ-
izing their retrieval plans, then one would expect them to show a mild
retrograde amnesia without sparing of older memories and which is most
apparent on tests of recall rather than recognition.

Frontal lobe lesions have also been found to affect performance on
relatively short-term memory tasks, producing disturbances that can
readily be understood as secondary to planning failures. Thus, patients
perform poorly on the Brown-Peterson task in which they are required to
recall triads of items, like words, after a delay during which they must
engage in an interfering activity (see Stuss & Benson, 1984). Normal
subjects probably rapidly alternate executing the interfering activity
and rehearsal whereas patients are unable to organize this rapid alter-
nation and so fail to rehearse. Patients with frontal lobe lesions also
fail to show release from proactive interference in the Brown-Peterson
task when there is a shift of semantic category in the words being presented although this deficit may only be seen in patients with more
marked recall problems (see Freedman & Cermak, 1986). This failure to
utilize a shift of set reflects another kind of planning difficulty that
affects memory. The idea that different frontal lobe lesions affect
distinct aspects of planning ability, which each have their characteristic effects on memory is supported by a study of Kapur (1985), who
found one patient to show normal release from the Brown-Peterson task
whilst making perseverative intrusion errors from earlier lists, and
another patient to show impaired release, but no intrusion errors.

All the above memory problems can easily be interpreted as secondary
to various kinds of planning failure caused by lesions in several frontal
lobe regions. But there are memory disorders, caused by frontal lobe
lesions, that seem to relate to kinds of information that is encoded
automatically and hence cannot be explained as secondary to planning
difficulties. In 1971, patients with frontal lobe lesions were found to
be very poor at judging which of two items they had seen most recently
despite retaining the ability to recognize the items normally (see Milner
et al., 1985). Since then Milner's group have found that patients are
impaired at a self-ordered pointing task and at judging the frequency
with which items have been presented (see Milner et al., 1985). If Hasher
and Zacks (1979) are right, these tasks do not require effortful encoding
for their successful performance in which case impairments on them might
represent a radically different type of memory disorder from one that is
secondary to a failure of planning elaborative and effortful processes.
Even if they are correct, however, this conclusion need not follow
because retrieval of recency, frequency and 'self-ordered' information
could require the execution of elaborate and effortful retrieval plans.
For example, recalling the order of two events probably involves setting
up a plan in which their relationship to one or more marker events is
compared. It remains to be seen therefore whether these failures of
certain aspects of contextual memory are similar or radically distinct
from the memory failures that more obviously result from failures of
planned and effortful processing. The issue may be resolved in two ways.
First, by studies of normal subjects, using dual task paradigms, to see
whether recency and frequency judgements depend on effortful retrieval
processes. Second, by more systematic studies of patients with frontal
lobe lesions to determine whether or not contextual memory deficits are

always accompanied by memory disorders that clearly are secondary to planning failures. For example, it has been suggested that dorsolateral frontal cortex lesions impair memory for item recency (Milner et al., 1985). If correct and recency memory deficits are caused by failures of effortful retrieval, then such lesions should also always cause memory disorders that are clearly secondary to failures of effortful processing.

THE ORGANIC AMNESIAS

The most studied organic memory disorder is amnesia and many people falsely believe that this syndrome is coterminous with organic memory disorders in general. As this syndrome has been reviewed in detail elsewhere recently (for example, see Mayes & Meudell, 1983; Squire, 1987) only a few major points will be made about it here. One major issue relates to why the disorder is of theoretical interest. Unlike the three previous kinds of memory deficit it is not caused by association neo-cortex lesions, but by damage to medial temporal lobe limbic system structures, structures in the medial diencephalon, or possibly to struct-ures in the cholinergic basal forebrain (see Mayes, 1987). Although it has been suggested by Mishkin (1982) that combined cingulate cortex and orbitofrontal cortex lesions can also cause amnesia there is currently no evidence for this suggestion from human studies and the available data from monkeys is subject to other interpretations. The current consensus is therefore that amnesia is not caused by lesions of the association neocortex. Furthermore, although patients who suffer from it have great difficulty in learning so as to be able to recall or recognize any new kinds of semantic or episodic information, and in recalling or recog-nizing much pre-traumatically acquired semantic and episodic information they may show normal intelligence and short-term memory. It seems likely therefore that the kinds of information for which amnesics show bad memory are largely stored in posterior association neocortex rather than in the structures damaged in amnesia and that amnesics' ability to process the kinds of information for which they have poor memory must be intact or nearly so because otherwise they would not have preserved intelligence. Is the syndrome an exception to the rule that lesions cause combined processing and storage deficits because it seems most natural to explain it as a selective storage failure? Before briefly discussing this issue in the context of the functional deficit(s) that underlie amnesia some other major points need to be made about the syndrome.

The first such point concerns whether amnesia is unitary or com-prises several elementary disorders. Some knowledge about this point is vital for determining what deficit(s) underlie amnesia. There is no doubt that verbal and non-verbal material-specific forms of the syndrome exist (see Milner, 1971), but these can be understood as disorders in which the same deficit either affects only verbal or only non-verbal information. More polemically, it has been argued by some that the basic deficit can be subdivided. Although these arguments are partially based on anatomical criteria the fact that lesions of several sites cause amnesia is not proof that the syndrome is heterogeneous because these sites could form part of a unitary functional circuit. Thus, it is well known that the medial temporal lobe limbic system structures, damaged in some amnesics, have two way connections not only with overlying association neocortex, but also with the medial diencephalic structures, damaged in other amnesics. Also, the cholinergic basal forebrain structures, lesions of which may sometimes cause amnesia, have two way connections with the limbic system structures, damaged in some amnesics. On anatomical grounds, therefore, it is possible to argue that amnesia is caused by damage to different parts of a functionally unified neural network or that this network has functional subdivisions, damage to each of which causes a slightly different memory impairment.

Three forms of subdivision have been proposed. First, some have argued that anterograde and retrograde amnesia are caused by distinct deficits, which normally co-occur (see Mayes, 1987 for a review). Some cases of isolated retrograde amnesia have been reported and although there are no convincing cases of totally isolated anterograde amnesia the retrograde and anterograde forms often correlate poorly with each other across patients. It is not known, however, whether lesions in separate sites are responsible for these effects. It has also proved hard to show that the cases of isolated retrograde amnesia are not caused by motivated forgetting rather than a lesion. With one such patient, however, Kapur et al. (1986) have reported that the isolated retrograde amnesia was accompanied by the ability to learn counterfactual associates like 'Telly Salvalas-tennis player' faster than control subjects. This finding suggests that the patient was genuinely unable to retrieve pretraumatically acquired facts even when the test was indirect. Isolated retrograde amnesia could therefore sometimes be caused by brain lesions, but whether these lesions are located within the region where larger lesions result in both anterograde and retrograde amnesia is unknown.

Second, it has been also claimed that limbic system and diencephalic lesions cause different kinds of amnesia (see Huppert & Piercy, 1979; Squire, 1981). Limbic system lesions purportedly cause abnormally fast forgetting in anterograde amnesia and retrograde amnesia with a steep temporal gradient whereas diencephalic lesions purportedly cause poor learning, but normal rate forgetting in anterograde amnesia and a retrograde amnesia of uncertain extent (see Mayes, 1987). Most research has been directed at rate of forgetting, but interpretation is hard because tests are subject to serious artefacts and their results may also be related to 'severity of amnesia'. Thus, recognition of patients and controls after a short delay has been matched by allowing the patients greater learning opportunity, but this has the effect of making the average item to test delay longer for patients and hence giving artificially low estimates of their forgetting rates (see Mayes, 1986). When average item to test delay is matched between patients and controls by modifying the standard procedure there is some evidence that even diencephalic amnesics forget pathologically fast (Mayes, 1988). Even if this finding is confirmed temporal lobe amnesics could still forget faster than diencephalic amnesics so that the two groups would show differing degrees of pathologically fast forgetting. One study that compared forgetting rates in patients with temporal lobe and diencephalic lesions after equivalent amounts of learning did find that the former patients forget significantly faster despite the apparent similarity in severity of amnesia between the groups (see Parkin & Leng, 1987). Although the study may be subject to a ceiling effect and hence needs replication, in conjunction with the finding of Mayes (1988), it does suggest that diencephalic and temporal lobe lesions increase forgetting rates for different reasons. At present, however, this issue is unresolved.

The third suggested subdivision of amnesia has been proposed by Mishkin (1982) on the basis of a monkey model of the amnesic syndrome. Mishkin's proposal is that severe, permanent amnesia requires lesions to both a hippocampal circuit and an amygdala one. The hippocampal circuit projects from the hippocampus via the fornix to the mammillary bodies and from there via the anterior thalamus to the cingulate cortex. The amygdala circuit projects to the dorsomedial thalamus and other medial thalamic nuclei and from these nuclei to the orbitofrontal cortex. Both these circuits contain back-projections so, as already indicated, it is uncertain whether the frontal regions play an important role in memory. Mishkin's work with monkeys demonstrates that conjoint lesions of the two circuits cause severe recognition impairments whereas damage to a single circuit only results in mild memory problems. Implicit in this view is the idea that the two circuits subserve distinct functions such that memory remains reasonably good provided one of these functions is still operating.

The issue of whether amnesia comprises several deficits is then still unresolved, but clearly needs to be in order to answer the question of what processing failure(s) cause the syndrome. Nevertheless, even if multiple, the deficits that cause amnesia may be closely related to each other. Their identification depends on proper characterization of the pattern of memory performance shown by amnesics, something that has been extensively researched in the past twenty years. This research has confirmed that amnesics show preserved learning and retention when explicit memory (recall and recognition) is not involved. Patients show good classical conditioning despite failing to recognize the training apparatus (Weiskrantz & Warrington, 1979) and learn and retain normally motor skills, such as the pursuit rotor, perceptual skills, such as reading mirror reversed words (Cohen & Squire, 1980), and possibly even cognitive skills, such as solving the Tower of Hanoi puzzle (Cohen, 1984). More importantly, amnesics show normal implicit memory for individual items (priming) for which their explicit memory is grossly impaired (see Mayes, 1987 for a review). For example, when subjects are shown words and later asked to complete their opening three letters with the first word that comes to mind, amnesics show as large a bias as their controls towards generating previously presented words (word-completion priming) despite being unable to recognize these words (Graf, Squire & Mandler, 1984). Priming like this, of items that are already in well-established memory might be explained as due to temporary activation of specific semantic memories especially as it tends to fade in a few hours. There is, however, more controversial evidence that some amnesics, if not all, show normal priming to previously novel information. For example, in normal subjects and at least some amnesics, word-completion effects are enhanced to an equal extent when unrelated word pairs are presented ('bird-stamp') and later, subjects perform word-completion with the first word cueing the first three letters of the second word ('bird-sta-') (Graf & Schacter, 1985). There is some evidence that amnesics can show normal priming both to novel target features on which attention is focussed during learning and to contextual features that fall on the periphery of attention during learning (see Mayes, 1987 for a review). As their explicit memory for such features is very poor this should throw some light on the causes of amnesia.

There is also some evidence that the explicit memory of amnesics for background spatiotemporal contextual information is disproportionately bad relative to their memory for target information. Such deficits are demonstrated when amnesic and control explicit memory for targets is matched by testing the latter under less favourable conditions and then examining context memory under the same conditions. It has been shown that some amnesics are disproportionately bad at memory for temporal order, at identifying the source of information, at identifying its spatial location and at identifying the mode of presentation of information (see Mayes et al., 1985 and Mayes, 1988 for reviews). Unfortunately, it is controversial whether these impairments are integral to the memory deficit or are results of incidental damage to the frontal lobes. Disproportionate contextual memory deficits have mainly been shown with amnesics, who have an aetiology of chronic alcoholism, and such patients are particularly likely to show incidental frontal lobe damage. As described in the last section, frontal lobe lesions cause impairments in memory for item recency and frequency and the amnesic recency judgement deficit correlates with extent of impairment on tests sensitive to frontal lobe lesions. There is even some evidence that the famous temporal lobectomy amnesic, H.M., who performs well on tests sensitive to frontal lobe lesions, is actually less impaired on memory for item recency and frequency than he is on target memory (Sagar, personal communication). The tests used to show this are similar to the ones that demonstrate contextual memory problems in patients with frontal lobe lesions. But as H.M. showed above chance recency and frequency judgements even when his recognition of target items was at chance, it is possible that his contextual memory was based on a form of implicit memory. If so, then all amnesics might show little impairment on these particular tests of recency and frequency memory.

Does the pattern of memory performance shown by amnesics that is outlined above support the view that the syndrome is caused by a storage failure? Although this remains a possibility the answer is probably no. Two hypotheses fit the data provided the syndrome is regarded as a unitary impairment. The first is the context-memory deficit hypothesis according to which amnesics have a selective impairment in processing and storing background spatiotemporal contextual information. This failure causes a secondary explicit memory failure for target information although such information is normally processed and stored because such memory depends on retrieving a target item's background context (see Mayes et al., 1985). The hypothesis predicts that amnesics should be disproportionately bad at remembering context and in an ad hoc fashion it can explain patients' normal intelligence, short-term memory and priming of familiar material by postulating that these activities do not require contextual processing. It has difficulty in explaining why amnesics show normal priming to novel contextual information if indeed they do. Once again, the hypothesis must assume that retrieval of contextual information is irrelevant for the priming of novel material. This seems implausible, particularly with the priming of novel contextual information and there is also preliminary evidence that even the priming of familiar material sometimes depends on retrieving background spatiotemporal context (Mayes, 1988).

The second hypothesis can explain preserved priming without difficulty because it supposes that amnesics show preserved implicit memory for all those kinds of information for which their explicit memory is bad. It argues that explicit memory depends on the more rapid, efficient or fluent processing of remembered information (as evinced by implicit memory) plus the judgement that processing is different from the way it would be with novel material. Amnesics are postulated to have an impairment of this judgemental process. The hypothesis depends on the universality of preserved priming in amnesics and cannot explain the disproportionate explicit memory deficits in contextual memory. It must assume that these deficits are either caused by incidental frontal lobe damage and hence are unrelated to amnesia or else that they indicate a second impairment distinct from the judgemental problem. Neither does it have any explanation for why amnesics show normal or, at least, less impaired explicit memory for older and greatly rehearsed pre-traumatic information. The context-deficit hypothesis, in admittedly ad hoc fashion, can argue that such memories have been 'decontextualized' through rehearsal and can be recalled without needing first to retrieve context. It is also hard to see on the basis of the inputs and physiology of the structures, damage to which causes amnesia, how lesions of them could secure a disturbance of judgement rather than one of the storage and processing of particular kinds of information.

Both the context-memory deficit and judgemental failure hypotheses propose that a single functional disorder underlies amnesia. But the former hypothesis, at least, is capable of adaptation so as to include two or more related deficits. If Mishkin (1982) is correct in suggesting that conjoint hippocampal and amygdala circuit lesions are required to produce severe, permanent amnesia, then evidence that he and his colleagues have collected from monkey lesion studies suggests a modification of the context-memory deficit hypothesis. It was found that hippocampal, but not amygdala, lesions impaired spatial memory whereas amygdala, but not hippocampal, lesions impaired temporal memory and the ability to make a cross-modal recognition judgements (see Mayes et al., 1985). Lesions of the two circuits could therefore cause different selective deficits in explicit context-memory, which in combination result in severe impairments of explicit memory for targets. An alternative adaptation of the hypothesis is based on the supposition that the distinction between temporal and diencephalic amnesia is valid. There is preliminary evidence that temporal amnesics perform worse than equivalently severe diencephalic amnesics at spatial memory whereas an opposite pattern of results obtains with temporal memory (see Parkin & Leng, 1987). These results need to be checked because the temporal memory deficit may have been caused by frontal lobe rather than diencephalic lesions.

DISORDERS OF SKILL AND CONDITIONING

There has been little research on the 'non-cognitive' memory disorders of skill and conditioning. It seems probable, however, that the locations of the lesions affecting these kinds of memory will vary depending on the type of skill or conditioning involved. For example, animal studies indicate that some forms of conditioning can occur in the spinal cord although with complex stimuli (such as words) the neocortex should be involved to some extent. Nevertheless, there is preliminary evidence that basal ganglia lesions are particularly likely to cause impairments of skill learning. Martone et al. (1984) found that patients with Huntington's chorea, who suffer from caudate nucleus atrophy, showed normal word recognition but were impaired at learning the skill of reading mirror-reversed words. In contrast, amnesic patients showed poor word recognition but acquired the skill normally. The interpretation of these results is not, however, straightforward because patients with Huntington's chorea suffer from involuntary movements and are likely to have difficulty controlling their eye movements. This disability could lead to secondary problems in learning to read mirror-reversed words in which case it would be exceeding the evidence to argue that the caudate nucleus lesions in the patients have prevented the storage of information vital to skill acquisition.

The possibility that skill acquisition deficits in Huntington's choreics are secondary to a motor control problem is less plausible in a second study. Heindel et al. (1987) trained patients and their controls on a pursuit rotor task in which they had to keep a stylus in contact with a small rotating disk. The patients with Huntington's chorea were impaired at learning this task even though their performance levels before training began were matched to those of their controls by making the task more demanding for the latter subjects. Interpreting an observed skill acquisition deficit as secondary to a motor control problem is also unlikely in the case of a study by Saint-Cyr et al. (1987). These workers found that Parkinson's disease patients, who have atrophy of the substantia nigra and probably sufer from secondary disruption of the caudate nucleus, are impaired at learning variants of the Tower of Hanoi problem despite showing relatively normal performance on standard tests of verbal memory. In contrast, amnesics showed an opposite pattern of relatively normal performance on the Tower of Hanoi problems and impaired verbal memory. It seems highly unlikely that the motor deficits of Parkinson's patients will affect the acquisition of a cognitive skill like the Tower of Hanoi.

Although there are still few studies of lesioned humans that support the view that the basal ganglia play a special role in the acquisition and retention of skills the position receives some support from the argument of Mishkin and Petri (1984) that habits are stored in the basal ganglia. A habit is a kind of memory that involves the formation of a link between stimulus elements and a particular response because that response is followed by reinforcement. It is clearly similar to a skill and like a skill it is supposed to increase in strength gradually over trials. Arguments that favour the view that habits are stored in the basal ganglia are therefore also likely to support the view that skills are stored in these structures. These arguments are partially based on general plausibility because there is a heavy, topographically organized projection from many neocortical sites onto the caudate nucleus, which then projects to other parts of the basal ganglia. Through a series of relays the projection eventually reaches neurons that control motor output and hence the basal ganglia can be seen to provide links between neocortically represented sensory elements and motor output. The idea that sensory information is sent to the basal ganglia is supported by metabolic studies in monkeys, which show that visual stimuli not only increase activity in visual cortex but also in the basal ganglia. Mishkin and his colleagues have further shown that slowly acquired visual pattern discriminations are not affected by the lesions that cause amnesia, but are affected by damage to parts of the caudate nucleus.

Although the evidence that the basal ganglia are involved in habit and skill formation is growing there is an older tradition that links these forms of memory to the cerebellum. Like the basal ganglia, the cerebellum also is well placed to mediate between sensory inputs and motor output and so play a role in skill processing and memory. In recent years, however, research on rabbits has suggested that parts of the cerebellum play a critical role in the acquisition and retention of certain kinds of classical conditioning. It has been shown by Thompson's group that lesions of the rabbit cerebellum can selectively affect the ability to acquire and retain CS-CR links without affecting UCS-UCR links (see Thompson, 1986). There is now preliminary evidence that cerebellar lesions can cause similar deficits in humans (O'Boyle, personal communication). In one patient with a selective lesion of the right cerebellar hemisphere a conditioned eyeblink response did not develop to a tone when the conditioning was mediated by the damaged half of the cerebellum. The patient showed a normal unconditioned eye blink response to a puff of air, however, and when the mode of stimulus presentation was changed so that conditioning was controlled by the intact cerebellum, then the learnt eye blink response developed normally. It can be tentatively concluded therefore that both skill memory and conditioning are primarily affected by basal ganglia and cerebellar lesions. It remains to be determined whether any aspects of these kinds of memory are ever affected by the cortical, limbic and diencephalic lesions that impair various aspects of explicit semantic and episodic memory.

CONCLUSIONS

The major conclusion that emerges from study of the five groups of organic memory disorders is that different kinds of information are stored in distinct brain regions. The brain comprises many separate modular units that process particular kinds of information. Probably as a direct result of processing activities the strength of connections between the neural elements that constitute the relevant units are changed. These changes underlie storage. Within the posterior association neocortex are many modules responsible for processing and storing interpreted sensory information. These modules process and store much of the information that constitutes semantic and episodic memory. Damage to some of these modules may impair short- and long-term memory for specific kinds of information. Such deficits do not necessarily support the existence of separate short-term storage systems because they may be caused by subtle processing disorders or disconnections between input and output systems. It is possible that lesions could damage neurons that merely prolong activity in processing modules so selective short-term memory storage deficits could exist. But such deficits have not yet been proved to exist and their interpretation might anyway be difficult because they are likely to have 'knock-on' effects that disrupt long-term memory for the same kinds of information.

Activation of posterior association cortex modules provides the processing necessary if storage changes are to occur. Coordination of processing across many such modules requires the planning provided by frontal association cortex modules. This planning ability of the frontal region may partly depend on the storage of procedures for flexibly performing motor and cognitive acts. If so, frontal lobe lesions should cause apraxias as well as planning deficits through the destruction of these programs. The creation of adequate semantic and episodic memories depends not only on the frontal cortex modules co-ordinating the processing of the posterior association cortex modules, but also on further processing by the limbic-diencephalic structures, affected in amnesics. These structures have strong two-way interconnections with both association cortices. Normal activity in them is vital for the creation and retrieval of (all but the most rehearsed) episodic and semantic explicit memories and may result in the processing and storage of various kinds of background context without the retrieval of which target information stored in the neocortex, cannot be explicitly remembered. This hypothesis is, however, only weakly supported and may prove to have little substance. Target information is stored as an interconnected set of attributes in the posterior association cortex with each attribute assigned to its own processing module. Lesions can affect specific kinds of semantic and episodic memory by disconnecting these modules from each other or destroying particular modules. In both cases, specific kinds of processing should be affected as well as storage. But this remains to be shown. Information, underlying skill memory and conditioning, is largely processed and stored in subcortical structures, like the basal ganglia and cerebellum. Finally, there is no compelling evidence that any organic memory disorder is ever caused by a selective storage deficit.

REFERENCES

Albert, M.S., Butters, N. & Brandt, J. (1981). Patterns of remote memory in amnesic and demented patients. Archives of Neurology, 38, 395-500.
Allport, D.A. (1985). Distributed memory modular subsystems and dysphasia. in: S. Newman & R. Epstein (eds.). Current Perspectives in Dysphasia. Edinburgh: Churchill Livingstone.
Baddeley, A.D. & Hitch, G. (1974). Working Memory. in: G.H. Bower (ed.). The Psychology of Learning and Motivation (Vol.8), New York: Academic Press.
Bauer, R.M. (1984). Autonomic recognition of names and faces in prosopagnosia: neuropsychological application of a guilty knowledge test. Neuropsychologia, 22, 457-469.
Cohen, N.J. (1984). Preserved learning capacity in amnesia; Evidence for multiple memory systems. in: L.R. Squire & N. Butters (eds.). Neuropsychology of Memory. New York: Guilford.

Cohen, N.J. & Squire, L.R. (1980). Preserved learning and retention of pattern analyzing skills in amnesia: dissociation of knowing how and knowing that. Science, 210, 207-210.

Davidoff, J. & Ostergaard, A.L. (1984). Colour anomia resulting from weakened short-term colour memory. Brain, 107, 415-430.

De Renzi, E. & Nichelli, P. (1975). Verbal and non-verbal short-term memory impairment following hemispheric damage. Cortex, 11, 341-354.

Freedman, M. & Cermak, L.S. (1936). Semantic encoding deficits in frontal lobe disease and amnesia. Brain and Cognition, 5, 108-114.

Friedrich, F.I., Glenn, C.G. & Marin, O.S.M. (1984). Interruption of phonological coding in conduction aphasia. Brain and Language, 22, 288-291.

Graf, P. & Schacter, D.L. (1985). Implicit and explicit memory for new associations in normal and amnesic subjects. Journal of Experimental Psychology: Learning, Memory and Cognition, 11, 501-508.

Graf, P., Squire, L.R. & Mandler, G. (1984). The information that amnesic patients do not forget. Journal of Experimental Psychology: Learning, Memory and Cognition, 10, 164-178.

Hasher, L.D. & Zacks, R.T. (1979). Automatic and effortful processes in memory. Journal of Experimental Psychology: General, 108, 356-388.

Heindel, W.C., Butters, N. & Salmon, D. (1987). Impaired motor skill learning associated with neostriatal lesions. Journal of Clinical and Experimental Neuropsychology, 9, 18.

Hirst, W (1985). Use of mnemonic in patients with frontal lobe damage. Journal of Clinical and Experimental Neuropsychology, 7, 175.

Huppert, F.A. & Piercy, M. (1979). Normal and Abnormal forgetting in organic amnesia: effect of locus of lesion. Cortex, 15, 385-390.

Kapur, N. (1985). Double dissociation between perseveration in memory and problem solving tasks. Cortex, 21, 461-465.

Kapur, K., Heath, P., Meudell, P. & Kennedy, P. (1986). Amnesia can facilitate memory performance: evidence from a patient with dissociated retrograde amnesia. Neuropsychologia, 24, 215-221.

Kinsbourne, M. (1972). Behavioural analysis of the repetition deficit in conduction aphasia. Neurology, 22, 1126-1132.

Martone, M., Butters, N., Payne, M., Becker, J.T. & Sax, D.S. (1984). Dissociations between skill learning and verbal recognition in amnesia and dementia. Archives of Neurology, 41, 965-970.

Mayes, A.R. (1986). Learning and memory disorders and their assessment. Neuropsychologia, 24, 25-39.

Mayes, A.R. (1987). Human organic memory disorders. in: H. Beloff & A. Colman (eds.). Psychology Survey (Vol.6). Leicester: BPS Publications.

Mayes, A.R. (1988). Recent developments in amnesia research. in: M.M. Gruneberg, P.E. Morris & Oborne, D.J. (eds.). Practical Aspects of Memory (Vol.2). Chichester: John Wiley & Sons.

Mayes, A.R. & Meudell, P.R. (1983). Amnesia in humans and other animals. in: A.R. Mayes (eds.). Memory in Animals and Humans. Wokingham: Van Nostrand Reinhold.

Mayes, A.R., Meudell, P.R. & Pickering, A. (1985). Is organic amnesia caused by a selective deficit in remembering contextual information. Cortex, 21, 167-202.

Milner, B. (1971). Interhemispheric differences in the location of psychological processes in man. British Medical Bulletin, 27, 272-277.

Milner, B., Petrides, M. & Smith, M.L. (1985). Frontal lobes and the temporal organization of memory. Human Neurobiology, 4, 137-142.

Mishkin, M. (1982). A memory system in the monkey. Philosophical Transactions of the Royal Society, 298B, 85-95.

Mishkin, M. & Peters, H.L. (1984). Memories and habits: Some implications for the analysis of learning and retention. in: L.R. Squire & N. Butters (eds.). Neuropsychology of Memory. New York: Guildford.

Parkin, A.J. & Leng, N.R.C. (1987). Comparative studies of human amnesia. in: H. Markowitsch (ed.). _Information Processing and the Brain._ Toronto: Hans Huber.

Saint-Cyr, J.A., Taylor, A.E. & De Lang, A.E. (1987). Procedural learning impairment in basal ganglia disease. _Journal of Clinical and Experimental Neuropsychology, 9_, 280.

Shallice, T. (1986). Impairments of semantic processing: multiple dissociations. in: M. Coltheart, R., Job & G. Sartori, (eds.), _The Cognitive Neuropsychology of Language._ Hillsdale, N.J.: Lawrence Erlbaum.

Shallice, T. & Warrington, E.K. (1979). Auditory verbal short term memory impairment and conduction aphasia. _Brain and Language, 4_, 479–491.

Shimamura, A.P., Salmon, D.P., Squire, L.R. & Butters, N. (1987). Memory dysfunction unique to Alzheimer's disease: impairment in word priming. _Journal of Clinical and Experimental Neuropsychology, 9_, 20.

Signoret, J.L. & Lhermitte, F. (1976). The amnesic syndromes and the encoding process. in: M.R. Rozenzweig & E.L. Bennett (eds.). _Neural Mechanisms of Learning and Memory._ Cambridge, Mass.: MIT press.

Squire, L.R. (1981). Two forms of amnesia: An analysis of forgetting. _Journal of Neuroscience, 1_, 635–640.

Squire, L.R. (1987). _Memory and the Brain._ Oxford: Oxford University Press.

Starr, A. & Barrett, G. (1987). Disordered auditory short-term memory in man and event related potentials. _Brain, 110_, 935–959.

Stuss, D.T. & Benson, D.F. (1984). Neuropsychological studies of the frontal lobes. _Psychological Bulletin, 95_, 3–28.

Thompson, R.E. (1986). The Neurobiology of learning and memory. _Science, 233_, 941–947.

Tranel, D. & Damasio, A.R. (1985). Knowledge without awareness: An autonomic index of facial recognition. _Science, 228_, 1453–1454.

Vallar, G. & Baddeley, A.D. (1984). Fractionation of working memory: neuropsychological evidence for a phonological short-term store. _Journal of Verbal Learning and Verbal Behaviour, 23_, 151–161.

Vallar, G. & Cappa, S.F. (1987). Articulation and verbal short-term memory: evidence from anarthria. _Cognitive Neuropsychology, 4_, 55–78.

Warrington, E.K. (1982). The fractionation of arithmetical skills: a single case study. _Quarterly Journal of Experimental Psychology, 34A_, 31–52.

Warrington, E.K. & Rabin, P. (1971). Visual span of apprehension in patients with unilateral cerebral lesions. _Quarterly Journal of Experimental Psychology, 23_, 423–431.

Weiskrantz, L. & Warrington, E.K. (1979). Conditioning in amnesic patients. _Neuropsychologia, 17_, 187–194.

ANARTHRIA AND VERBAL SHORT-TERM MEMORY

R Logie, R Cubelli, S Della Sala, M Alberoni and P Nichelli

INTRODUCTION

The nature of coding in verbal short-term memory has been a topic of some considerable debate. Much of the evidence for phonological coding in normal adults is based on the phonological similarity effect; the finding that sequences of items that are phonologically similar to one another are less well recalled than items that are phonologically dissimilar (Conrad, 1964).

One important issue concerns the role of sub-vocal articulation in phonological coding. Support for an involvement of articulation comes from experiments where subjects are required to vocalize aloud an irrelevant word (e.g. ...the the the...) while attempting to retain verbal sequences. Under these conditions, known as articulatory suppression, the verbal material is less well recalled. A more interesting finding is that the phonological similarity effect is removed by this technique, but only when the sequence for recall is presented visually (Baddeley, Lewis & Vallar, 1984). The interpretation of this finding is that articulation is necessary for translating visually presented material into a phonological code. Articulatory suppression is thought to act to prevent this translation, thus removing the effects of phonological similarity. If the sequence for recall is presented aurally, suppression has an overall effect on recall of the material, but the phonological similarity effect remains intact. It appears that the basis for this code is unlikely to be acoustic. Conrad (1973) reported that congenitally deaf children who were rated as good speakers show a clear effect of phonological similarity on shortterm verbal memory performance. Deaf children who are poor speakers do not show the effect. These findings strongly suggest articulatory coding is involved in effects of phonological similarity.

A second source of evidence for the role of articulatory coding comes from the finding that lists of polysyllabic words such as 'hippopotamus' and 'Mississippi' tend to be less well recalled than lists of monosyllabic words such as 'bus' or 'clock'. Further, the crucial variable appears to be how long the words take to pronounce rather than the number of syllables or letters. Thus lists of bisyllabic words such as 'typhoon' or 'Friday' take longer to pronounce and are less readily recalled than are lists of words such as 'bishop' or 'wicket' which are also bisyllabic but take much less time to pronounce (Baddeley, Thomson & Buchanan, 1975). This word length effect occurs with both auditory and visual presentation of the words. However, articulatory suppression removes the effect of word length for both modes of presentation.

Finally, Salame and Baddeley (1982) have shown that recall of visually presented digit sequences is disrupted by simultaneous present-

203

ation of irrelevant speech. The disruption is greater where the irrelevant speech is phonologically similar to the digits for recall (e.g. 'tun', 'woo', 'tee', 'sore' and so on).

This body of evidence has been incorporated by Baddeley and his colleagues within the notion of an articulatory loop system, thought to be responsible for effects of both phonological similarity and word length on serial verbal recall (e.g. Baddeley, 1986). The concept of the loop has also been useful in the study of adult reading (Baddeley & Lewis, 1981) and counting (Logie and Baddeley, 1987). The suggestion is that the articulatory loop consists of two components, a passive phonological store and an articulatory rehearsal process. The phonological similarity effect is thought to reflect confusion among items contained in this store. The phonological store is also thought to be accessed directly by speech. This accounts for the effect of irrelevant speech (Salame & Baddeley, 1982) by suggesting that the digits for recall are coded in the phonological store, but that irrelevant speech has privileged access to this store, thereby disrupting its contents.

The word length effect is thought to reflect the articulatory rehearsal process, in that the longer the words are, the less readily they can be rehearsed. Articulatory suppression is thought to involve the rehearsal mechanism, thereby preventing rehearsal of the material for recall. Since rehearsal is employed whether the material for recall is presented visually or aurally, articulatory suppression undermines the word length effect for both presentation modalities. Articulatory rehearsal is also thought to be involved in translating visually presented material into a phonological code. Thus information from visual presentation enters the phonological store via articulatory rehearsal. Articulatory suppression is thought to prevent this recoding, thus removing the effect of phonological similarity with visual presentation. Since speech has direct access to the store, no recoding of information occurs via articulatory rehearsal and thus with auditory presentation the phonological similarity effect is immune from effects of articulatory suppression. The rehearsal process is also responsible for refreshing the contents of the store which is itself subject to decay or displacement with new material (see Vallar & Baddeley, 1984; Baddeley, 1986).

One aspect of the function of the articulatory loop is the extent of its involvement in making judgements of phonology. Baddeley and Lewis (1981) have shown that suppression has no effect on judgements as to whether two visually presented letter strings are phonologically similar (e.g. oshun-ocean). This suggests that the articulatory loop is not involved in making judgements of homophony. This allows for phonological coding of visually presented material without the need for articulation. However, judgements as to whether two words rhyme does appear to be affected by suppression. Besner (1987) has concluded that phonological coding in reading does not require articulation, but that where some operation on that code is required, subvocal articulation may well be involved. By operation, he includes maintenance of the information. He also suggests that rhyme judgements involve segmentation of the phonological code to determine whether one component of a word rhymes with one component of another word. This segmentation constitutes an operation on phonology. This accounts for the presence of an effect of articulatory suppression on rhyme judgements, but not on homophone judgements or on the process of normal reading.

There are a number of interesting questions concerning the nature of the articulation involved in rehearsal. For example, to what extent is the rehearsal mechanism merely a component of speech production? One suggestion is that the articulatory loop acts as an output buffer for speech production. Indeed, Ellis (1980) reported striking similarities between the phonological errors found in short-term memory tasks and errors observed in the production of speech. However, it is likely to be the articulatory rehearsal process which is involved in speech production rather than the phonological store. Evidence for this view comes from a number of case studies of patients with short-term memory deficits (e.g. Shallice & Butterworth, 1977; Shallice & Warrington, 1974; Vallar & Baddeley, 1984) who show evidence of a deficit in the phonological store but no difficulty in articulation (Baddeley, 1986, p 100) and who have normal speech.

SPEECH PRODUCTION AND SHORT-TERM MEMORY

A second question concerns the extent to which mechanisms for speech production are necessary for adequate functioning of the articulatory loop. One approach to this question is to study patients who have generally intact linguistic abilities but who have lost the ability to speak through damage to the systems responsible for control of the speech muscles. Such patients are generally termed anarthric. In less 'pure' cases, dysarthric patients are individuals whose speech is severely impaired, but who nonetheless have a residual capability for speech production in the absence of language impairment. Baddeley and Wilson (1985) reported one case of an anarthric patient, GB, who had normal language comprehension and could communicate very efficiently by means of a typewriter-like keyboard. His ability to produce sound was limited to a single inspiratory cry. However he exhibited clear phonological similarity effects with both auditory and visual presentation. He was also capable of making judgements as to whether a visually presented word and non-word would sound alike when pronounced (e.g. ocean-oshun). This suggested that he could recode visually presented material into a phonological code. Finally, he showed clear effects of word length with auditory presentation, indicating the use of sub-vocal rehearsal. Baddeley and Wilson reported similar findings for five cases of dysarthric patients who could be considered less 'pure' than GB. It appeared that these patients showed the pattern of results obtained from subjects with normal speech, and did not perform as normal subjects under articulatory suppression. Baddeley and Wilson concluded that use of the speech musculature was not necessary for adequate functioning of the articulatory loop, and in particular was not necessary for subvocal rehearsal.

However, the report of patient GB was not quite as clear-cut as it seemed initially. The anarthria resulted from a severe closed head injury and Baddeley and Wilson reported the damage as being '...surprisingly focal and central... not affecting the cortex', but gave no further details as to the site of damage. It is common for damage resulting from closed head injury to be rather diffuse, and GB showed signs of frontal lobe impairment in both spontaneous behaviour and formal testing using both a category generation task and a modified version of the Wisconsin Card Sorting Test. More important, from a theoretical point of view, GB was not tested for the effects of word length with visual presentation. Given the importance of the modality of presentation in its interaction with suppression, this makes the interpretaton of GB's impairment somewhat more complex.

More recently Vallar and Cappa (1987) reported two case studies of anarthria. Case GF was diagnosed as having 'locked-in syndrome' presumably due to a pontine infarction. He was alert but could not speak or make any muscle movements other than eye movements and eyelid closure. He also had some residual head movement that allowed him to communicate by pressing on a transducer connected to a letter board and typewriter. A CT scan showed a severe cerebellar atrophy prevailing on the left side. The left sylvian fissure was slightly larger than the right. The second case, MDC, was anarthric following 'bi-opercular syndrome' due to bilateral ischemic strokes in the Rolandic area. She could utter only inarticulate moans but could communicate by sign language and by writing. A CT scan indicated an atrophic dilatation of the paracentral sulci on the left with a hypodense area involving the anterior portion of the temporal lobe and the fronto-parietal operculum on the right.

While Baddeley and Wilson concentrated on purely verbal material, Vallar and Cappa extended the study to include picture-word rhyme matching as well as phonological judgements, effects of phonological similarity and of word length. The Vallar and Cappa results were not as straightforward as those of Baddeley and Wilson. Patient GF showed the standard phonological similarity effect with both auditory and visual presentation, while patient MDC showed effects of phonological similarity only with auditory presentation. The word length effect was shown by MDC with auditory, but not with visual presentation. For GF, there was no effect of word length with auditory presentation, but this patient was not tested with visual presentation. Vallar and Cappa suggested that a possible interpretation for these apparently anomalous results lies in the response method used by the two patients. In the test for word length, GF responded by pointing with his apparatus, to words on the letter board, thus employing a recognition procedure. Typically, the word length effect is tested by means of a recall procedure (Baddeley, Thomson & Buchanan, 1975). However, Baddeley and Wilson used essentially the same recognition procedure with patient GB and obtained a clear effect of word length with auditory presentation. Patient MDC was able to write her responses. Vallar and Cappa interpreted these findings by suggesting that MDC appeared to use articulatory rehearsal with auditory, but not with visual presentation. These authors suggest that MDC suffers from a deficit in phonological coding of visual material which occurs prior to articulatory rehearsal. Thus articulatory rehearsal is available with auditory presentation, but not with visual presentation. This would also explain the presence of a phonological similarity effect with auditory but not with visual material.

The case of GF is somewhat more complex, since phonological similarity occurs with both visual and auditory presentation, we would expect the word length effect to appear also. According to the model, phonological similarity with visual presentation ought to involve articulatory rehearsal and hence show an effect of word length. It is unfortunate that Vallar and Cappa did not test this patient for the word length effect with visual presentation. It may be that the difference in response mode resulted in this finding. However, it clearly merits further investigation.

TWO CASE STUDIES OF ANARTHRIA

Recently we have been able to study a further two cases of anarthric patient. Della Sala, Logie and Alberoni (manuscript in preparation) studied case LB, a well educated 72 year old woman who showed a complete lack of articulate speech following a stroke. An NMR scan showed an ischemic lesion in the middle third of the pons. She was alert and although she could not speak, she had no deficit in language comprehension. She was capable of appropriate gestures in response to questions. She was suffering from severe right hemiplegia and was confined to a wheelchair. She communicated by pointing; spelling out words on an alphabet letter board. She could also write slowly, but legibly, with her left hand. Her comprehension of spoken and written language was well preserved, writing from dictation and spontaneous writing appeared intact and she showed no difficulties with mental calculations. Her general intelligence was normal, as were her visuo-spatial abilities.

She could make accurate phonological judgements by discriminating syllable pairs such as pa-ba or ca-da. She could also make rhyme judgements that involved matching a picture and a word or a picture and a non-sense word which rhymed with a picture name. She produced a number of errors when asked to match two pictures according to whether or not the names rhymed. However, we later asked our patient LB as to which names she had used for the pictures. In the cases where she had previously made an error, it was evident that most errors were due to her choice of alternative picture names.

She could also make homophone judgements. This involved a task originally devised by Sartori (1984). In Italian, there is a complete lack of homophonous words, but it is possible to find some expressions which are spelled in identical ways, but if written as two words rather than one, change their meaning considerably. For example, in Italian the word for 'heavenly' is divino, but di vino means 'of wine'. A phrase such as 'heavenly mystery' is written mistero divino, which sounds the same and is spelled the same as mistero di vino which means 'mystery of wine'. The patient had very little difficulty with this task. LB showed a clear phonological similarity effect wih both auditory and visual presentation. Her span (4) was lower than normal.

The effect of word length was also tested using auditory and visual presentation of sequences of two and five syllable words. We used three different methods for testing retrieval. In one case, LB was given a board on which were written in block capitals, the set of ten words of a given length. LB was instructed to point to the words immediately after presentation, in their correct serial order. In order to prevent the use of location cues, the pointing board was kept face down during present-ation. This method of retrieval was adopted by Baddeley and Wilson for patient GB. It was also used by Vallar and Cappa for patient GF, who you will remember, did not show effects of word length. The second method of retrieval involved the subject spelling out the words by pointing to letters on her alphabet board. For the five syllable words, LB was allowed to spell out only the first two syllables of the word, e.g. 'ippo' for ippopotamo. The third method involved the subject writing down the recalled words. As with spelling, she was required to write only the first two syllables of the five syllable words. Unfortunately, it was only possible to test the patient with auditory presentation using this method of recall.

The effect of word length was clear for both auditory and visual presentation with a pointing response that involved spelling out the words. The effect with auditory presentation for written recall was also very clear. However, the result for pointing to whole words was very weak, and it appears that the lack of a word length effect with the Vallar and Cappa patient, GF, may have been due to the use of this recog-nition procedure for recall. We shall return later to this point. Fin-ally, LB also showed an effect of unattended speech on recall of visually presented digit sequences.

The major thrust of the discussion so far has centred on whether the speech muscles are necessary for the adequate functioning of the articu-latory loop. We have discussed a number of issues that suggest the pic-ture is not completely clear-cut, but on the whole it appears that the articulatory loop can function adequately (in the cases of GB and of LB) without the use of peripheral speech musculature. However, there is one important aspect that remains to be adequately explored; the relationship with the control processes necessary for speech, rather than physical speech output.

A major advance in the evidence for a separate phonological store came from patients who appeared to have an impairment in their ability to store phonological information, but nonetheless had normal articulation (Shallice & Warrington, 1974; Vallar & Baddeley, 1984). The anarthric patients that we have described so far appear to have an intact phonological store and intact articulatory rehearsal processes, in the absence of speech output. That is, the control processes for articulation appear to be intact even if the physical speech output is not. There has been a lack of patients who appear to have an intact phonological store, but do not have intact subvocal rehearsal. The discovery of such patients would complete the appropriate double dissociation between phonological store and subvocal articulation and greatly increase our understanding of short-term verbal memory function.

Cubelli and Nichelli (manuscript in preparation) have tested an anarthric patient, CM, a 23 year old student who suffered a cerebrovascular accident which resulted in a complete inability to utter speech sounds. She was diagnosed as having 'locked-in syndrome' and a CT scan indicated a possible hypodense area in the pontine region. An NMR scan confirmed a bilateral pontine lesion in the median and paramedian portion of the ventral pons, anterior to the fourth ventricle. As with LB, CM's comprehension was unimpaired for both written and spoken language. She had above average intelligence and visuo-spatial abilities. She could also write adequately to dictation and spontaneously. Phonological discrimination was normal. She was normal on tasks which involved matching an aurally presented word with its written version, and matching non-words one of which was in lower case, and the other in upper case. Her digit span was 5 for both auditory and visual presentation, which is marginally lower than normal. She showed a clear effect of phonological similarity with both auditory and visual presentation. The word length effect with visual presentation was also very clear. However, there was no evidence of a word length effect with auditory presentation. This last dissociation was replicated using a more intensive procedure. She did show a clear effect of unattended speech.

The dissociation between the presence of the standard phonological similarity effect with visual presentation and the lack of a word length effect with auditory input was also shown by Vallar and Cappa's patient GF. Case CM and GF shared the same neurological picture and lesion site. Vallar and Cappa attributed this unpredicted result to methodological bias, and some support for this interpretation came from patient LB. However, this cannot account for CM's performance since she was capable of writing her responses.

Cubelli and Nichelli decided to study further CM's subvocal articulation using a technique devised by Hintzman (1967). Hintzman analysed the errors produced by normal subjects on immediate repetition of visually presented nonsense syllables. He argued that the pattern of errors could be due only to subvocal articulation rather than phonological storage or processing. Specifically, when comparing substitution errors that involved phonemes with the same phonological features, these occurred much more frequently with phonemes having closer rather than more distant articulation points. For example, within unvoiced stop consonants the bilabial target 'P' was more frequently substituted by alveolar 'T' than by the velar consonant 'K'. Cubelli and Nichelli adapted Hintzman's task for the rules of Italian pronunciation, using sequences of phonologically similar nonsense syllables (e.g. PAV, TAV, KAV, DAV etc.). They found that CM produced substitution errors that were quite unlike those that might be predicted from Hintzman's normal subjects. If anything, there was a tendency for the more distant items to be confused (i.e. PAV for KAV) than the items involving more similar articulation patterns (i.e. PAV for TAV). This task has yet to be carried out with normal Italian subjects, but this omission is unlikely to undermine the suggestion that CM did not have normal subvocal articulation.

CM's free recall performance was very similar to that of a group of control subjects under articulatory suppression. This was true of both the overall level of recall and the shape of the serial position function. That is, CM showed a normal recency effect as do normal subjects under suppression (Richardson & Baddeley, 1975). In addition, she showed no forgetting in a version of the Brown-Peterson task (e.g. Brown, 1958) involving retention of consonant trigrams. This mimics the Vallar and Baddeley (1982) finding that articulatory suppression does not cause short-term forgetting in normal subjects, with visually presented material.

In most cases it appears as though CM's verbal short-term memory is operating like that of normal subjects under suppression and further supports the distinction between subvocal rehearsal and phonological storage. However, there is one rather curious finding that does not appear to fit this description; specifically her results for the effects of phonological similarity and of word length. Under articulatory suppression, normal subjects do not show the word length effect with either visual or auditory presentation. CM shows no word length effect with auditory presentation as might be expected. However, she does show a word length effect with visual presentation. She also shows phonological similarity effects with both auditory and visual presentation. Under suppression, normal subjects show phonological similarity only with auditory presentation. This pattern of results suggests that visually presented information is gaining access to the phonological store via some form of articulation, but that such articulation does not occur with auditory presentation.

On the basis of these results, Cubelli and Nichelli propose a dissociation between the articulatory coding involved in translating into a phonological code, visually presented verbal material, and an articulatory rehearsal process that is used to enhance memory performance. They suggest that the word length effect with visual presentation reflects the operation of the articulatory coding process, a process that also allows access to the phonological store. In contrast, they suggest that the lack of a word length effect with auditory presentation reflects damage to the mechanism that allows subvocal rehearsal. They further suggest that the articulatory rehearsal process is the component that is involved in speech output. This notion would suggest that case MDC (Vallar & Cappa, 1987) who shows a pattern of results for word length that is complementary to that for CM, is likely to have a complementary deficit. That is, MDC's deficit would be in the articulatory recoding process that is involved in giving visual information access to the phonological store. MDC's articulatory rehearsal mechanism would be intact. This would also account for the lack of a word length effect with visual presentation, but the presence of an effect of word length with auditory presentation. Presumably in normal adults, the effect of articulatory suppression is to prevent the use of both articulatory rehearsal and articulatory coding since under suppression normal subjects show no effects of word length with either visual or auditory presentation. This dissociation between subvocal rehearsal and articulatory coding makes some intuitive sense, since two different functions seem to be involved and it would appear to make a case for further fractionation of the articulatory loop. This necessarily complicates the model, but removes the need for locating MDC's impairment in the phonological recoding process as suggested by Vallar and Cappa. In addition, it would be difficult to incorporate the pattern of CM's deficit within the current version of the articulatory loop.

CONCLUSIONS

The study of patients with anarthria is largely concerned with the relationship between speech and verbal short-term memory. It appears that the control processes for speech constitute an integral component of verbal short-term memory. The data from patients GB and LB appear to suggest that the absence of speech output does not necessarily imply an impairment of the articulatory loop although there may be some reduced capacity. However, in the case of LB, GF and CM, digit span was somewhat lower than one might expect on the basis of their age and educational level. Also, there is evidence to suggest that overt speech enhances memory span (Murray, 1965). This is true even when auditory feedback is masked by white noise (Salame & Baddeley, 1983).

An alternative suggestion to the role of subvocal articulation as a memory process comes from work by Reisberg, Rappaport and O'Shaughnessy (1984). They demonstrated an enhanced memory span through the use of finger tapping, with each finger associated with a different number. When subjects were subsequently asked to suppress the use of this strategy by drumming their fingers on the table, they showed effects analogous to those of articulatory suppression. Reisberg et al. suggested that subvocal articulation was an example of subjects capitalising on the characteristics of the speech system as an aid to memory. Similarly finger tapping used the sequencing of muscle actions as a memory aid. According to this view articulation appears to be a motor-based control system, crucial for the adequate functioning of verbal short-term memory and for enhancing memory span. Therefore it can be considered an integral component of that system. An important distinction with the Reisberg et al. 'Digit Digit-Span' is that normal adult subjects appear to use subvocal articulation spontaneously. As such further exploration of the relationship between speech and memory is likely to be aided rather than undermined by further development of the articulatory loop hypothesis.

REFERENCES

Baddeley, A.D. (1986). Working Memory. Oxford: Oxford University Press.
Baddeley, A.D. & Lewis, V.J. (1981). Inner active processes in reading: the inner voice, the inner ear and the inner eye. in: A.M. Lesgold & C.A. Perfetti (eds.). Interactive Processes in Reading. Hillsdale N.J.: Erlbaum.
Baddeley, A.D., Lewis, V.J. & Vallar, G. (1984). Exploring the articulatory loop. Quarterly Journal of Experimental Psychology, 36A, 233-252.
Baddeley, A.D., Thomson, N. & Buchanan, M. (1975). Word length and the structure of short-term memory. Journal of Verbal Learning and Verbal Behavior, 14, 575-589.
Baddeley, A.D. & Wilson, B. (1985). Phonological coding and short-term memory in patients without speech. Journal of Verbal Learning and Verbal Behavior, 24, 490-502.
Basso, A. & Capitani, E. (1979). Un test standardizzato per la diagnosi dell'acalculia: descrizione e valori normativi. Rivista di Applicazioni Psichologiche, 1, 551-564.

Basso, A., Capitani, E. & Vignolo, L.A. (1979). The influence of rehabilitation on language skills in aphasic patients. A controlled study. Archives of Neurology, 36, 190-196.

Besner, D. (1987). Phonology, lexical access in reading and articulatory suppression: a critical review. Quarterly Journal of Experimental Psychology, 39A, 467-478.

Brown, J. (1958). Some tests of the decay theory of immediate memory, Quarterly Journal of Experimental Psychology, 10, 12-21.

Conrad, R. (1964). Acoustic confusions in immediate memory. British Journal of Psychology, 55, 75-84.

Conrad, R. (1973). Some correlates of speech coding in the short-term memory of the deaf. Journal of Speech and Hearing Research, 16, 375-384.

De Renzi, E. & Vignoli, L.A. (1962). The Token Test: a sensitive test to detect receptive disturbances in aphasics, Brain, 85, 665-678.

Dunn, L.M. (1965). The Peabody Picture Vocabulary Test. Circle Pines, Minnesota: American Guidance Services Inc..

Ellis, A.W. (1980). Errors in speech and short-term memory: the effect of phonemic similarity and syllable position. Journal of Verbal Learning and Verbal Behavior, 19, 624-634.

Hintzman, D.L. (1967). Articulatory coding in short-term memory. Journal of Verbal Learning and Verbal Behavior, 6, 312-316.

Logie, R.H. & Baddeley, A.D. (1987). Cognitive processes in counting. Journal of Experimental Psychology: Learning, Memory, and Cognition, 13, 310-326.

Murray, D.J. (1965). Vocalisation of presentation and immediate recall with varying presentation rates. Quarterly Journal of Experimental Psychology, 17, 47-56.

Reisberg, D., Rappaport, I. & O'Shaughnessy, M. (1984). Limits of working memory: The digit digit-span. Journal of Experimental Psychology: Learning, Memory, and Cognition, 10, 203-221.

Richardson, J.T.E. & Baddeley, A.D. (1975). The effect of articulatory suppression in free recall. Journal of Verbal Learning and Verbal Behavior, 14, 623-629.

Salame, P. & Baddeley, A.D. (1982). Disruption of short-term memory by unattended speech: implications for the structure of working memory. Journal of Verbal Learning and Verbal Behavior, 21, 150-164.

Salame, P. & Baddeley, A.D. (1983). Differential effects of noise and speech on short-term memory. Proceedings of the Fourth International Congress on Noise as a Public Health Problem. Milan: Centro di Recerche di Studi Amplifon.

Sartori, G. (1984). La lettura. Processi normali e dislessia. Bologna: Il Mulino.

Shallice, T. & Butterworth, B. (1977). Short-term memory impairment and spontaneous speech. Neuropsychologia, 15, 729-735.

Shallice, T. & Warrington, E.K. (1974). The dissociation between long-term retention of meaningful sounds and verbal material. Neuropsychologia, 12, 553-55.

Vallar, G. & Baddeley, A.D. (1982). Short-term forgetting and the articulatory loop. Quarterly Journal of Experimental Psychology, 34, 53-60.

Vallar, G. & Baddeley, A.D. (1984). Fractionation of working memory: Neuropsychological evidence for a phonological short-term store. Journal of Verbal Learning and Verbal Behavior, 23, 151-161.

Vallar, G. & Cappa, S.F. (1987). Articulation and verbal short-term memory: Evidence from anarthria. Cognitive Neuropsychology, 4, 55-78.

RETROGRADE AMNESIA IN KORSAKOFF'S SYNDROME:

AN EXPERIMENTAL AND THEORETICAL ANALYSIS

Daniela Montaldi and Alan J. Parkin

INTRODUCTION

Retrograde amnesia (RA), loss of memory for the pre-morbid period, is a primary characteristic of Korsakoff's Syndrome. Without exception, published reports of this disorder indicate an RA extending back between 25 and 35 years into the pre-morbid period (see Parkin, 1984 for a review). A critical feature of this RA is that it follows Ribot's Law (1882): severity of memory loss is an inverse function of the age of any given memory, i.e. the more recent a memory is the more likey it is to be impaired (e.g. Albert et al., 1979). The presence of these temporal gradients in Korsakoff's Syndrome presents a major challenge to theorists and their explanation is essential to any proper account of this intriguing memory disorder.

ASSESSING RETROGRADE AMNESIA

Assessing RA is no easy matter because the remote memories of individuals are highly varied thus making it difficult to devise standardised tests. Nonetheless a number of authors have produced RA tests (e.g. Sanders & Warrington, 1971; Albert et al., 1979) and used them to assess both normal and amnesic patients. These tests have been based on information that is assumed to be common to all people within a given culture. Various types of material have been used, one of the most popular being famous faces. Among these tests the most commonly used is the Boston Remote Memory Test (BRMT).

A prerequisite for any RA test is that it must assess the patient's memory for different time periods - for convenience remote memory is usually divided into decades or, occasionally, half decades. In this way it will be possible to detect any temporal gradients. Devising such a test is fraught with difficulties. One problem is that any difference in impairment as a function of decade might be an artefact of item difficulty. For example, the presence of a temporal gradient might be partly or wholly attributable to the use of harder items when testing memory for more recent decades. This difficulty can be overcome by pilot work which ensures that, in the normal population, the items selected to represent each decade are of equivalent difficulty (although here one must ensure that such flat functions are not due to a ceiling effect). Another problem is devising test items which are representative of one specific decade. Many people and events remain in the public eye for several decades (a phenomenon Weiskrantz has termed 'public rehearsal'), and correct identification of these cannot be construed as 'decade specific' memory. In order to provide decade-specific items one must therefore avoid the confounding influence of public rehearsal. The best control for this is, wherever possible, to pilot material on subjects who were not alive during the time period addressed by certain items. The degree to which these subjects can identify the items gives a valid index of public rehearsal.

RETROGRADE AMNESIA IN KORSAKOFF'S SYNDROME - AN EXPERIMENT

The present chapter reports a study of RA in a group of British Korsakoff patients. Existing RA tests (e.g. Albert et al., 1979) were unsuitable for cultural reasons so it was necessary to devise a new test. The test addresses memory for the five decades beginning 1936-1945. For each decade there were three decade-specific (DS) faces and three public-ally rehearsed (PR) faces. The items were selected using the methodological procedures outlined above. Examples of DS faces are Douglas Bader, Mark Phillips, examples of PR faces are Winston Churchill, Elvis Presley. For each test item there were two versions, no-context (NC) and context (C). In the former the target was presented without any obvious contextual cue (e.g. General Montgomery in casual clothes), whilst in the latter there was a strong contextual element (e.g. General Montgomery in uniform peering out of a tank).

The provision of contextual cues enabled us to establish the extent to which Korsakoff RA might represent a deficit in contextual encoding. Accounts of the Korsakoff anterograde deficit have centred on contextual encoding as a key explanatory factor (e.g. Mayes et al., 1985) but, to date, there has been little investigation of this factor in accounts of RA.

The subjects were 12 patients with Korsakoff's Syndrome (mean age 60.3 years) and 23 normal controls (mean age 61.3 years). The subjects were first shown the faces in the NC condition and required to name them. All the faces were then repeated in the C condition.

The results of the experiment are shown in Figure 1. For control subjects the PR faces were identified more easily than the DS faces and for both PR and DS faces there was considerable improvement with the provision of contextual cues. Performance across the decades was fairly even although there was a small but significant lower level of perform-ance in the earliest decade. Figure 1 shows that this drop is due to the difficulty of the DS condition. This may have arisen because the subjects were too young to remember some of these faces. For Korsakoff patients performance was significantly better on PR compared with DS faces. As one might expect the performance across decades showed a marked temporal gradient reaching its asymptote in the fourth decade after which perform-ance showed a degree of improvement. There was also an interaction between context and decade. Figure 1 shows that there is a substantial effect of contextual cueing in the early decades but this is reduced systematically until it is virtually non-existent at the fourth decade. There is then a small contextual effect in the most recent decade.

DISCUSSION ·

Our data replicate previous studies of Korsakoff RA using famous faces tests (i.e. Albert et al., 1979, Marslen-Wilson & Teuber, 1975). The patients show a marked temporal gradient which reaches asymptote in the penultimate decade. This decade corresponds to the time period during which the patients suffered their Wernicke's episodes. The upturn in performance found for the most recent decade indicates the patients'

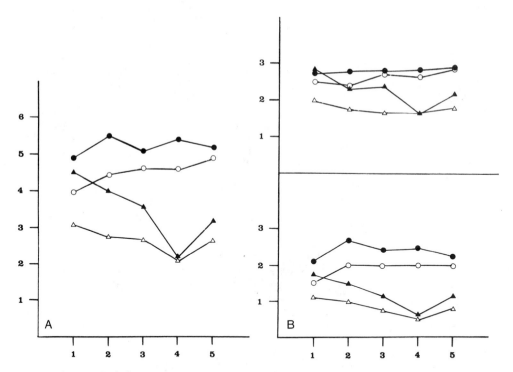

Figure 1 (a) shows performance on the famous faces test. Circular symbols show control data, triangular symbols show Korsakoff data. Hollow symbols show performance without context, filled symbols performance with context; (b) shows the data broken down into PR faces (upper panel) and DS faces (lower panel) - key is the same as Figure 1.

residual learning ability in the Korsakoff state. This upturn cannot be attributed to differential item difficulty because the same trend is not shown by the controls in the DS condition (its non-appearance in the PR condition could be due to a ceiling effect). To our knowledge this is the first demonstration of residual learning of famous faces in Korsakoff's Syndrome that exceeds performance in the asymptote of the premorbid period.

The most interesting feature of the data is the gradual weakening of the contextual effect until there is no effect at all for faces in the decade 1965-1975. One interpretation of temporal gradients in Korsakoff's Syndrome derives from the so-called continuity hypothesis (Ryback, 1971). This asserts that chronic alcohol consumption has a gradually worsening effect on cognitive function. From this perspective the temporal gradient could reflect the gradual worsening of memory processes during the premorbid period. Thus, more recently formed memories are more degraded and provide less basis for significant contextual enhancement. This process culminates in the most recent premorbid period (i.e. that preceding the Wernicke's episode) where the operation of memory is so poor that it precludes any contextual effect.

There are, however, problems with attributing the RA to the effects of chronic alcoholism. Experimental studies of RA in non-Korsakoff alcoholics have shown that they have only mild memory deficits (Albert et al., 1980; Cohen & Squire, 1981). If the continuity hypothesis were correct, there should have been more evidence of impairment in this group. One could, however, argue that chronic alcoholics used in these studies may have less severe problems than those who develop Korsakoff's Syndrome.

The above possibility is diffficult to evaluate because one cannot normally gather information about the state of a Korsakoff patient's premorbid memory before the onset of Wernicke's Disease. A unique exception to this has been provided by patient PZ (Butters, 1985). This man, a university professor, drank extremely heavily all his adult life but nonetheless had a distiguished academic career. A few years prior to developing Korsakoff's Syndrome PZ wrote his autobiography thus providing a concrete indication that his memory for the past was intact at that time point. However, subsequent testing has shown that he can recall little of the content of his autobiography. The data from PZ might be accommodated by arguing that PZ's pre-morbid memory was not as good as his autobiographic recall implies, but this is an extremely weak argument.

A strong version of the continuity hyothesis asserts that RA stems from the effects of brain damage that have occurred over the chronic alcoholic period. In neuropathological terms we must therefore attribute RA to the cerebral atrophy characteristic of alcoholics (e.g. Lishman, 1982). We cannot attribute it to diencephalic damage because this occurs only at the acute Wernicke's stage. This being so, we would not expect to observe RA in patients who had suffered diencephalic damage similar to that of Wernicke's Disease who did not have an alcoholic aetiology. Unfortunately, the literature is unclear on this point.

Patient BY (Winocur et al., 1984) had bilateral thalamic lesions which gave rise to a severe anterograde amnesia. However, on two tests of remote memory he performed normally. Similarly, the diencephalic case NA has been shown to be free of remote memory impairment (Cohen & Squire, 1981). Von Cramon et al. (1985) studied six cases of midline thalamic infarction. They found severe anterograde disruption but only one case appeared to have a clear retrograde impairment. In contrast, Graff-Radford et al. (1984) studied four patients who had become amnesic following midline thalamic infarction and found that these patients had extensive RA when assessed on the BRMT. Similarly, the thalamic tumour case of McEntee et al. (1976) also showed extensive RA. Finally, Ignelzi and Squire (1976) found extensive RA in a case of cystic craniopharyngioma of the third ventricle which ameliorated with drainage.

Collectively these data indicate that extensive RA can be found in diencephalic amnesics without an alcoholic aetiology, but that a severe retrograde impairment cannot be predicted with any certainty unless the disorder is confounded with chronic alcoholism. This suggests that there may be more than one component to the RA associated with diencephalic amnesics. Support for this idea comes from a study by Shimamura and Squire (1986) who found a correlation between the severity of Korsakoff anterograde impairment and scores on the more recent decades of a remote memory test. Recall of older remote memories, in contrast, did not correlate with anterograde amnesia. The differential representation of earlier and more recent remote memories has been addressed by Cermak (1985). He argues that, with the passage of time, remote memories transform from having an 'episodic' quality (i.e. being event specific) to becoming general knowledge or part of 'semantic' memory (cf. Tulving, 1985).

If we accept this framework it is possible to argue that the midline diencephalic lesions disrupt a system that mediates both the retrieval of pre-morbid episodic memories and the formation of new episodic memory - the idea being that it is more parsimonious to attribute two correlated deficits to a common underlying lesion. This system might invariably be damaged in Korsakoff's Syndrome, but only damaged in a limited proportion of non-alcoholic diencephalic amnesics. The next question concerns the nature of the psychological deficit. Case PZ plus RA in non-alcoholic diencephalic amnesics suggests that the deficit must arise from a sudden disruption of remote memory. Addressing this point Parkin and Leng (1989) suggested that the contextual processing deficit thought to underlie the anterograde deficit in Korsakoff's Syndrome might also contribute to the retrograde deficit, i.e. that the processes establishing contextual relations among new memories might also maintain contextual relations among existing memories. The present study, which examined the effects of context on remote memory in Korsakoff's Syndrome, provides a test of this theory but the results go in the opposite direction to what one might expect. If the temporal gradient represents the loss of memories that are increasingly dependent on context specific information for recall, we should have expected contextual enhancement to be greatest for memories formed in the more recent parts of the pre--morbid period. The reverse trend was observed with context having most effect on the most remote and least impaired memories.

It should be noted, however, that the interactive effects of context and temporal gradient obtained here relate only to Korsakoff patients. One speculation is that contextual factors might have a different effect on non-alcoholic diencephalic amnesics - i.e. they might show proportionally more contextual enhancement in more recent pre-morbid periods. If so, this would ease the explanatory problem because one could then explain the absence of contextual enhancement effects in Korsakoff's in terms of the degraded memorial representations formed as a result of alcoholism. Alternatively the processing deficit underlying the sudden onset of retrograde amnesia in diencephalic amnesia per se may have a different cause - one which, at present, we are unable to explain apart from arguing that it may be related to the factors underlying anterograde impairment.

REFERENCES

Albert, M.S., Butters, N. & Brandt (1980). Patterns of remote memory in amnesic demented patients. Journal of Studies on Alcohol, 41, 1071-1081.
Albert, M.S., Butters, N. & Levin, J. (1979). Temporal gradients in the retrograde amnesia of patients with alcoholic Korsakoff's disease. Archives of Neurology, 38, 495-500.
Butters, N. (1985). Alcoholic Korsakoff's Syndrome: Some unresolved issues concerning aetiology, neuropathology and cognitive deficits. Journal of Clinical and Exerimental Neuropsychology, 7, 181-210.
Cermak, L.S. (1985). The episodic-semantic distinction in amnesia. in: L.R. Squire & N. Butters (eds.). Neuropsychology of Memory. New York: Guildford Press.
Cohen, N. & Squire, L.R. (1981). Retrograde amnesia and remote memory impairment. Neuropsychologia, 19, 337-356.
Graff-Radford, N.R., Eslinger, P.J., Damasio, A.R. & Yamada, T. (1984). Non-hemorrhagic infarction of the thalamus: Behavioural, anatomic and physiological correlates. Neurology, 34, 14-23.
Ignelzi, R.J. & Squire, L.R. (1976). Recovery from anterograde and retrograde amnesia after percutaneous drainage of a cystic craniopharyngioma. Journal of Neurology, Neurosurgery and Psychiatry, 39, 1231-1235.
Lishman, A. (1981). Cerebral disorder in alcoholism. Brain, 104, 1-20.
Marslen-Wilson, W.D. & Teuber, H.L. (1975). Memory for remote events in

anterograde amnesia. Recognition of public figures from newsphotos. Neuropsychologia, 13, 353-364.

Mayes, A.R., Meudell, P.R. & Pickering, A. (1985). Is organic amnesia caused by a selective deficit in remembering contextual information? Cortex, 21, 167-201.

McEntee, W.J., Biber, M.P., Perl, D.P. & Benson, F.D. (1976). Diencephalic amnesia: a reappraisal. Journal of Neurology, Neurosurgery and Psychiatry, 39, 436-441.

Parkin, A.J. (1987). Memory and Amnesia: An Introduction. Oxford: Basil Blackwell.

Parkin, A.J. & Leng, N.R.C. (1989). Comparative studies of the amnesic syndrome. in: H. Markowitsch (ed.). Information Processing by the Brain: Views and Hypotheses from a Physiological Perspective. Toronto: Hans Huber, in press.

Ribot, T.H. (1882). Diseases of Memory. New York: Appleton.

Ryback, R. (1971). The continuum and specificity effects of alcohol on memory. Quarterly Journal of Studies on Alcohol, 32, 995-1016.

Sanders, H.I. & Warrington, E.K. (1971). Memory for remote events in amnesic patients. Brain, 94, 661-668.

Shimamura, A.P. & Squire, L.R. (1986). Korsakoff's Syndrome: A study of the relation between anterograde amnesia and remote memory impairment. Behavioural Neuroscience, 100, 165-170.

Tulving, E. (1985). How many memory systems are there? American Psychologist, 40, 385-398.

Von Cramon, D.Y., Hebel, N. & Schuri, U. (1985). A contribution to the anatomical basis of thalamic amnesia. Brain, 108, 993-1008.

Winocur, G., Oxbury, S., Roberts, R., Agnetti, V. & Davis, C. (1984). Amnesia in a patient with bilateral lesions to the thalamus. Neuropsychologia, 22, 123-143.

REY'S AUDITORY VERBAL LEARNING TEST - A REVIEW

Alison Peaker and Lesley E Stewart

INTRODUCTION

Memory dysfunction is a common problem in both organic and functional disorders and is frequently the reason for referral for psychological assessment. It is clearly necessary for the clinician to have access to reliable and accurate tests to assess the nature and severity of memory deficits in order that the patient can be appropriately treated and the effectiveness of any therapy monitored.

At present, one of the most frequently used tests for clinical memory assessment is the Wechsler Memory Scale. However, this scale has been criticised on a number of points (Prigatano 1978). The test was standardised on a relatively small and restricted sample, the available norms are limited, and no age-corrected scores for the individual subtests are provided. The test is biased towards verbal functions, and the practice of combining scores from all 7 subtests to obtain the memory quotient may mask important patterns of deficit. Research on the Scale's efficiency in detecting memory deficits has produced mixed results and this led Prigatano (1977) to conclude that the WMS is not a good neuropsychological screening instrument. It must be said that Russell's revision of the WMS (Russell, 1975) and the WMS-R (Wechsler, 1987) incorporate changes which address many of these criticisms.

In recent years researchers and clinicians have been turning to alternative memory assessment procedures and Rey's AVLT is one of the tests which has appeared more frequently in the literature. This test has been used in the evaluation of a wide range of disorders and in an increasing number of empirical investigations. It has been used in studies of neuropsychological deficits following localised brain damage (Glosser, Kaplan & Loverme, 1982, Speedie & Heilman, 1983, Damasio et al., 1985), studies of memory functions in the cortical and subcortical dementias (Delwaide, Devoitille & Ylieff, 1980; Folstein & Whitehouse, 1983; Butters et al., 1986; Crols et al., 1986), and in exploring the cognitive deficits associated with tardive dyskinesia (Wolf, Ryan & Mosnaim, 1983), fragile-X syndrome (Madison, George & Moeschler, 1986), low level mercury exposure (Uzzel & Oler, 1986), hydrocephalus (Graff-Radford & Godersky, 1986; Ogden 1986), epilepsy (Mungas et al., 1985) and hemiparkinson's disease (Starkstein et al., 1987). The AVLT has also been used in studies of acute mountain sickness (White, 1984), attention deficit disorder and reading disability (Felton et al., 1987), and hyperlexia (Richman & Kitchell, 1981), and in studies of changes in cognitive function following anaesthesia (Flatt, Birrell & Hobbes, 1984), treatment with gangliosides (Miceli et al., 1977) and treatment with lithium (Christodoulou et al., 1981).

The aims of this chapter are firstly to review the literature concerning the AVLT to establish whether the apparent popularity of the test is warranted and secondly to bring together some of the findings of the studies looking at the test in clinical populations.

DESCRIPTION OF THE AVLT

The AVLT was first developed by Rey (1941, 1964) and more recently described by Lezak (1983). It is a serial learning test which involves two lists of 15 concrete nouns, List A and List B. List A is read to the subject a total of 5 times, with immediate recall being tested after each presentation. List B is then read and again the subject is requested to recall as many words as possible. This is followed by delayed recall of List A (trial VI). Finally an optional auditory yes/no recognition test may be given which consists of the previously presented word lists randomly embedded amongst semantically or phonetically related words. Lezak suggests that a 30 minute delayed recall trial can be administered to obtain further information on retention of material.

In the published research using the AVLT a number of variations to the standard procedure are reported. The number of recall trials may vary, with some authors using only three (Christadoulou et al., 1981; White, 1984), some using six (Madison, George & Moeschler, 1986) and others omitting the delayed recall trial (eg. Uzzel & Oler, 1986). Another procedural variation involves omitting the interference list (e.g. Miceli et al., 1981). Both the number and order of words may be changed: White (1984) used a 20 word list whilst Squire and Shimamura (1986), Shimamura et al., (1987) and Mungas (1985) changed the order of words at each presentation, in contrast to the usual procedure. The rate of presentation of words also differs depending on the source reference used. Rey (1964) and Taylor (1959) suggested that an interval of 1 second should separate each word but instructions provided by Lezak (1983) advised a rate of 1 per second. White (1984) presented words every 2 seconds. Mungas et al. (1985) modified the AVLT to an even greater degree by forming 2 new word lists, composed of 8 categories of 2 words each, with 4 categories containing concrete words and 4 containing abstract words. In addition, each category contained 1 high frequency and 1 low frequency word. They also provided an additional delayed recall trial of the second list and 2 cued recall trials using phonemic/-graphemic or semantic cues. To give a measure of long term retention some authors request a final free recall trial of list A after 15 minutes (Miceli et al., 1981) or 1 hour (Ivnik, Sharbrough & Laws, 1987). Others simply delay recall on trial VI for 40 minutes (Regard & Landis, 1984). An alternative form of the recognition test was described in Lezak (1976) and was used by some authors (Query & Megran, 1983, 1984: Ryan, Rosenberg & Mittenberg, 1984). They presented their subjects with a brief printed story and asked them to circle all the words they recognised from list A. Ivnik, Sharbrough and Laws, (1987) postponed the recognition test until after their long term recall and used their own 30 word list form. Squire and Shimamura (1986) and Shimamura et al. (1987) described a recognition form of the AVLT in which there were no free recall trials, but rather the subject was given a recognition test after each of the 5 presentations of the list.

Although the AVLT, in its basic form, is deceptively short and easy to administer, it provides detailed information about an individual's memory functioning. The number of words recalled on Trial I is a simple measure of immediate memory span for words. Unlike other memory tests the AVLT also examines learning ability. Scores on Trials I through to V form a learning curve, and the slope of this curve, or a comparison of recall on Trial I with the highest number of words subsequently recalled, provides a measure of verbal learning. Recall on Trial VI, following the interpolated list, gives a measure of delayed recall, and when compared with performance on Trial V may reveal difficulties in the retention of newly learned information or a susceptibility to proactive interference. A comparison of recall on Trial I with that on List B may be of clinical interest. Higher recall on Trial I than on List B may be a result of proactive inhibition, whereas the opposite pattern might suggest that the poorer initial performance was related to difficulties in changing response set rather than memory dysfunction per se (Lezak, 1983). Recall pattern can be examined for the presence or absence of primacy and recency effects - another potential index of sensitivity to proactive inhibition. Intrusion errors may also provide valuable information. Intrusions from List A on recall of List B, or from List B on Trial VI, give evidence of proactive interference, while extra-list intrusions can reveal a tendency to make semantic or phonetic confusion errors or confabulatory responses. Lezak (1983) suggests that intrusions and free associations in recall reflect a breakdown in self-monitoring functions. The tendency for a subject to repeat a word from the list more than once during recall may also relate to self monitoring functions. Rey (1964) recommends recording the number of repetitions and whether they are queried by the subject or passed unquestioned. The recognition test allows the examiner to compare free recall and recognition performance, and hence to isolate the role of retrieval difficulties and encoding or retention difficulties. A comparison of the numbers of words recognised from List A with those recognised from List B may reveal differences in the retention of overlearned material and once-presented information. The nature of the errors made on the recognition test may also be evaluated as, again, these may highlight semantic or phonetic confusion. An examination of a subject's pattern of recall may provide information on qualitative aspects of their performance such as their use of memory strategies and their subjective organisation of the material. Rey advises timing the response to give an indication of the 'rhythm' of recall. The possibilities raised by some of the recent modifications of the test may add to the richness of information which it can provide.

VALIDITY AND RELIABILITY

In order for the AVLT to be regarded as a valid test, it must be demonstrated that it does in fact measure verbal learning and memory. The relationship between the AVLT and other measures of cognitive and mnestic ability was examined by Ryan, Rosenberg and Mittenberg (1984) who, in a sample of psychiatric and neurological patients, factor analysed AVLT scores with three Verbal and three Performance WAIS-R subtests, and the Wechsler Memory Scale subtests of Mental Control, Digit Span, Paired Associate Learning, Logical Memory and Visual Reproduction. The AVLT scores included in their analysis were the sum of words recalled on Trials I to V, recall on Trial VI and the number of words correctly identified on the story form of the recognition test. Four factors emerged which accounted for 75.4% of the variance. The AVLT measures loaded on Factor 1 which was interpreted as a verbal learning and memory factor since it also had high loadings from Paired Associates and Logical Memory which are believed to measure verbal learning and short-term verbal memory respectively. The AVLT variables did not load on Factor 3 which was viewed as a verbal-comprehension and expression factor, nor on Factor 2, regarded as a perceptual organisation factor. Factor 4, an attention-concentration factor with loadings from Mental Control and Digit Span which has been extracted in previous factor analyses of the WAIS and WMS combined, (e.g. Larrabee et al., 1983) was not associated with the AVLT. These results would suggest that the AVLT provides information different from that provided by tasks of attention-concentration and verbal intelligence.

In considering the reliability of a test, there are 3 aspects which should be examined - internal consistency, inter-rater agreement and test-retest reliability. Split-half reliability is not a concern of the AVLT, due to the nature of the test. Inter-rater reliability has not been investigated to date. However, unlike the WMS and in particular the Logical Memory and Visual Reproduction subtests, the role of subjective judgement in scoring the AVLT is minimal. The main study of the test-retest reliability (Lezak, 1982) investigated the reliability and stability of some commonly used tests, including the AVLT. Most of the normal male volunteers were administered the AVLT at approximately 6 month to one year intervals. Lezak then compared performance over the test period for 4 AVLT measures: Trial I, Trial V, Trial B and Trial VI. Despite the presence of practice effects, particularly on the Trial V and VI scores, coefficients of concordance were respectable, ranging between .53 and .73. In a more recent study similar results were obtained using a proposed alternative form of the AVLT (see below). In this study Ryan et al. (1986) retested a mixed sample of inpatients after a mean interval of 140 minutes and found that reliability coefficients were highly significant.

RETESTING AND ALTERNATIVE FORMS

In clinical practice retesting of a patient's memory function is often necessary to assess whether any change has occurred. The AVLT is particularly useful for this purpose because of the richness of information which it provides. However, as the test involves repeated presentations of the same word list, the subject may retain some of the information over the retest interval. The confounding influence of practice effects may lead to an underestimation of any decline in memory function or give an incorrect impression of stability. Existing research demonstrates that savings influence scores on repeat testing. Lezak (1982) noticed a significant improvement in performance on the delayed recall trial when subjects were retested at 6 month and 1 year intervals. In Crawford, Stewart and Moore's (in press) study of the equivalency of an alternative word list (see below), those subjects receiving the same version at retest approximately 4 weeks later showed a significant improvement in performance, with savings occurring mainly on the first few trials. Similarly, Miceli et al. (1977) report an improvement over a 4 week period for patients receiving a placebo. This effect was particularly noticeable for the total score of Trials I to V.

Practice effects can be due to either or both of two factors. One is that the improvement in performance may be attributed purely to subjects remembering specific items from the test. Alternatively, it could be argued that there is a metamemoric influence - in addition to remembering the actual stimulus materials, previous exposure to the test requirements and demands may lead to an improvement in performance at retesting as subjects adopt the optimal strategy for remembering. In Lezak's study the effects of these two factors could not be disentangled as the same version of the AVLT was used at retesting. However, Crawford, Stewart and Moore controlled for the confounding effect of savings by administering a different form of the test to half of the group at retest. From their results it would appear that when metamemoric factors are examined in isolation, they do not contribute to any significant improvement in performance, and that practice effects are a result of retention of material from previous presentations.

Because the subject may retain some of the learned information the AVLT may not be entirely satisfactory for serial testing and a parallel form of the test would be highly desirable. With this in mind, Ryan et al. (1986) attempted to develop an alternate form of the test. They administered the original and parallel form in counterbalanced order to a group of 85 patients referred to a psychology department for assessment. The mean test-retest interval was 140 minutes. They reported that their alternate version was significantly more difficult than the original AVLT on Trials IV, V and VI and the total of Trials I through to V. Crawford, Stewart and Moore, suggested that this may have been a consequence of using Lezak's alternative word list (List C) as a replacement for List A. Analysis of list C with Thorndike and Lorge's (1944) word count indicated that it contained more low frequency words than List A. It has been consistently demonstrated that low frequency words tend to produce lower scores in free recall (e.g. Anderson & Bower, 1972). In contrast, the alternate form recognition test was found to be easier than the original. Again this could be explained by differences in word frequency between the original form and the parallel version: although low frequency words result in lower scores in free recall, they tend to produce higher scores on recognition tests (Anderson & Bower, 1972).

The alternate form proposed by Crawford, Stewart and Moore appears to be more satisfactory. For the new version they constructed 2 lists of 15 concrete nouns with each word being individually matched with a word from the original AVLT for word length, serial position and, using Thorndike and Lorge's word count, frequency of occurrence in English usage. The new recognition test was formed by replacing original AVLT words with their equivalents from the new lists. Words which were semantically or phonetically related to the new list were then inserted in the serial positions occupied by words semantically or phonetically related to the original AVLT, and the balance between semantically and phonetically related words was maintained. They compared two matched groups of subjects, one of which had received the original AVLT and the other the putative parallel version. Analysis of the results revealed that there were no significant differences between the groups on recall for Trials I to VI, recall of List B, a learning measure based on the ratio of performance on Trials I and V or recognition test performance.

The evidence suggests that when the same version of the test has been repeatedly used the interpretation of retest data is likely to be confounded by practice effects. In both research and clinical settings it would be advisable to use one of the proposed alternate forms for such purposes. Although independent confirmation of the equivalency of the alternative lists developed by Crawford, Stewart and Moore would be welcome, the preliminary evaluation suggests that it can be used with confidence.

RELATIONSHIP TO DEMOGRAPHIC VARIABLES

The influences of age, educational status, intellectual ability and sex of the subject on memory test performance have been well researched. However, there have been few studies which have investigated the association of such factors with the various AVLT scores.

Studies examining the performance of young versus old subjects on memory tasks have invariably reported an age related decline in performance. In particular ageing appears to be associated with a decrement in the rate of acquisition and the efficiency of retrieval of new information from memory. In a review of the effects of advancing age on memory Poon (1985) notes that age differences are most apparent when the task requires spontaneous organisational processes. As this is clearly a requirement of the AVLT, it is to be expected that older subjects will perform at a lower level on some aspects of the test. The preliminary studies with the AVLT confirm this expectation, although there is disagreement about the nature and extent of the influence of age. Query and Berger (1980) found that in a sample of patients with a variety of psychophysiological disorders (n=143) increasing age was associated with lower scores on the story form of the recognition test. Delayed recall (Trial VI) and learning (Trial I subtracted from the highest number recalled on subsequent trials) did not show an age related decline. In a larger sample of male general hospital patients, Query and Megran (1983) observed an overall age-related decline in all of the three measures examined in the previous study, with the greatest effect being on recall, and the least on learning. In Query and Megran's sample the relationship with age was curvilinear, with an increase in performance around the age of 35. This was most marked for the measure of learning, and less clear in the recall and recognition data. Wiens et al. (1988) presented results for 3 age groupings: 20 to 29, 30 to 39 and over 40 years. Despite the restricted age range, they reported that a number of AVLT components were negatively correlated with increasing age.

Higher levels of education appear to be associated with improved performance on some measures, and this interacts with the effects of ageing. Query and Berger found that in data from a sample of general hospital patients higher educational status protected against the age-related decline in learning and recognition performance. Recall was not related to educational level. In Query and Megran's study, education was found to relate to higher learning ability in their group of younger men (30-34 years), but conversely related to higher recall and recognition in their group of older men (50-54 years). The authors suggested that this could be a result of differences in methods of education over the years, with a change in the emphasis on rote learning. In the Wiens et al. study the only effect of education upon AVLT performance was found on trial V where those subjects with 16 years of education recalled a greater number of words than those with 12 years.

As with educational level, intellectual ability is known to correlate highly with performance on memory tests (Eysenck, 1977). Three of the studies cited above found that recognition scores were related to IQ. However, Wiens et al., state that recognition scores were high for all their IQ groups (the range was 80-139) and suggest that this may indicate a ceiling effect. In the Query and Berger study the recall and learning measures were not associated with IQ, whereas Query and Megran found that both learning and recognition correlated with IQ at both of their age groups. The present authors analysed data from Crawford, Stewart and Moore and found that higher intellectual ability, as measured by the National Adult Reading Test (Nelson, 1982), was significantly associated with performance on Trial I, Trial V, and the list form of the recognition test. Wiens et al. (1988) presented normative data for six IQ groups ranging from 80 to 139. They noted that performance on the learning trials is consistent for all IQ groups apart from the highest group who showed superior recall ability on all 5 trials. Except for the two extreme IQ groups, the number of words learned (V-I) was fairly similar for all groups; they suggested that the highest group demonstrated a ceiling effect on this measure. The total number of words recalled increased linearly for all groups, as did the percentage of words recalled as trial VI; the exception to this was the 80-89 FSIQ group who had the highest mean recall score of 99.5%. The authors suggested that it is possible that these subjects compensated for fewer words learned by more words remembered.

There have been few studies to date which have investigated the possibility of sex differences on AVLT performance. It is generally noted that females tend to have superior verbal abilities and that they may perform at a higher level on some aspects of memory tasks (eg Wilkie & Eisdorfer, 1977; Ivison, 1986). In view of this, it seems likely that sex differences would exist on some of the AVLT measures, although they may not be of a sufficient magnitude to affect the interpretation of an individual's performance. Wiens et al. (1988) found no significant differences between males and females on most AVLT variables although it should be noted that only 13% of the sample was female. The exception to this was a tendency for females to make fewer false identifications during the recognition test than males.

The association between demographic variables and cognitive functioning is complex, and further research is needed to explore the parameters which influence performance on the various AVLT measures.

NORMS

At present there are very few studies which present normative data for the AVLT. Lezak (1983) provides norms adapted from Rey (1964) for Trials I to V for five groups of adults divided according to age and social class (manual labourers, professionals, students, elderly labourers aged 70-90 years and elderly professionals aged 70-88 years). These norms are limited in practice as many individuals cannot be easily assigned to one of the five categories. In addition, Rey provided information on the mean number of errors and repetitions, recognition performance (including the number of false identifications) and centile scores for overall recall and overall recognition performance. Taylor (1959) also reports Rey's data and gives percentile scores for Trials I, III and V for adults and children. More detailed data for performance at various ages is provided by Query and Megran (1983) but account is not taken of IQ and social class. They administered the AVLT to a group of in-patients (n=677) in a general hospital and presented the results for Trials I, V, VI and the story form of the recognition test. This paper provides norms for the age range 15-69, in 5 year age intervals with the exception of the 15-24 group. In a recent publication Wiens, McMinn and Crossen, (1988) argue that the norms provided by Lezak and by Query and Megran may be inadequate for a number of reasons (procedural variations, cultural and educational differences, and the unspecified medical conditions of subjects) and have developed norms presented according to age, education and IQ, based on data collected from 222 healthy job applicants (age range 19 to 51 years). Mean scores are given for Trials 1 to VI, trial B, the story form of the recognition test, a learning score, percentage of words recalled on Trial VI, errors, repetitions and the total number of words recalled on Trials I to V. These authors point out that their norms should be used with caution as older age groups and females are underrepresented in their sample. They also suggest that the size of the sample should be expanded and propose a pooling of data with other researchers who are currently using the AVLT and WAIS-R.

To date there are no norms for the list form of the recognition test, for the strength of recency effects, or for the various other AVLT measures which may prove to have clinical validity.

Some authors have suggested guidelines for interpreting AVLT performance on the basis of their clinical experience. Lezak (1983) notes that a loss of more than three words from Trial V to Trial VI is an abnormal amount of shrinkage and could reflect retention or retrieval problems. She also suggests that in normal subjects few words, if any, are lost from Trial VI to a 30 minute delayed recall trial. On the basis of their work with thousands of patients, Ivnik, Sharbrough and Laws, (1987) have provided some tentative guidelines for interpreting the percentage loss between Trial V and a delayed recall Trial 1 hour later. They suggest that normal forgetting is less than or equal to 30% and that a loss of 30 - 45% indicates that, although memory problems may not be apparent to others, the individual may complain of 'memory frustrations'. They state that a loss of 45 - 60% may be regarded as 'handicapping' and that more than 60% forgetting may become 'disabling' and can interfere with every-day life. From the results reported by Uzzel and Oler (1986) intrusions and repetitions seem to be rare. They found that the frequency of such errors averaged less than one in both their control group and in a group of subjects with low level mercury poisoning.

EVALUATION OF RESEARCH WITH THE AVLT

The increasingly frequent use of the AVLT in research and in clinical practice suggests that workers have confidence in the properties of the test. The foregoing discussion indicates that the test is reasonably psychometrically sound, but has not considered whether the scores are clinically meaningful. In evaluating the research and clinical value of the AVLT there are a number of predictions and claims which can be examined.

1. As a test of memory the performance of individuals who are known to have memory problems should be poorer than that of individuals who do not have such problems.

2. As a test of verbal memory there should be a clear discrepancy between the performance of individuals with left hemisphere damage and those with right hemisphere damage. As verbal memory functions are mediated by the dominant hemisphere it is to be expected that patients with left hemisphere damage will show reduced scores, and those with right hemisphere damage will show relatively little impairment.

3. One of the unique features of the AVLT is that it provides a range of scores which are believed to reflect experimentally validated aspects of memory functioning. If this is valid then it should be possible to differentiate between different types of memory dysfunction on the basis of the AVLT scores.

4. The increasing use of the AVLT seems to have been partially a result of the assumption that it provides more detailed and more sensitive measures of memory processes than do other verbal memory tests. If this is the case, then an examination of studies using the AVLT in conjunction with other memory tests should reveal any advantages of one test over another.

Patients with Memory Impairment Compared with Patients with Normal Memory Functions

There have been only two studies which have specifically addressed the issue of whether patients with memory dysfunction perform at a lower level than those with normal memory functioning. Rosenberg et al. (1984) compared the performance of memory-impaired and non-memory-impaired patients on AVLT Trials I to VI and the story form of the recognition test. Memory impairment was defined as a discrepancy of at least 12 points between WAIS Full Scale IQ and WMS MQ or a MQ of less than 85. They reported that the group designated as having normal memory functions performed at a level comparable with the published norms, but that the impaired group performed significantly worse on all measures. Coughlan and Hollows (1984) examined the sensitivity of various memory tests in differentiating patients with generalised cerebral dysfunction, and hence likely to have memory impairment, from normal controls. They used a modification of the AVLT which provided a score based on the total number of words recalled over the 5 trials. Using a cut-off score which was 2 standard deviations below the mean of their control group, they were able to identify over 40% of the patients. However, this procedure also classified 16% of depressed patients and 4% of normal controls as memory impaired. This disappointing result may have been partly due to the practice of totalling scores over the 5 trials, which may have masked significant group differences on some trials.

Other studies can be examined with this question in mind. Both Squire and Shimamura (1986) and Shimamura et al. (1987) found that the performance on their modification of the AVLT of patients with memory dysfunctions (eg. Korsakoff's syndrome, amnesia due to anoxia or ischaemia, Alzheimer's disease and patients receiving bilateral ECT) was significantly lower than those from normal controls, alcoholics or depressed patients. Similar results are reported by Butters et al. (1986) for Korsakoff's and Alzheimer's patients compared with normal controls. O'Brien and Lezak (cited in Lezak, 1983) found that the number of words lost from Trial V to the post-interference trial was significantly higher in traumatically brain-injured patients than in normal controls. This study is consistent with the evidence reported by Lezak (1983) which suggested that a drop of more than three words from Trial V to Trial VI may reflect retention or retrieval problems.

Taken in total these studies suggest that certain AVLT scores are sensitive to independently classified memory impairment, and to the performance of patient groups which are known to have memory deficits.

Right vs Left Brain Injury

Miceli et al. (1981) looked at two AVLT scores, the total number of words recalled on Trials I to V and the number recalled after 15 minutes, in patients with either left or right localised lesions. Those with left hemisphere lesions performed significantly worse than those with right hemisphere lesions on both measures. Similarily, in a study comparing a non-verbal version of the test with the verbal version, O'Brien and Lezak (cited in Lezak, 1983) found that predominantly left brain damaged subjects had poorer retention of the verbal material than the non-verbal material, whereas predominantly right brain damaged subjects showed the opposite pattern.

The results of two studies comparing patients with focal left or right temporal lobe epilepsy are also consistent with the notion that the AVLT is sensitive to verbal memory deficits associated with dominant hemisphere dysfunction. Mungas et al. (1985) used a complex variation of the AVLT methodology, involving delayed recall of List B and phonemic and semantic cued recall of List A as well as immediate and post-interference free recall trials. They found that, while recall of the first 5 trials did not discriminate between the two groups, substantial differences in favour of the right temporal lobe epilepsy group emerged on the delayed recall trials, particularly the phonemic cued recall trial. Interestingly, they found that this pattern only emerged for recall of List A and suggested that there may have been psychometric differences between the two lists. This result might also reflect the difference in retention of overlearned material (List A) and once-presented information (List B). The second study of focal left or right temporal lobe epilepsy (Ivnik, Sharbrough & Laws, 1987) reported the scores for AVLT Trials I to V, List

B recall, free recall after 1 hour, a 'percent forgotten' score and a recognition score obtained from the number of words recognised from a printed list of 30 words. Assessment which also included the WAIS and the WMS, was carried out before and after temporal lobectomy. Before the operation none of the AVLT measures differentiated the two groups. After the operation however, there were significant differences between the two groups on all these measures, with the left lobectomy group performing significantly worse than the right lobectomy group.

The negative findings of Uzzel and Oler (1986) and Villardita (1987) would also support the hypothesis that the AVLT is sensitive to impairment of verbal memory functions. In their study of neuropsychological functioning in individuals with elevated mercury levels, Uzzel and Oler found that scores on Trial I, Trial V and the story form of the recognition test were not significantly different from those achieved by normal control subjects. As the authors note, this is not surprising as verbal memory is known to be relatively unaffected by chronic low level mercury exposure. Villardita (1987) compared right brain damaged patients with cognitively intact controls on the total number of words recalled over the 5 AVLT trials and a delayed free recall trial 20 mins later. The right brain damaged patients performed as well as the controls, suggesting that the functions measured by the AVLT are largely mediated by the dominant hemisphere.

Other reports are also in agreement. Starkstein et al. (1987) found that the average number of words correctly recalled by patients with Parkinson's disease with predominantly right-sided symptoms was lower than the number recalled by patients with predominantly left-sided symptoms, although this difference failed to reach significance. In their case report, Speedie and Heilman (1983) report scores for two patients with left dorsomedial nucleus lesions as well as for their patient with a similar right sided lesion. The scores show that the performance of the patients with left lesions was characterised by an early plateau in rate of acquisition, massive loss after interference and defective recognition scores. In contrast the right damaged patient's performance was comparable with the published norms.

These preliminary studies suggest overwhelmingly that AVLT scores are sensitive to verbal memory deficits associated with dominant hemisphere damage.

Differentiation Between Different Types of Memory Dysfunction

Because the AVLT provides detailed information on memory processes it may have clinical utility in discriminating between different types or degrees of memory impairment.

Squire and Shimamura (1986) noted that AVLT recall scores allowed some discrimination between their amnesic groups. Patients with Korsakoff's syndrome were the most severely impaired, anoxic and ischaemic patients performed at an intermediate level and patients receiving ECT were least impaired. Similar findings are reported by Shimamura et al. (1987), who administered their modified AVLT to patients with Alzheimer's disease, Huntington's disease, Korsakoff patients and controls. Again all patient groups were impaired, and again some discrimination between the groups was possible on the basis of the severity of the deficit. The Korsakoff's and Alzheimer's patients were similarily impaired on the recall and recognition tests and the patients with Huntington's disease performed significantly better, although still at a worse level than the controls. Butters et al. (1986) found that the delayed recall trial scores discriminated between Korsakoff's syndrome and Huntington's disease patients, with the former group being more severely impaired. In addition their recognition form of the test, involving recognition tests after each of 5 presentations, differentiated between the two groups, both on the grounds of severity of memory deficit, and by the type of errors made on this task. The Korsakoff's patients made both false positive and false negative errors, whereas the Huntington's disease patients tended to err on the side of false positives only, thus suggesting that the mechanisms behind the defective performance differed in the two groups.

A detailed study of the sensitivity of several of the AVLT scores to different aspects of memory and learning disorder is reported by Mungas (1983). In this study the AVLT was administered to five diagnostic groups – a) a group of amnesic patients with severe memory impairment considered to be unrelated to intellectual ability or concentration impairment, b) a group of patients with severe head injuries resulting in significant impairment of concentration as well as memory deficits, c) a group of patients with schizophrenia, and hence with memory deficits resulting from initial organisation or information processing difficulties, d) patients with childhood onset Attention Deficit Disorder, and e) a group of non-psychotic, non-neurological psychiatric patients. The AVLT scores examined were word span on Trial I and List B, recall on Trials I to V, the number lost from Trial V to VI, the percent lost over these two trials, word order position and a measure of subjective organisation.

Measures of word span did not differentiate between the groups. In order of increasing sensitivity, the measures of learning which discriminated between the groups best were the number of words recalled on Trial V, the number recalled on the delayed recall trial and the percentage lost. The amnesic groups consistently performed at a significantly lower level than all other groups, the head injured group performed better than the amnesics but worse than the other three groups and the schizophrenic, Attention Deficit Disorder and non-psychiatric groups performed at similar levels. Mungas concludes that these measures, and especially the percentage lost index show a strong relationship with the severity of primary learning deficit, and that this should have important clinical significance.

The presence or absence of serial position effects also permitted some discrimination between the groups. Group differences were apparent in the frequency of recall of words 1, 2, 3, 6 and 8 which may be interpreted as a primacy effect. Generally the amnesic group, being most sensitive to interference, recalled these words significantly less often than the other groups. The head injured patients showed a moderate diminution of the primacy effect. The recency effect was apparent in the data from all groups. The degree of subjective organisation was examined through the consistency of recall sequences from one trial to the next. On this measure the amnesic, schizophrenic and Attention Deficit Disorder groups did not differ, with each group showing no change in the degree of consistency across trials. The non-psychotic group showed a significant increase in consistency across trials, and the head-injured group showed a significant decrease. Mungas notes that subjective organisation has been found to relate to recall in intact subjects, and he suggests that this measure may be useful for assessing the role of disordered thinking or impaired information processing in memory disorders.

The clinician is frequently required to make decisions as to whether an individual is depressed or whether there is an organic basis to the presenting picture. The use of memory tests in such circumstances is common, and it is generally accepted that depressed patients may show impaired immediate memory, but intact delayed recall and recognition memory (e.g. Henry et al., 1973; Sternberg & Jarvik, 1976). There have been three studies which have examined the effect of depressed mood on AVLT scores. Coughlan and Hollows (1984) used a modification of the AVLT with groups of neurological, depressed and control subjects and tested for group differences on the total number of words recalled over the five trials. In this study severity of depression was not associated with the AVLT scores, but the depressed subjects were more likely to be classified as 'impaired' on the basis of cut-off scores than the normal controls. Similarily, Query and Megran (1984) compared the performance of alcoholic and depressed subjects and concluded that both conditions affected scores, but in different ways. They found that depressed subjects were impaired on Trial I scores, but unimpaired on Trial VI or the story form of the recognition test. The type of errors made on the recognition test proved to discriminate between normal and depressed subjects (Chiulli et al., 1985, cited in Wiens et al., 1988). They found that depressed subjects made significantly more phonemic errors than their normal controls. These studies suggest that the AVLT may have value in differentiating depression from organic impairment, although further research is needed to define any distinct patterns of functioning across the various AVLT measures in these two groups.

Only one study has explored the effect of anxiety on AVLT scores. Wiens, McMinn and Crossen (1988) found that in their normal sample the Speilberger State and Trait Anxiety Scale scores did not correlate with any of the AVLT scores. They suggest that this was not due to an absence of anxiety in their sample, and note that replication of this result would increase clinicians' confidence in the validity of test scores.

Comparison With Other Memory Tests

Squire and Shimamura (1986) examined the suitability of various memory tests for characterising amnesic patients. They concluded that the AVLT had advantages over delayed prose recall and paired associate learning, in that the latter two tests tended to be too difficult to provide information about the severity of the deficit - all the amnesic patients in this study scored close to zero on these tests. As noted above, the AVLT scores allowed some discrimination between the groups. The AVLT also seemed to be better suited to assessing the severity of memory impairment than Warrington's Recognition Test for words and a continuous recognition test for verbal material. The authors conclude that for assessing the degree of memory impairment the 'auditory-verbal test is excellent, because it obtains repeated scores and tracks performance over a wide range of ability'.

Christodoulou et al. (1981) found that a simplified version of the AVLT was more sensitive than Wechsler's Paired Associates task in detecting the effects of lithium on memory functioning. Whereas Squire and Shimamura argued that the AVLT seemed to be easier than the other test, Christodoulou et al. suggest that it is more difficult as their subjects tended to perform at a uniformly high level on the associate learning task. They note that the fact of the 15 words being logically unrelated may make the task more taxing, and hence avoid ceiling effects. These conflicting views may be reconciled when consideration is made of the fact that the AVLT is a complex test involving fairly basic memory functions, such as rote learning, at one level, and more complex functions such as organisational processes, at another. As a result it might be expected that the test would provide useful information about the functioning of subjects who are fairly severely impaired as well as of those who are cognitively intact.

In the study of cognitive deficits following temporal lobectomy discussed above, Ivnik, Sharbrough and Laws, (1987) found that some of the WMS scores, as well as all of the AVLT scores, were sensitive to the group differences, but they note that when a stricter statistic for assessing the significance of group differences was used (omega-square) the AVLT analyses fulfilled the criteria more frequently than the analyses from other tests. They recommend that research in this area should be continued with the 'AVLT and other tests that permit a more detailed evaluation of the components of learning and memory'.

If future research confirms the findings from these studies it would seem that the AVLT has advantages over other tests in its sensitivity to different levels of impairment and its focus on different aspects of verbal memory and learning processes.

LIMITATIONS AND FUTURE DIRECTIONS

The studies reviewed above suggest that the AVLT is psychometrically robust. The problems associated with practice effects on retesting appear to have been overcome now that an alternative form is available. The test has promising clinical validity in assessing the nature and severity of memory dysfunctions. Scores which are of particular interest are those based on learning over the five presentations, the loss of information on Trial VI, delayed free recall scores, recognition performance, serial position effects and the subjective organisation measure examined by Mungas. The AVLT would seem to have advantages over other memory assessment procedures in that it taps the abilities of both the severely impaired and the more able subject, and allows an analysis of the contribution of particular aspects of memory processes to test performance.

The literature on the AVLT is limited, with most of the papers being published in the last seven or eight years. As a result many of the findings are tentative and a number of areas have yet to be explored. Further studies examining the factor structure of AVLT scores in the context of other memory and neuropsychological test data are needed. It may be of interest to include some of the less well researched AVLT derived measures, such as the frequency and type of intrusion errors, in such analyses to investigate their construct validity. These measures have not been included in studies examining the reliability of the test to date, and this is another area of uncertainty. Similarily, the results of clinical studies using the AVLT, while providing valuable information on the clinical validity of the test, have not been rigorously confirmed and there are some areas which have yet to be researched. The majority of studies have looked at scores relating to span, learning, retention and recognition, and have not explored the potential of quantifying recency effects, subjective organisation, memory strategies and intrusion errors. As well as confirming the findings of earlier studies, future research should concentrate on exploring the utility of other scores in clarifying the nature of memory impairments in different clinical groups.

As regards the test itself, there is scope for further development. It is notable that many authors modify the test procedures, and in several instances the AVLT is used more as a methodology than as a standardised test. While retaining the list learning format researchers have introduced a range of variations, such as giving phonemic and semantic cued recall trials (Mungas et al., 1985), re-ordering the words on each presentation (Squire & Shimamura, 1986; Shimamura et al., 1987), developing recognition forms of the test (Butters et al., 1986; Squire & Shimamura, 1986; Shimamura et al., 1987) and changing the content of the lists to include categories and to examine differences in recall of concrete and abstract, and high and low frequency words (Mungas et al., 1985). Studies also differ in whether they include or omit the interference list and the delayed recall trial, and in the length of the interval before delayed recall is requested. Authors vary on the type of recognition test which they use, and the equivalency of the list and story forms, and any advantages of auditory versus visual presentations should be clarified, as they may impose different demands on the subject. The list form of the recognition test has the disadvantage of including only semantically or phonetically related words, and does not allow a comparison of the frequency of confusion errors with confabulations. In this respect, the story form may be more useful, although it would be relatively straightforward to retain the list format and include words unrelated to those presented for the learning trials.

The number of studies employing modifications of the AVLT testifies to the test's flexibility, and the results of these studies have indicated that some of the modifications have clinical validity and merit further study. However, one consequence of the differences in practice is that direct comparison between studies can be difficult, and authors should take care to clearly describe the procedures they have used. The clinician should also be aware of this point when referring to the literature to aid interpretation of an individual subject's performance.

Lesser variations in the administration of the test may also be a source of extraneous influence on test scores. Word presentation rate may vary in different studies as the two main sources give different instructions. Rey recommends that the words be presented with 1s intervals between each and Lezak recommends that the words be read at a rate of one per second. Wiens, McMinn and Crossen (1988) note that this may have effects on scores, with slower rates allowing more rehearsal time. Examiners may also vary in the length of time they allow for recall, and in how persistent they are in asking the subject whether they can remember any more words. These aspects of administration tend not to be reported in research studies and there are few guidelines to follow, although Rey (1964) suggested that one minute should be given for recall after the first presentation and one and a half minutes for subsequent trials. Although there is no empirical evidence indicating that these factors are cause for concern, it would be advisable for researchers to adhere to Rey's guidelines in future studies.

The instructions and feedback given to the subject may be of importance - for example, whether they are told that there will be 5 learning presentations, warned of subsequent delayed recall trials, informed of repeats in their recall and told the number of words correctly recalled at the end of each trial. These factors could influence test performance, either negatively, by causing distraction and interference, or positively, by providing encouragement and in allowing the subject to develop strategies appropriate to the task. Delayed recall scores may be affected by the nature of the activities carried out during the delay interval. Interference effects or test fatigue may affect subsequent recall and this may vary depending on whether the intervening period is filled with other verbal or visuospatial tasks or inactivity.

In many respects it appears that the increasing use of the AVLT has preceded the development of suitably rigorous guidelines for its administration. Again, further research is required to demonstrate any effects of variations in administration and set out agreed guidelines.

Another interesting possibility for further research is the development of a non-verbal analogue of the test. The earliest report of such a adaptation appears in Meyer and Simmel (1947) who presented 15 pictures from the Stanford-Binet Picture Vocabulary Test for 5 or 6 trials, with verbal recall after each presentation. Taylor (1959) also described this variation and suggested that the pictures be named as they are presented. More recently, a similar procedure was described by Lezak (1983) with the addition of an interference task (paragraph recall) and post-interference recall. She reported the results of a study by O'Brien and Lezak which suggested that this type of test is sensitive to right hemisphere dysfunction. As Taylor noted, this procedure is not purely non-verbal, but rather a combination of verbal and pictorial material. Regard and Landis (1984) described a variation which may be less biased towards verbal functions. They presented 15 figures one at a time, and measured recall through the subject's drawn reproductions. A non-verbal counterpart of the AVLT would be a valuable research and clinical instrument, and future research might aim to determine whether it is most appropriate for the subject to respond verbally or through drawings, and whether abstract shapes or easily verbalisable pictures should be used as stimuli.

For research purposes Rey's AVLT should be a valuable addition to the batteries currently used to assess and define the nature and severity of memory impairments in different diagnostic groups. However, for use in clinical practice certain other issues must be addressed. Firstly, the procedures which prove to be of the greatest clinical relevance need to be defined and standardised instructions for their administration set out. Secondly, in order to draw meaningful conclusions from the performance of an individual the clinician requires access to normative data which takes into account any subject variables which can affect scores. As noted above, the available norms are limited, and further research is required to develop a more comprehensive data base. The proposal made by Wiens, McMinn and Crossen, (1988) that researchers pool information on Trial I, V and VI and Recognition by age and IQ represents a major advance in this direction. Preliminary studies suggest that as well as further work on these scores norms may be required for the subjective organisation measure, the strength of primacy effects, and the number and type of recognition errors. Regression equations based on the predictive value of various demographic variables may be an alternative and more economical method of gaining an estimate of the expected level of functioning to compare with actual performance.

REFERENCES

Anderson, J.R., & Bower, G.H. (1972). Recognition and retrieval processes in free recall. Psychological Review, 79, 97-123.
Butters, N., Wolfe, J., Granholm, E. & Martone, M. (1986). An assessment of verbal recall, recognition and fluency abilities in patients with Huntington's disease. Cortex, 22, 11-32.
Christodoulou, G.N., Kokkevi, A., Lykourase, D. Stefanis, C. & Papadimitriov, G.N. (1981). Effects of Lithium on memory. American Journal of Psychiatry, 138, 847-848.
Coughlan, A.K. & Hollows, S.E. (1984). Use of memory tests in differentiating organic disorder from depression. British Journal of Psychiatry, 145, 164-167.
Crawford, J.R., Stewart, L.E. & Moore, J.W. Demonstration of savings on the AVLT and development of a parallel form. Journal of Clinical and Experimental Neuropsychology, in press.
Crols, R., Saerens, J., Noppe, M. & Lowenthal, A. (1986). Increased GFAp levels in CSF as a marker of organicity in patients with Alzheimer's disease and other types of irreversible chronic organic brain syndrome. Journal of Neurology, 233, 157-160.
Damasio, A.R., Eslinger, P.J., Damasio, H., Van Hoesen, G.W. & Cornell,

S. (1985). Multimodal amnesic syndrome following bilateral temporal and basal forebrain damage. Archives of Neurology, 42, 252-259.

Delwaide, P.J., Devoitille, J.M. & Ylieff, M. (1980). Acute effects of drugs upon memory of patients with senile dementia. Acta Psychiatrica Belgica, 80, 748-754.

Eysenck, M.W. (1977). Human Memory: Theory, Research and Individual Differences. Oxford: Permagon.

Felton, R.H., Wood, F.B., Brown I.S. & Campbell, S.K. (1987). Separate verbal memory and naming deficits in attention deficit disorder and reading disorder. Brain and Language, 31, 171-184.

Flatt, J.R., Birrell, P.C. & Hobbes, A. (1984). Effects of anaesthesia on some aspects of mental functioning of surgical patients. Anaesthesia and Intensive Care, 12, 315-324.

Folstein, M.F. & Whitehouse, P.J. (1983). Cognitive impairment of Alzheimer disease. Neurobehavioral Toxicology and Teratology, 5, 631-634.

Glosser, G., Kaplan, E. & Loverme, S. (1982). Longitudinal neuropsychological report of aphasia following left-subcortical haemorrhage. Brain and Language, 15, 95-116.

Graff-Radford, N.R., Damasio, H., Yamada, T., Eslinger, P.J. & Damasio, A.R. (1985). Nonhaemorrhagic thalamic infarction. Clinical, neuropsychological and electrophysiological findings in four anatomical groups defined by computerized tomography. Brain, 108, 485-516.

Graff-Radford, N.R. & Godersky, J.C. (1986). Normal pressure hydrocephalus. Onset of gait abnormality before dementia predicts good surgical outcome. Archives of Neurology, 43, 940-942.

Henry, G.M., Weingartner, H. & Murphy, D.L. (1973). Influence of affective states and psychoactive drugs on verbal learning and memory. American Journal of Psychiatry, 130, 966-971.

Ivison, D. (1986). Anna Thompson and the American liner New York: some normative data. Journal of Clinical and Experimental Neuropsychology, 8, 317-320.

Ivnik, R.J., Sharbrough, F.W. & Laws, E.R. (1987). Effects of anterior temporal lobectomy on cognitive function. Journal of Clinical Psychology, 43, 128-137.

Larrabee, G.J., Kane, R.L.P., Schuck, J.R. (1983). Factor analysis of the WAIS and Wechsler Memory Scale: an analysis of the construct validity of the Weschsler Memory Scale. Journal of Clinical and Experimental Neuropsychology, 5, 159-168.

Lezak, M.D. (1976). Neuropsychological Assessment. Oxford: Oxford University Press.

Lezak, M.D. (1982). The test-retest stability and reliability of some tests commonly used in neuropsychological assessment. Paper presented at 5th European conference, INS, Deauville, France, June 1982.

Lezak, M.D. (1983). Neuropsychological Assessment. (2nd Edit.). Oxford University Press.

Madison, L.S., George, C. & Moeschler, J.B. (1986). Cognitive functioning in the fragile-X syndrome: a study of intellectual, memory and communication skills. Journal of Mental Deficiency Research, 30, 129-148.

Meyer, E. & Simmel, M. (1942). The psychological appraisal of children with neurological defects. Journal of Abnormal and Social Psychology, 42, 193-205.

Miceli, G., Caltagirone, C. & Gainotti, G. (1977). Gangliosides in the treatment of mental deterioration: a double blind comparison with placebo. Acta Psychiatrica Scandinavica, 55, 102-110.

Miceli, G., Caltagirone, C., Gainotti, G., Masullo, C. & Siweri, M.C. (1981). Neuropsychological correlates of localised lesions in non-aphasic brain-damaged patients. Journal of Clinical Neuropsychology, 3, 53-63.

Mungas, D. (1983). Differential sensitivity of specific parameters of the Rey Auditory Verbal Learning Test. Journal of Consulting and Clinical Psychology, 51 (6), 848-855.

Mungas, D., Ehlers, C., Walton, N. & McCutchen, C.B. (1985). Verbal learning differences in epileptic patients with left and right temporal lobe foci. Epilepsia, 26, 340-345.

Nelson, H.E. (1982). The National Adult Reading Test: Test Manual. Windsor: NFER Nelson.

Ogden, J.A. (1986). Neuropsychological and psychological sequelae of shunt surgery in young adults with hydrocephalus. Journal of Clinical and Experimental Neuropsychology, 8, 657-679.

Poon, L.W. (1985). Differences in human memory with ageing: nature, causes and clinical implications. in: J.E. Birren & K.W. Schaie (eds.) Handbook of the Psychology of Ageing. (2nd Edit.), New York: Van Nostrand Reinhold Company.

Prigatano, G.P. (1977). The Wechsler memory scale is a poor screening test for brain dysfunction. Journal of Clinical Psychology, 33, 772-777.

Prigatano, G.P. (1978). Wechsler memory scale: a selective review of the literature. Journal of Clinical Psychology, 34, 816-832.

Query, W.T. & Berger, R.A. (1980). AVLT memory scores as a function of age among general medical, neurologic and alcoholic patients. Journal of Clinical Psychology, 36, 1009-1012.

Query, W.T. & Megran, J. (1983). Age related norms for AVLT in a male patient population. Journal of Clinical Psychology, 39, 136-138.

Query, W.T. & Megran, J. (1984). Influence of depression and alcoholism on learning, recall and recognition. Journal of Clinical Psychology, 40, 1097-1100.

Regard, M. & Landis, T. (1984). Transient global amnesia: neuropsychological dysfunction during attack and recovery in two 'pure' cases. Journal of Neurology, Neurosurgery and Psychiatry, 47, 668-672.

Rey, A. (1941). L'examen psychologique dans les cas d'encephalopathie traumatique. Archives de Psychologie, 28, 286-340.

Rey, A. (1964). L'examen Clinique en Psychologie. Paris: Presses Universitaires.

Richman, L.C. & Kitchell, M.M. (1981). Hyperlexia as a variant of developmental language disorder. Brain and Language, 12, 203-212.

Rosenberg, S.J., Ryan, J.J. & Prifitera, A. (1984). Rey Auditory Verbal Learning Test performance of patients with and without memory impairment. Journal of Clinical Psychology, 40, 785-787.

Russell, E.W. (1975). A multiple scoring method for the assessment of complex memory functions. Journal of Consulting and Clinical Psychology, 43, 800-809.

Ryan, J.J., Geisser, M.E., Randall, D.M. & Georgemiller, R.J. (1986). Alternate form reliability and equivalency of the Rey Auditory Verbal Learning Test. Journal of Experimental and Clinical Neuropsychology, 8, 611-616.

Ryan, J.J., Rosenberg, S. & Mittenberg, W. (1984). Factor analysis of the Rey Auditory Verbal Learning Test. The International Journal of Clinical Neuropsychology VI, 4, 239-241.

Shimamura, A.P., Salmon, D.P., Squire, L.R. & Butters, N. (1987). Memory dysfunction and word priming in dementia and amnesia. Behavioral Neuroscience, 101, 347-351.

Speedie, L.J. & Heilman, K.M. (1983). Anterograde memory deficits for visuospatial material after infarction of the right thalamus. Archives of Neurology, 40, 183-186.

Squire, L.R. & Shimamura, A.P. (1986). Characterising amnesic patients for neurobehavioral study. Behavioral Neuroscience, 100, 866-877.

Starkstein, S., Leiguarda, R., Gershanik, O. & Berthier, M. (1987). Neuropsychological disturbances in hemiparkinson's disease. Neurology, 37, 1762-1764.

Sternberg, D.E. & Jarvik, M.E. (1976). Memory functions in depression. Archives of General Psychiatry, 33, 219-224.

Taylor, E.M. (1959). The Appraisal of Children With Cerebral Deficits. Cambridge, MA: Harvard University Press.

Thorndike, E.L. & Lorge, I. (1944). The Teacher's Word Book of 30,000 words. New York: Teachers College Columbia University.

Uzzel, B.P. & Oler, J. (1986). Chronic low-level mercury exposure and neuropsychological functioning. Journal of Clinical and Experimental Neuropsychology, 8, 581-593.

Villardita, C. (1987). Verbal memory and semantic clustering in right brain damaged patients. Neuropsychologia, 25, 277-280.

Wechsler, D. (1987). Wechsler Memory Scale - Revised Manual. San Antonio: The Psychological Corporation.

White, A.J. (1984). Cognitive impairment of acute mountain sickness and acetazolamide. Aviation, Space and Environmental Medicine, 55, 589-603.

Wiens, A.N., McMinn, M.R. & Crossen, J.R. (1988). Rey Auditory-Verbal Learning Test: development of norms for healthy young adults. The Clinical Neuropsychologist, 2, 67-87.

Wilkie, F.L. & Eisdorfer, C. (1977). Sex, verbal ability, and pacing differences in serial learning. Journal of Gerontology, 32, 63-67.

Wolf, M.E., Ryan, J.J. & Mosnaim, A.D. (1983). Cognitive functions in tardive dyskinesia. Psychological Medicine, 13, 671-674.

MEASURING MEMORY IMPAIRMENT AFTER BRAIN DAMAGE : THE INFLUENCE OF
PERCEPTUAL PROBLEMS

Janet Cockburn, Barbara A Wilson and Alan D Baddeley

INTRODUCTION

Impairment of memory skills is a frequent and well recognised consequence of acquired brain damage. Both clinical and experimental studies indicate the extent, frequency and persistence of memory deficits
after closed head injury. Brooks (1984) cited a series of investigations
in Glasgow that compared the performance of severely head-injured patients with non-head-injured control subjects. These found that the head-
injured patients scored significantly lower on tests of both verbal and
non-verbal material, involving recall, recognition and relearning. Lezak
(1979), investigating recovery of memory after traumatic brain injury,
found wide variability in the extent of measurable recovery, with indications that few patients would improve their verbal learning ability in
the first three years post trauma. She further suggested that, with
increasing time post injury, other dysfunctions, that had not been immediately influential, might compromise the recovery of efficient memory
skills.

Less interest has been shown to date in the impairment of memory
performance after stroke. However, Wade, Parker and Hewer (1986) assessed the memory ability of 138 patients three months after an acute stroke
and found poor verbal recall in 29 per cent and poor visual recall in 14
per cent. It is not clear from their paper whether these two groups were
mutually exclusive or whether some patients were significantly impaired
for both visual and verbal memory. Of, perhaps, more clinical interest,
they also noted a marked reduction in measured daily living skills in
those with poorer memories. They concluded that, with regard to stroke,
'more research is needed to confirm the frequency of memory disturbance,
to delineate the processes involved, and to determine its importance.'

Although head-injury and stroke provide the majority of patients
seen for assessment following acquired brain damage, there are also
studies documenting the presence and severity of memory impairment after
tumour removal (Wilson, 1981) and herpes simplex encephalitis (Wilson,
1987). There are, in addition, extensive reports of memory deficits
following surgery to ameliorate the effects of temporal lobe epilepsy
(e.g. Milner, Corkin & Teuber, 1968); as a concomitant of Korsakoff's
Syndrome (Butters, 1985; Kopelman, 1986) and Alzheimer-type dementia
(Morris & Kopelman, 1986).

These studies cover a wide range of deficits, both in type and severity. There is also considerable variation in the purpose of the investigations. Some, such as Milner et al. (1968), concentrate on detailed
single-case analysis that documents impairment and attempts to locate

parts of the brain responsible for specific functions. Others are epidemiological, reporting a pattern of behaviour seen to a greater or lesser extent in a number of people with broadly similar aetiology, (e.g. Wade et al., 1986). It is only relatively recently, however, that considerable interest has been shown in the measurement of memory deficits as they affect performance in everyday life, with a view both to documenting the frequency of their occurrence and to investigating the success of remediation strategies (Kapur & Pearson, 1983; Wilson, 1982). Difficulties in remembering what one has been told, what one should be doing, where to go and how to get there prove serious impediments to a person's ability to respond to rehabilitation and to cope with everyday life (Wilson & Moffatt, 1984; De Renzi, 1982; Newcombe, 1985; Gianutsos & Matheson, 1987). Identification of such difficulties is an important factor in the provision of appropriate remediation.

The term 'memory' can be seen to cover a number of skills. Forgetting what you have been told is qualitatively different from forgetting the route to a house you have visited once before but both are in some way dependent on 'memory'. Theoretical concepts, such as the working memory model proposed by Baddeley (Baddeley, 1986; Baddeley & Hitch, 1974), of a central executive that controls slave systems such as the articulatory loop and the visuo-spatial sketchpad, suggest that there are at least two partially independent subsystems for processing to-be remembered material. Whichever is activated will depend on the nature of the task. The articulatory loop processes language-based stimuli whereas the visuo-spatial sketchpad is, as its name suggests, concerned with visually mediated material. This theory is supported by studies of normal subjects' behaviour which suggest independent pictorial and lexical memories converging on a common semantic system (Newcombe, 1985). It is suggested that one sub-system may reinforce another or, in the case of selective damage, may operate alone.

Since global amnesia is relatively rare and a degree of selective loss that may be evident in specific situations or only with certain types of material is more common (Wilson & Moffatt, 1984), the clinical relevance of a theory that postulates separate mechanisms for processing verbally or visually mediated material is evident. Much of the work in the area of memory loss has concentrated on localisation of lesions which produce particular deficits. The work of Milner and her associates (e.g. Milner, 1970) suggests a strong asymmetry of temporal lobe function, with damage on the left resulting in impaired recall of verbal material, such as short stories and word lists. Damage to the right temporal lobe affects recall of such material as geometric drawings, faces and tunes. Immediate recall, however, appears to be affected not by temporal but by parietal lobe lesions (Warrington & Weiskrantz, 1973), although evidence for participation of the right parietal lobe in short-term storage of nonverbal material is less strong than for the role of the left with verbal material (Kolb & Whishaw, 1985). The implication from these findings is that in normal memory the temporal and parietal lobes have a complementary function which may be upset as a result of selective damage.

MEASURING MEMORY IMPAIRMENT

Such findings, although of considerable importance in furthering our understanding of the neurological and neuropsychological substrates of memory function, may not be of much immediate value to the clinician who is required to assess and treat patients with diffuse lesions and/or a multiplicity of problems of which impaired memory may be only one. It is generally recognised that the majority of patients referred for clinical assessment after brain damage are unlikely to suffer from highly specific deficits resulting from isolated lesions. Consequently, investigation of memory problems cannot be divorced from assessment for other cognitive deficits (Brooks & Lincoln, 1984). Although many different tests of 'memory' exist, their value in clinical assessment appears to be limited. Parkin (1987) argued that memory tests designed to evaluate theories of memory are not generally suitable for measuring differences between individuals. Erickson and Scott (1977), when reviewing tests available for measuring memory in clinical settings, found that many of the available tests were 'practically unusable with patients with language or perceptual-motor impairments'. Newcombe (1985) criticised the reliance of clinicians on memory scales since these imply that 'memory' is an unitary concept on which a numerical value can be put. She further commented on the failure of memory tests to relate to functional competence outside the laboratory.

Probably the most widely used scale of memory assessment in clinical use is the Wechsler Memory Scale (Wechsler, 1945). It is heavily weighted towards the measurement of verbal memory skills, with only one of its seven component parts having a primarily non-verbal element. This can result in an overestimate of memory impairment in patients with a language disturbance or an underestimate in those with primarily non-verbal deficits. This was shown by Wilson (1982) who reported on a patient with a Wechsler memory quotient of 96, suggesting a mild memory deficit, who had profound problems with learning and remembering his way around.

A more recent test developed specifically for clinical use (Randt, Brown & Osborne, 1980) claims to provide a quantitative measure of mild to moderate memory loss, using material relevant to everyday memory. It focuses on transfer to and retrieval from long-term memory of specific items, such as a short story and pictures of easily recognisable objects, and places only limited reliance on previously overlearnt information. It does, however, appear to be highly loaded on verbal memory skills, with no obvious measure of non-verbal or visuo-spatial memory. In addition the 'clinical' group of subjects consisted of people who had subjectively complained of memory loss but who were without focal neurological deficit or prior history of depression requiring treatment. This would appear to be a very dissimilar symptomatology to that generally found in subjects referred for clinical assessment of memory impairment.

The recently published Warrington Recognition Memory Battery (Warrington, 1984) was designed to provide a standardised measure of memory deficit that would be valid across a wide age range of the adult population. Arguing that the Wechsler Memory Scale, in its reliance on a global memory quotient, disguises the possible influence of other cognitive variables, Warrington intended this test to identify the material specific memory deficits that are seen more frequently in a brain-injured population. It has been acclaimed as being particularly useful in discriminating between right and left hemisphere damage (Parkin, 1987) because it uses comparable techniques for assessment of verbal and non-verbal memory. However, the test does not identify people with deficits of delayed memory. It also places a considerable load on attention capacity during the initial presentation of the material, which renders it less suitable for a number of brain-injured subjects. Moreover, the viewpoint that memory for faces is selectively impaired in patients with right hemisphere lesions and memory for single words selectively impaired in those with left hemisphere damage may be something of an over-simplification.

Recently considerable interest has been shown in providing measurements of memory loss and of preserved abilities that relate directly to functional needs and competence in daily life. Much of this has been in the form of questionnaires and checklists, such as the study undertaken by Sunderland, Harris and Baddeley, (1983) of memory difficulties noticed by people who had suffered a head-injury and/or those observed in them by their relatives. They found that relatives of subjects whose head-injury was recent, and also of those where it had occurred at least two years previously, reported significantly more memory lapses than did relatives of a control group with orthopaedic injuries. Observations of memory deficits correlated better with standardised tests of verbal memory than with visual memory tests, suggesting that it is more difficult to be aware of visual errors committed by another person in everyday life. The generally low correlations between checklist or questionnaire responses and standardised test results have sometimes been taken as a criticism of these more subjective techniques. It may be, however, that such studies are emphasising the differences between 'memory' as defined and used in everyday life and 'memory' as measured in the laboratory.

The Rivermead Behavioural Memory Test (RBMT - Wilson, Cockburn & Baddeley, 1985) was developed in order to bridge the gap between laboratory tests of memory and self-rating questionnaires. It aims to provide an objective measure of the memory skills needed to function adequately in everyday life, to indicate the people whose memory problems will impede them and to predict the areas in which these impairments will be likely to be a handicap. The component items were chosen partly on the basis of observation by psychologists and therapists at Rivermead of commonly occurring lapses and partly in response to the findings of Sunderland and his colleagues. There are twelve items which draw on visual, visuo-spatial and verbal memory skills in immediate, delayed and prospective conditions. The population on whom the test was standardised consisted of patients admitted to Rivermead Rehabilitation Centre over a two year period with acquired brain damage and locally recruited non-brain-injured control subjects. With very few exceptions the patients included in the study were in the early stages of rehabilitation following a stroke or a head injury and had not been admitted specifically for remediation of memory problems. Subsequent analysis indicated that over 60% of them scored below the fifth percentile for non-brain-injured subjects on the RBMT.

The items in the RBMT were designed to measure different aspects of memory. Remembering a route round a room does not tap the same processes as remembering the gist of a newspaper article or remembering to ask about one's next appointment. However, statistical analysis indicated that all the items were positively correlated with one another, although none, apart from obvious pairings such as immediate and delayed story recall, were higher than r=0.5. Cluster analysis was similarly uninformative, yielding no obvious clusters of visual or verbal memory, of learning new material or of prospective memory. These findings suggested that perhaps the different aspects of memory were not easy to distinguish in a short test. However, the sample was clearly heterogeneous, with patients' scores ranging from failure on all items and performance at chance level on both parts of the Recognition Memory Test to scores as high as those produced by any control subject. It was also confounded by a mixture of aetiologies. Previous studies (e.g. Milner, 1971) indicated that there would be a dissociation in performance between subjects who had suffered from a left as opposed to a right CVA in performance on individual test items, if not on overall score. Surprisingly, there were very few differences. Only remembering a new name and retaining the gist of a short story were significantly more difficult for subjects who had had a left CVA than for those whose stroke had affected the right hemisphere. None of the items was significantly more difficult for those with a right CVA (Table 1). In contrast, there was no significant difference between the

TABLE 1

DIFFERENCES ON RBMT ITEMS BETWEEN LEFT AND RIGHT CVA PATIENTS

Item	Left CVA Mean	S.D.	Right CVA Mean	S.D.	t	p
Names	1.06	0.89	1.60	0.67	-2.93	**
Belonging	1.06	0.88	1.33	0.79	-1.38	NS
Appointment	1.30	0.85	1.45	0.80	-0.78	NS
Pictures	1.79	0.48	1.81	0.51	-0.14	NS
Immediate route	1.59	0.70	1.31	0.84	1.58	NS
Delayed route	1.47	0.79	1.26	0.86	1.10	NS
Message	1.38	0.74	1.19	0.86	1.04	NS
Orientation	1.50	0.79	1.40	0.80	0.52	NS
Date	1.32	0.91	1.19	0.92	0.63	NS
Faces	1.44	0.75	1.24	0.85	1.11	NS
Immediate story	1.38	0.90	1.74	0.54	-1.91	NS
Delayed story	1.48	0.83	1.86	0.42	-2.24	*
Total	16.33	6.33	17.17	5.13	-0.57	NS

Key: ** p<0.01; * p<0.05; NS not significant.

two groups on the Warrington Recognition Memory for Words but those with a right CVA were just significantly worse than those with a left CVA on the Recognition Memory for Faces. This does not accord with Warrington's findings for her original sample that the left hemisphere group was significantly worse than the right on recognition memory for words.

The patients at Rivermead who had suffered a head injury, and whose damage was in general more diffuse than that of the stroke patients, were performing at a lower level overall and with greater variability of scores on all the tests but were not selectively more impaired on either predominately verbal or visual tasks.

RELATIONSHIP BETWEEN PERCEPTUAL AND MEMORY IMPAIRMENT

These findings raised that possibility that there might be more appropriate classifications for investigating the presence of specific memory problems than side of lesion. Most of the patients had come to the centre at a relatively early stage in their recovery from illness or injury and memory impairment was only one aspect to be considered when assessing their needs for rehabilitation. It seemed possible that the RBMT, which set out to measure the extent of everyday memory problems, might be sensitive to the influence of other factors that were recognised as impeding recovery. Impaired visual perception, in view of its documented adverse effect on rehabilitation (Diller, 1974), appeared an important variable to consider. The Rivermead Perceptual Assessment Battery (RPAB - Whiting et al. 1984), which had also been developed and standardised at Rivermead, was in routine use in the Occupational Therapy department and data were available for approximately two-thirds of the patients who had participated in the memory study. As the RPAB does not provide a global score of perceptual impairment, one item was chosen that had been shown to discriminate well between control subjects and patients with moderate to severe perceptual problems (Cockburn et al. 1982). This is a three-dimensional copying task in which subjects have to choose the

TABLE 2

EFFECT OF PERCEPTUAL PROBLEMS ON RBMT TEST SCORE

Item	Unimpaired Mean	S.D.	Impaired Mean	S.D.	t	p
Names	1.23	0.89	0.95	0.86	1.61	NS
Belonging	1.24	0.82	1.05	0.82	1.18	NS
Appointment	1.28	0.81	1.02	0.90	1.46	NS
Pictures	1.72	0.56	1.50	0.82	1.51	NS
Immediate route	1.60	0.69	0.98	0.86	3.93	***
Delayed route	1.50	0.77	0.81	0.82	4.28	***
Message	1.30	0.81	0.88	0.91	2.40	*
Orientation	1.43	0.79	0.98	0.88	2.73	**
Date	1.42	0.85	0.89	0.92	3.00	**
Faces	1.45	0.77	0.75	0.87	4.27	***
Immediate story	1.42	0.83	1.50	0.77	0.50	NS
Delayed story	1.56	0.74	1.50	0.77	0.41	NS
Total	17.08	5.49	12.86	6.26	3.43	***

Key: *** p<0.001; ** p<0.01; * p<0.05; NS not significant.

appropriate blocks from an array in order to copy the model set in front of them.

Patients in the memory study who also had RPAB scores were classified as having 'normal perception' if their three-dimensional copying score met the RPAB criterion for normality of falling within two standard deviations of the control subjects' score. There were 60 patients so classified. The remaining 44 were considered to be perceptually impaired. RBMT scores were reanalysed according to presence/absence of perceptual impairment (Table 2). There was a highly significant difference on total score, made up primarily from differences on immediate and delayed route recall and face recognition but scores on orientation, date and message items also contributed to the difference. This supports the viewpoint that a diagnosis of poor response to rehabilitation resulting from impaired memory cannot be made on the basis of a memory test score alone without exploration of other possible contributory factors. The patients with poor perceptual scores were not significantly worse than those with 'normal' perception on the other RBMT items and scored marginally better overall on the story recall.

Not surprisingly, there was no significant difference in Memory for Words scores between the two groups, while those in the perceptually impaired group had lower Recognition Memory for Faces scores than those in the unimpaired group. There was also no significant difference between the two groups on Mill Hill Synonyms (Raven, 1958), indicating that they had been performing at a similar cognitive level premorbidly, but the perceptually impaired group had significantly lower Raven's Matrices scores (Raven, 1960) than the unimpaired group. There are at least two possible factors to consider here. One is that there is a discernible perceptual element in the skills required to complete the Matrices (Gainotti et al. 1986). It may be that this test should not be used as the only measure of current level of cognitive function with people who are suspected of having some perceptual impairment, or that the material should be presented in such a way as to minimise the perceptual element, as Gainotti et al. suggested. The other possibility to consider is that patients attending for rehabilitation who have perceptual problems have more severe general cognitive impairment than those who do not. This may endorse earlier findings that poor perceptual skills are an adverse prognostic factor in rehabilitation (Lorenze & Cancro, 1962; Taylor et al. 1971).

DISCUSSION

It is interesting to compare the aetiology of the two subgroups of patients in this study. Both the head injured patients and those who had suffered a sub-arachnoid haemorrhage were distributed approximately equally between perceptually impaired and unimpaired groups, possibly reflecting the hemisphere most affected by the damage. So too, however, were the patients who had suffered a right CVA, for which this cannot have been the explanation. There were quite different patterns of item performance and overall score for people whose damage was located by CT scan as being in the same cerebral hemisphere. This shows quite clearly that, at least for this test, there are other factors than side of lesion to be considered when interpreting the results. This is not to deny that cases exist of visual memory disorder in the absence of perceptual deficit. However, in the sample reported here, only one person, a young head-injured man with a compound depressed fracture in the right parietal area, failed the visually mediated tasks - the immediate and delayed route and the face recognition - while scoring normally on the RPAB. This would suggest that a visual memory deficit per se is much rarer than memory disorder compounded by perceptual problems.

Although these findings raise implications for treatment, more work needs to be done to identify the most appropriate strategies to be adopted. It may be advisable initially to treat the underlying perceptual problem rather than concentrate on the memory deficit, e.g. by use of visual scanning techniques, although evidence for the successful generalisation of such training methods to everyday life is not strong. Other work, such as the remediation programmes being developed by Ian Robertson and his colleagues at the Astley Ainslie Hospital, Edinburgh may give us more information on the methods that are most likely to succeed.

ACKNOWLEDGEMENT

This work was funded by a MRC project grant held by Barbara Wilson.

REFERENCES

Baddeley, A.D. (1986). Working Memory. Oxford: Oxford Science Publications.
Baddeley, A.D. & Hitch, G.J. (1974). Working Memory. in: G. Bower, (ed.) Recent Advances in Learning and Motivation Vol VIII. New York: Academic Press.
Brooks, D.N. (1984). Closed Head Injury. Oxford: Oxford University Press.
Brooks, D.N. & Lincoln, N.B. (1984). Assessment for Rehabilitation. in: B.A. Wilson and N. Moffat (eds.) Clinical Management of Memory Problems. London: Croom Helm.
Butters, N. (1985). Alcoholic Korsakoff's Syndrome: some unresolved issues concerning aetiology, neuropathology and cognitive deficits. Journal of Clinical and Experimental Neuropsychology, 7, 181-210.
Cockburn, J., Bhavnani, G., Whiting, S. & Lincoln, N. (1982). Normal performance on some tests of perception in adults. British Journal of Occupational Therapy, Feb. 67-68.

De Renzi, E. (1982). Disorders of Space Exploration and Cognition. Chichester: Wiley.

Diller, L. (1974). Studies in Cognition and Rehabilitation in Hemiplegia. Rehabilitation Monograph no.50. New York: New York University Medical Centre.

Erickson, R.C. & Scott, M.L. (1977). Clinical memory testing: a review. Psychological Bulletin, 84. 1130-1149.

Gainotti, G., D'Erme, P., Villa, G. & Caltagirone, C. (1986). Focal brain lesions and intelligence: a study with a new version of Raven's Coloured Matrices. Journal of Clinical and Experimental Neuropsychology, 8, 37-50.

Gianutsos, R. & Matheson, P. (1987). The rehabilitation of visual perceptual disorders attributable to brain injury. in: M. Meier, A. Benton & L. Diller (eds.) Neuropsychological Rehabilitation. London: Churchill Livingstone.

Kapur, N. & Pearson, D. (1983). Memory symptoms and memory performance in neurological patients. British Journal of Psychology. 74. 409-415.

Kolb, B. & Whishaw, I.Q. (1985). Fundamentals of Human Neuropsychology. (2nd Edit.) New York: Freeman.

Kopelman, M.D. (1986). Clinical Tests of Memory. British Journal of Psychiatry, 148, 517-525.

Lezak, M.D. (1979). Recovery of memory and learning functions following traumatic brain injury. Cortex, 15, 63-72.

Lorenze, E.J. & Cancro, R. (1962). Dysfunctions in visual perception with hemiplegia: its relation to activities of daily living. Archives of Physical Medicine, 43, 514-517.

Milner, B. (1970). Memory and the medial temporal regions of the brain. in: K. Pribram & D.E. Broadbent (eds.) Biology of Memory. New York: Academic Press.

Milner, B. (1971). Interhemispheric differences in the localisation of psychological processes in man. British Medical Bulletin: Cognitive Psychology, 27, 272-277.

Milner, B., Corkin, S. & Teuber, H-L. (1968). Further analysis of the hippocampal amnesic syndrome: 14-year follow-up study of H.M. Neuropsychologia, 6, 215-234.

Morris, R.G. & Kopelman, M.D. (1986). The memory deficits in Alzheimer-type Dementia: A review. in: P.T. Smith & R.A. Boakes (eds.) Human and Animal Memory. London: Lawrence Erlbaum.

Newcombe, F. (1985). Rehabilitation in clinical neurology: neuropsychological aspects. in: J.A.M. Fredericks (ed.) Handbook of Clinical Neurology vol.2 (46): Neurobehavioural Disorders Amsterdam: Elsevier.

Randt, C.T., Brown, E.R. & Osborne, D.P. (1980). A memory test for longitudinal measurement of mild to moderate deficits. Clinical Neuropsychology, 2, 184-194.

Raven, J.C. (1958). Mill Hill Vocabulary Scale. (2nd edition). London: H.K. Lewis.

Raven, J.C. (1960). Guide to the Standard Progressive Matrices. London: H.K. Lewis.

Sunderland, A., Harris, J. & Baddeley, A.D. (1983). Do laboratory tests predict everyday memory? a neuropsychological study. Journal of Verbal Learning and Verbal Behaviour, 22, 341-357.

Taylor, M.M., Schaeffer, J.N., Blumenthal, F.S. & Grisell, J.L. (1971). Perceptual training in patients with left hemiplegia. Archives of Physical Medicine and Rehabilitation, 52, 163-169.

Wade, D.T., Parker, V. & Hewer, R.L. (1986). Memory disturbance after stroke: frequency and associated losses. International Rehabilitation Medicine. 8. 60-64.

Warrington, E.K. (1984). Recognition Memory Test. Windsor: NFER-Nelson.

Warrington, E.K. & Weiskrantz, L. (1973). An analysis of short-term and

long-term memory defects in man. in: J.A. Deutsch (ed.) The Physio-
     logical Basis of Memory. New York: Academic Press.
Weschler, D. (1945). A standardised memory scale for clinical use. Jour-
     nal of Psychology, 19, 87–95.
Whiting, S., Lincoln, N., Bhavnani, G. & Cockburn, J. (1984). The River-
     mead Perceptual Assessment Battery: An Objective, Standardised Test
     for Occupational Therapists. Windsor: NFER–Nelson.
Wilson, B.A. (1981). Teaching a patient to remember names after removal
     of a left temporal lobe tumour. Behavioural Psychotherapy, 9, 338–
     334.
Wilson, B.A. (1982). Success and failure in memory training following a
     cerebral vascular accident. Cortex, 18, 581–594.
Wilson, B.A. (1987). Rehabilition of Memory. New York: Guilford Press.
Wilson, B.A., Cockburn, J. & Baddeley, A.D. (1985). The Rivermead Behav-
     ioural Memory Test. Reading: Thames Valley Test Co.
Wilson, B.A. & Moffat, N. (1984). Rehabilitation of memory for everyday
     life. in: J. Harris & P. Morris (eds.) Everyday Memory, Actions and
     Absentmindedness. London: Academic Press.

INVESTIGATIVE METHODS IN PAEDIATRIC NEUROPSYCHOLOGY

Peter Griffiths

INTRODUCTION

A branching out of clinical neuropsychology into that area concerned with developmental disorders of known or suspected neurological origin is foreseeable. The beginnings of this diversification are already evident in the titles of several major texts published in recent years (e.g. Gaddes, 1980; Hynd & Obrzut, 1981; Rourke et al., 1983; Obrzut & Hynd, 1986). Indeed, Barkley (1983) has gone so far as to anticipate the emergence of a fully-individuated specialty to which he gave the name 'child clinical neuropsychology'. The alternative expression 'paediatric neuropsychology' has crept into the literature at least once (Stoddart & Knights, 1986) and this has a certain appeal compared with the former, not simply on the grounds of phraseological parsimony, but because it directly parallels the traditional medical subdivision of 'paediatric neurology' (Gordon, 1976).

At the theoretical core of a subdiscipline of paediatric neuropsychology must rest the assumption that certain cognitive and behavioural disorders in childhood are partly, if not wholly, explicable in terms of organic or constitutional factors. This follows from the existing tenets of neuropsychological science and is axiomatic in relation to disorders where hard neurological signs are evident and brain damage demonstrable - head injury, focal epilepsy or anoxic syndromes, for instance. However, there also exists a large number of diagnostic categories, including infantile autism, attention dysfunction/hyperkinesis and developmental dyslexia, for which the concept of 'damage' (in the sense of, for example tissue infarction) is manifestly inappropriate but where insufficient is known about the nature of their relationship to brain structure for alternative models to have emerged.

Uncertainty about the status of non-acquired developmental disorders should not preclude them from the domain of neuropsychological inquiry. Nevertheless, the idea that brain factors other than damage might exert a limiting influence on specific aspects of development - or act as a 'constraint on learning' (Hinde, 1973) - must be acknowledged as being primarily a working hypothesis awaiting validation rather than a general principle. For instance, in developmental dyslexia only a handful of studies exist that attempt to provide direct evidence about possible links between literacy difficulties and atypical neurological organization (for a review, see Galaburda, 1983). There is always a risk of conviction being allowed to compensate for a dearth of facts; and the criticism, voiced by Taylor and Fletcher (1983), that unwarranted conclusions have occasionally been drawn about brain function solely on the basis of psychological measures cannot be escaped. Thus, the status of the 'organic' hypothesis in relation to the aetiology of learning disorders is, for the present, an insecure one.

There are undoubted technical and ethical difficulties involved in validating psychometric findings against neurological criteria in children who are not suffering from manifest neuropathology. While these considerations should not curtail the construction of neuropsychological tests appropriate for children and the collection of parametric data (e.g. Spreen & Gaddes, 1969), it must be accepted that the validation of cognitive and behavioural measures against known neurological criteria will inevitably be a protracted process. It might be a matter of time before the opportunity arises – say, in the form of a patient with a rare neurological lesion – to undertake such exercises (e.g. Griffiths & Woodman, 1985). In the interim, the narrow boundaries of theoretical knowledge about brain-behaviour relationships in children must be carefully observed and respected.

The clinical psychologist working in a paediatric neurology setting enjoys a privileged position in having access both to patients with a wide range of conditions and a multi-disciplinary service structure. Thus, in addition to patient care, opportunities abound for elaborating and refining child neuropsychological theory and methodology. Few of the investigative procedures in this field are routine and, despite the emergence of the specialist texts mentioned above, theoretical synthesis is a long way off. In fact, some major neuropsychological source books omit a discussion of childhood disorder altogether (e.g. Walsh, 1978; Beaumont, 1983). Against this background of patchy knowledge and under-developed methodology, the 'modus operandi' adopted by the pioneer paediatric neuropsychologist is most likely to be the single case-study or small-sample approach (Kazdin, 1982).

In the early stages of neuropsychology with adult patients the dominant role of the clinician was a neuro-diagnostic one, psychological tests being devised or adapted primarily for the purpose of localizing cerebral lesions or establishing whether the aetiology of presenting symptons was functional or organic (McFie, 1975). However, the emerging specialty of paediatric neuropsychology need not necessarily recapitulate the evolution of adult neuropsychology. With the recent, rapid advances in non-invasive neurological diagnostic techniques – such as computerized remote-sensing of brain morphology and cortical activity (Jabbour, 1977; Heiss & Phelps, 1983) – the earlier activity of localizing brain lesions on the basis of psychometric test results has been rendered largely redundant. Kopelman (1981) proposed that machines such as the CT scanner would displace the psychologist as a diagnostician, but this is an extreme view and only tenable if the goal of neuro-psycho-diagnosis is narrowly (and archaically) defined as the making of inferences about brain damage on the basis of psychological test data (see Herbert, 1964). Now that modern imaging techniques have become commonplace in the neurological examination, much of the future endeavour of applied neuropsychology – both adult and child – will probably centre on ascertaining sensory, motor and cognitive defects specifically related to known underlying cerebral derangement; developing and refining clinical measuring instruments; monitoring recovery of function following CNS insult or trauma; quantifying the behavioural effects of surgical or pharmacological treatment; and evaluating rehabilitation programmes.

The challenge for paediatric neuropsychology will be to devise investigative methods at a rate commensurate with advances in clinical neurology. Already a methodological dichotomy in child neuropsychological assessment procedures is identifiable. On the one hand may be found the multi-test battery approach represented by screening devices such as the Halstead-Reitan or Luria-Nebraska neuropsychological batteries for children (Teeter, 1986); on the other, the more theory-driven (or hypothetico-deductive) individualized approach discussed by Rourke et al., (1983). These two approaches are not seen as exclusive, but as having complementary parts to play in clinical assessment. In the early stages of the development of an emergent subdiscipline such as paediatric neuropsychology, investigative methods are likely to be derivative, and also representative of these two approaches. It would therefore be natural for existing procedures in adult neuropsychology to be identified as one potential source of information-gathering methods suitable for clinical use with children. The Halstead-Reitan Battery exemplifies how a battery-type procedure originally devised for adult patients has been modified for use with children. The alternative, individualized approach to the assessment of childhood neuropsychological problems might equally draw upon techniques already explored with adult patients, especially in its initial stages of development.

Three case-studies follow, each describing the evaluation of a child suffering from a discrete neurological syndrome. The particular assessment and management questions raised were tackled by means of an individualized approach that capitalized on procedures first applied to adult subjects. Each case illustrates how methods originally devised for the older patient might be adapted for the benefit of the younger.

METHODS AND RESULTS

Study One - Attentional Disorder in a Child with Microcephaly

Short attention span is a customary accompaniment of classical hyperactivity (Barkley, 1981). However, defective attention can exist in the absence of gross motor disturbance in a child of any age or can persist in the older child as a residual symptom of an earlier, full-blown hyperactive disorder. The current edition of the Diagnostic and Statistical Manual of Mental Disorder (American Psychiatric Association, 1980) outlines a taxonomic scheme that allows for attentional deficiency both with and without hyperactivity, but only qualitative and observational criteria are given to aid the clinician in making the differential diagnosis. The overt features of florid hyperactivity are so characteristic that recourse to more detailed procedures for assessing motor behaviour (e.g. Hutt & Hutt, 1964) may be unnecessary; but where hyperkinesis is absent, the symptoms indicative of attentional defect may present themselves in an altogether more subtle manner. The comment by Dulcan (1986) that psychological testing is superfluous in diagnosing attentional deficit disorder is a curious one given the essentially cognitive - and covert - nature of the processes involved. Arguably, in formulating the diagnosis, a sensible precaution would be to confront the child with a task that makes specific demands on the ability to sustain attention as there is no guarantee of impairment being revealed in more informal situations such as the playroom or consulting room interview. Despite the centrality of attention in all intellectual activity, it is a paradox that no measure for children is currently available commercially in the UK.

The Matching Familiar Figures Test has been mentioned as an experimental measure suitable for possible clinical use - although only as a non-specific index of impulsivity rather than one of prolonged attention (Aaron, 1981). A task which holds rather greater promise for the measurement of concentration is the Continuous Performance Test (Rosvold et al., 1956). It conforms to a traditional vigilance paradigm (Mackworth, 1969). Random letters are presented singly to the subject except that, at unpredictable intervals, the letter 'A' is succeeded by an 'X'. The

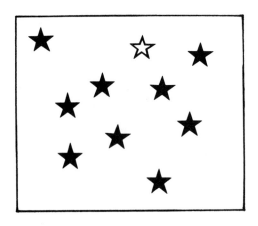

Figure 1. An example of the modified Visual Transients Test. The unfilled star indicates the stimulus which must be identified.

subject is required to detect these pairings, the total period of time spent on the task being determined by the experimenter. While the Continuous Performance Test generally fulfils the requirements of a measure suitable for clinical use with children, the letter stimuli and the task's demands on memory limit its applicability to the older, literate age group. For the younger or mentally retarded child, a vigilance task based on non-symbolic stimuli and having the potential memory confound removed would be preferable.

One task originally devised for adults that satisfies these criteria is the Visual Transients Test (Phillips & Singer, 1974). This is a simple signal detection measure in which the target is an asterisk that appears suddenly in a pre-selected position within a random array of similar stimuli. The subject responds to the target by pointing. This task was modified in order to provide an index of sustained attention in a young, borderline mentally retarded boy with microcephaly. Asterisks were located in different positions on a VDU screen by means of a micro-computer program. After 6 seconds of this display the computer presented a single askerisk in one of the quadrants of the screen and the subject was instructed to point to the 'new star in the sky' (see Figure 1. Target stimulus is unfilled). The screen was then cleared and a different array of similar density was shown, the target asterisk appearing in another quadrant according to a balanced, randomized sequence. A total of twenty-five trials was given in each epoch.

The patient was a 6 year 6 month old boy with IQ scores consistently in the upper 70's on serial testing. His head circumference was well below the 2nd percentile on chronological age norms. Although diminished in size, his brain appeared morphologically normal on a CT scan except for small ventricles. Chromosome studies revealed an aberrant 46XY ring-4 karyotype (Carter et al., 1969). His parents described him as inattentive and teachers reported an inability to concentrate in the classroom. On clinical examination he was not motorically hyperactive, but his gaze was apt to wander and he had to be frequently re-directed to the task in hand. In order to quantify this apparent attentional dysfunction, he was tested on the modified Visual Transients Task described above and his results compared with those from a like-aged group of 10 normally developing control children.

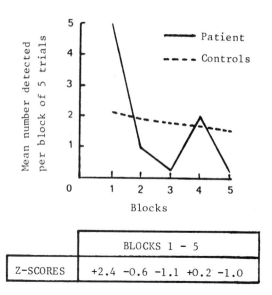

	BLOCKS 1 - 5				
Z-SCORES	+2.4	-0.6	-1.1	+0.2	-1.0

Figure 2. Performance of a microcephalic child
and aged matched control group (n=10) on the
modified Visual Transients Test. The patients'
Z-scores are shown underneath the graph.

The graph in Figure 2 is an example of the findings obtained from a
block of 25 trials. It depicts the relative signal detection performance
over time of the microcephalic child and the controls. Discrepancies are
given beneath as Z-scores. Similar results were found on repeated test-
ings, providing experimental corroboration of the clinical and anecdotal
evidence. The patient's data suggest that he was able to sustain attention for short periods only. After an initial phase of good signal
detection, the remainder of the vigilance period was characterized by
erratic performance. Compared with the control children, the patient
appeared markedly deviant in this ability (see Z-scores, Figure 2).
Despite their somewhat low average detection rate, the non-neurologically
impaired children were at least able to sustain attention over the 25
trial test period, whereas the patient failed to concentrate consistently. Combining the findings of the standardized IQ tests with those
from the Visual Transients Test, the most likely formulation of this
child's developmental problems is that retarded intelligence and attentional dysfunction were both functional correlates of his microcephaly.
A diminution in the overall size of the cerebrum can perhaps best be
regarded as a global brain malformation, but the mechanism by which the
ring-4 chromosome anomaly expresses itself to produce this phenotypic
aberration remains a matter for speculation.

Study Two – Topographical Disorientation in a Child with Septal Agenesis

Not every malformation of the CNS involves a generalized growth
disorder of the brain such as microcephaly. Occasionally structures
within the brain are selectively malformed. Midline structures seem to
be especially susceptible to intra-uterine growth failure and the psychological effects of agenesis of the largest of these organs, the corpus
callosum, have begun to be documented (e.g. Milner & Jeeves, 1979). A
rarer midline malformation syndrome is that of septo-optic dysplasia. In
this condition, the ·septal area of the limbic system fails to grow,

usually along with the optic chiasm and the anterior portion of the corpus callosum. Customarily the pituitary gland is under-active (Hale & Rice, 1974).

Results from studies of rats with surgically-induced septal lesions have suggested that the septum plays an important role in mediating whole-body spatial behaviour such as maze learning (Fried, 1972). The opportunity to investigate this hypothesis in a human subject arose when a 13 year old girl with septo-optic dysplasia was referred for neuropsychological assessment. Optic nerve hypoplasia had rendered her totally blind, however the cerebral hemispheres were intact and her Verbal IQ was above average at 122. The main presenting symptom was an inordinate inability to learn place-to-place routes within familiar, everyday settings such as home and school. Her topographical disorientation was so severe that her parents reported her incapable of finding her way from one room to another at home and at her residential school for the blind she required constant guidance from other pupils when changing classrooms for different academic subjects and activities. She had failed to benefit from several years of mobility training and teaching staff considered her navigational problems to be excessive even in relation to those normally exhibited by the congenitally blind.

This apparent specific learning disability was investigated formally by means of a route-finding task, the construction of which was inspired by one originally devised for the study of adults who had sustained localized brain-damage as a result of wartime missile wounds (Semmes et al., 1950). To measure the patient's ability to learn simples routes, a floor-maze in the form of a 'Union Flag' pattern was made out of raised rubber strips. Three small, hand-held tactile maps of the same pattern were then cut out of thick card and mounted on hardboard. Each bore a route indicated by sandpaper strips superimposed on the card, the task for the subject being to feel the maps and to reproduce the routes accurately by walking through the floor-maze (see Figure 3 for example).

The navigational performance of the child with septo-optic dysplasia was compared with that of a congenitally blind, CA-matched control whose condition was aetiologically different (Leber's amaurosis). Four repeated, map-assisted learning trials were given to each subject for each route. A fifth trial was attempted from memory. If an error were made at any choice-point, one penalty mark was recorded and the child directed along the correct path and allowed to continue. The results for the two children are given in Figure 4.

It can be seen from Figure 4 that the control child's data conformed to a normal learning curve and that minimal forgetting was present on the memory trial. By contrast, the child with septo-optic dysplasia failed utterly to benefit from practice and remembered virtually nothing of the topographical information contained in the maps. The results from this formal neuropsychological investigation thus confirmed the impression gained by her caretakers that she suffered from an atypical navigational deficiency - even in relation to her blind peers. It has been argued elsewhere, first, that the cognitive deficit could be explained in terms of the patient's congenital neurological lesion and, second, that the absence of the septal area would render the achievement of independent mobility by training methods virtually impossible (Griffiths & Hunt, 1984). Nothing in the child's more recent history has arisen to gainsay this somewhat pessimistic prognosis.

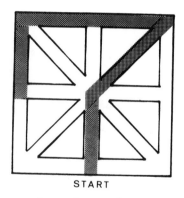

START

Figure 3. Floor plan of the maze
used in study two.

Study Three — Language Lateralization in a Child with Temporal Lobe
Epilepsy

Malformations of the brain result from little understood influences
on growth process during the embryological period. Post-natally, however, the brain still remains at risk of damage from hostile external
agents. The temporal lobes are particularly vulnerable and liable to
incur damage as a result of oedema accompanying, for example, viral
encephalopathy. The ensuing lesion can give rise to an epileptogenic
focus. In addition to seizures, conduct and personality disorders are
common sequelae (Gordon, 1976).

A 7 year old boy with unilateral temporal lobe epilepsy was referred
for neuropsychological investigation, the central question being which
cerebral hemisphere was dominant for language. Electroencephalography
revealed a seizure focus in the left anterior temporal lobe. Meningitis
at 8 months of age was assumed to have been responsible for the lesion.
He manifested many of the classic behaviours of the syndrome including
impulsivity and fluctuating attention, but of primary interest neuropsychologically was the fact that he was left-handed in the absence of
any family history of sinistrality.

Little is known about the cerebral organization of non-familial
left-handers, but one theory states that in some of these a dynamic
rearrangement of function occurs following early injury to the left
hemisphere (Levy & Gur, 1980). In these so-called 'pathological' left-
handers, the functionally plastic brain in early childhood is thought to
compensate for lateralized damage in the left hemisphere by developing
language and motor skills predominantly in the right. Following amytal
testing of left-handers with and without early left hemisphere damage,
Rasmussen and Milner (1975) produced some evidence to support this
theory. They found that within a sample of non-pathological left-handers
only 15% had right hemisphere speech representation, whereas 51% of pathological left-handers showed this pattern.

The investigation of the patient in the present case-study was at an
early stage and amytal testing was rejected on ethical grounds as being
too stressful a method for determining cerebral dominance. Instead, non-
invasive dichotomous perception techniques were chosen as a means of
providing some initial indications. Dichotic listening and split visual-
field procedures have been used extensively in the study of adult neuropsychological patients and in the experimental study of childhood learning disorder. The majority of the latter have employed verbal stimuli;

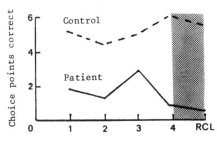

Figure 4. Performance of a blind child with
septal agenesis and a blind-matched control on
the route-finding task used in study two.

but in some, responses to non-verbal stimuli have been explored (e.g.
Smith & Griffiths, 1987). The application of dichotomous perception tech-
niques to clinical assessment problems with children is increasing (e.g.
Pohl, 1979).

The epileptic patient was tested on four visual hemifield tasks in
which the stimuli were competing, tachistoscopically-presented letters,
digits, words and arrowheads. The arrowhead task was derived from one
originally devised for adult brain-damaged patients in which the orientations of straight lines had to be judged (Benton, 1969). In respective
tasks, two pairs of letters, two pairs of digits, one pair of consonant-
vowel-consonant words and one pair of arrowheads oriented in different
directions were flashed simultaneously to each visual field. The exposure duration was 5 milliseconds throughout. The child was instructed to
try and detect all the stimuli. An oral response was required, except
for the arrowhead task in which a matching-to-sample procedure was used.
In addition, the child was tested on a dichotic listening measure in
which the stimuli were one to four pairs of spoken digits.

An analysis by competing stimulus pairs was performed on the data
derived from each of the five tests. The results, expressed as percentage correct scores, are shown in Table 1. The columns relate to
whether both or neither stimuli of each simultaneously-presented pair
were reported, or only those relayed to the left or right sensory field.
Comparing the child's detection rates in the left-only and right-only
columns of Table 1, it can be seen that, for the verbal items, substantially more left-field stimuli were detected, whereas, for the difficult-
to-verbalize stimuli (arrowheads), the results were equivocal. This left
hemi-field advantage for verbal dichotomous material runs counter to prediction; however, it may be explicable in terms of the child's known left
hemisphere lesion and non-familial left-handedness. The experimental
findings lend support to the view that language functions had developed
in the child's right cerebral hemisphere following the early encephalo-
pathic illness, this unconventional organization presumably having arisen
as a compensatory reaction to localized damage in the left temporal area.
The unclear findings from the arrow orientation task suggest either bi-
hemispheric processing of spatial information, or a retention of this
capacity by the intact right hemisphere but at a much diminished level.

Throughout his life, the patient's seizures had resisted remediation
by anti-convulsant medication. In the event of persistent intract-
ability, the option of surgical resection of the damaged lobe remains

TABLE 1

	STIMULUS	MODALITY	BOTH	LEFT	RIGHT	NEITHER
1.	Letters	Visual	30.0	30.0	17.5	22.5
2.	Digits	Visual	83.0	13.0	2.5	2.5
3.	Words	Visual	50.0	30.0	10.0	10.0
4.	Arrows	Visual	56.3	25.0	18.7	0.0
5.	Digits	Auditory	3.5	87.0	7.8	1.7

(Falconer, 1971). A decision to operate would not be taken solely on the basis of data derived from dichotic listening and visual hemifield tests. In the final analysis, amytal testing would be necessary. The neuro-psychological measures desribed above, however, are simple for the clinician to administer (the intra-subject design obviates the need for testing of control subjects) and are not intrinsically stressful for children, even those as young as the boy described here. Amytal testing would be one method of establishing the criterion validity of the dichotomous perception tests and, if neurosurgery were performed, the degree of post-operative language retention would be the ultimate validation. For the moment, the lateralization indices obtained by non-invasive methods are strongly suggestive of the patient having developed language in the right cerebral hemisphere and point towards the probability of language being largely spared were a left temporal lobectomy eventually performed.

DISCUSSION

The three case studies summarized above illustrate how investigative methods devised primarily for studying adult patients may profitably be applied to the assessment of children with neurologically-based disorders. Modifications to either stimulus materials, testing procedures or both were necessary in all three cases in order to adjust the demand characteristics of the task to the developmental level of the child. However, many of these changes were comparatively minor.

For each subject, an individualized as opposed to a battery-type approach to the quantification of neuropsychological variables was adopted, each study representing a miniature experiment. In keeping with conventional neuropsychological research paradigms, the independent variable was the presence or absence of a neurological lesion and the dependent variable performance level on a cognitive task. In attempting to determine the effect of the various lesions on the chosen outcome measures, simple control procedures were adopted; however, the specificity of these effects must remain an open question given the limitations of the studies and their essential purpose, namely, to provide clues to the solution of clinical problems. For instance, in Study One, it would be foolhardy to suggest vigilance performance was related uniquely to microcephaly. Poor performance on a protracted signal detection task may be a feature of intellectual retardation whatever the aetiology, although generalizations of this kind await empirical validation. The Visual Transients Task as a method for assessing vigilance could find immediate application in clinical practice. For instance, the identification of hyperactive children who respond favourably to treatment by stimulant medication remains a trial-and-error procedure, as does establishment of the optimal therapeutic dose (Taylor, 1983). A vigilance measure like the Visual Transients Test might prove a valuable adjunct to the rating scales (Barkley, 1981), mobility indices (Kavale, 1982) and clinical judgments that are customarily used in evaluating drug treatments.

In the paediatric neuropsychology setting, opportunities can arise for the clinician to make a significant contribution to general neuropsychological theory in addition to making improvements to existing methodology. The child described in Study Two demonstrates this point. She represented a rare chance to explore the role of the septal area in the control of movement at the human level. Hitherto, only comparative data were available, and these from studies of artificially lesioned animals. The findings obtained from Study Three also have implications for theory. In particular, they speak to the issue of functional plasticity in the young brain and corroborate the view that, following unilateral damage, functions can be selectively spared by means of a mechanism that promotes their elaboration in the undamaged hemisphere (cf. Dennis & Whitaker, 1976).

In deciding what investigative methods to adopt, the practitioner working with children is faced with a choice between the battery approach – which featured prominently in the early days of adult neuropsychology – and the individualized approach as illustrated by the above studies. The relative merits and demerits of each have been discussed by Rourke and Adams (1984). The battery approach has the advantage of being wide-ranging in scope. Its use minimizes the chance of the clinician missing an important dysfunction in the cognitive make-up of the patient; and, unquestionably, it has a central role to play in diagnostic screening. By contrast, the advantage of the individualized approach is that it allows for specific hypotheses to be set up, then tested by procedures that approximate to the design and conventions of the formal scientific experiment. Part of the challenge of the individualized approach is that novel and creative solutions to data-gathering problems may have to be devised. It may occur that information will be sought about variables for which no measures are readily available or which exist in other fields such as adult or experimental neuropsychology. The future of assessment methodology in paediatric neuropsychology will probably lie in an amalgam of these two approaches. A dual-stage process can be envisaged in which information is obtained initially on a broad front by means of norm-referenced, multi-test batteries – then more narrowly by means of miniature experiments or quasi-experiments that are devised on an individualized basis and which address specific hypotheses.

REFERENCES

Aaron, P.G. (1981). Diagnosis and remediation of learning disabilities in children: a neuropsychological key approach. in: G.W. Hynd & J.E. Obrzut (eds.), Neuropsychological Assessment and the School-Age Child. New York: Grune & Stratton.
American Psychiatric Association. (1980). Diagnostic and Statistical Manual of Mental Disorders, (3rd Edit.). Washington: American Psychiatric Association.
Barkley, R. (1981). Hyperactive Children: A Handbook for Diagnosis and Treatment. New York: Guilford.
Barkley, R. (1983). Neuropsychology: introduction. Journal of Clinical Child Psychology, 12, 3-5.
Beaumont, J.G. (1983). Introduction to Neuropsychology. Oxford: Blackwell.
Benton, A.L. (1969). Disorders of spatial orientation. in: P. Vincken & G. Bruyn (eds.), Handbook of Clinical Neurology, Vol.3. Amsterdam: North Holland.

Carter, R., Baker, E. & Hayman, D. (1969). Congenital malformations associated with a ring-4 chromosome. Journal of Medical Genetics, 6, 224-227.

Dennis, M. & Whitaker, H.A. (1976). Language acquisition following hemi-decortication. Brain and Language, 3, 404-433.

Dulcan, M.K. (1986). Comprehensive treatment of children and adolescents with attention deficit disorders: the state of the art. Clinical Psychology Review, 6, 539-569.

Falconer, M.A. (1971). Anterior temporal lobectomy for epilepsy. in: V. Logue (ed.). Operative Surgery, Vol. 14. London: Butterworth.

Fried, P.A. (1972). Septum and behaviour: a review. Psychological Bulletin, 78, 292-310.

Gaddes, W.H. (1980). Learning Disabilities and Brain Function. New York: Springer-Verlag.

Galaburda, A. (1983). Developmental dyslexia: current anatomical research. Annals of Dyslexia, 33, 41-53.

Gordon, N. (1976). Paediatric Neurology for the Clinician. London: SIMP, Heinemann.

Griffiths, P. & Hunt, S. (1984). Specific spatial defect in a child with septo-optic dysplasia. Developmental Medicine and Child Neurology, 26, 391-400.

Griffiths, P. & Woodman, C. (1985). Conjugate lateral eye movements and cognitive mode. Neuropsychologia, 23, 257-262.

Hale, B.R. & Rice, P. (1974). Septo-optic dysplasia: clinical and embryological aspects. Developmental Medicine and Child Neurology, 16, 812-820.

Heiss, W.D. & Phelps, M.E. (1983). Positron Emission Tomography of the Brain. Berlin: Springer-Verlag.

Herbert, M. (1964). The concept and testing of brain damage in children: a review. Journal of Child Psychology and Psychiatry, 5, 197-216.

Hinde, R.A. (1973). Constraints on Learning. London: Academic Press.

Hutt, S.J. & Hutt, C. (1964). Hyperactivity in a group of epileptic brain-damaged children. Epilepsia, 5, 334-351.

Hynd, G.W. & Obrzut, J.E. (1981). Neuropsychological Assessment and the School-Age Child. New York: Grune & Stratton.

Jabbour, J.T. (1977). Atlas of CT Scans in Paediatric Neurology. London: Kimpton.

Kavale, K. (1982). The efficacy of stimulant drug treatment for hyperactivity. Journal of Learning Disabilities, 15, 280-289.

Kazdin, A.E. (1982). Single Case Research Designs. Oxford: OUP.

Kopelman, M. (1981). Psychological aspects of neurology. British Journal of Hospital Medicine, Oct., 367-379.

Levy, J. & Gur, R.C. (1980). Individual differences in psychoneurological organization. in: J. Herron (ed.). Neuropsychology of Left Handedness. New York: Academic Press.

Mackworth, J.F. (1969). Vigilance and Habituation. Harmondsworth: Penguin.

McFie, J. (1975). Assessment of Organic Intellectual Impairment. London: Academic Press.

Milner, A.D. & Jeeves, M.A. (1979). A review of behavioural studies of agenesis of the corpus callosum. in: I.S. Russell, M.W. Van Hof and G. Berlucchi (eds.). Structure and Function of Cerebral Commissures. London: Macmillan.

Obrzut, J.E. & Hynd, G.W. (1986). Child Neuropsychology, Vol. 2. London: Academic Press.

Phillips W.A. and Singer W. (1974). Function and interaction of On and Off transients in vision: I - Psychophysics. Experimental Brain Research, 19, 493-506.

Pohl, P. (1979). Dichotic listening in a child recovering from acquired aphasia. Brain and Language, 8, 372-379.

Rasmussen, T. & Milner, B. (1975). Clinical and surgical studies of the cerebral speech areas in man. in: K.J. Zulch, O. Creutzfield & G.C. Galbraith (eds.), Cerebral Localization. Berlin: Springer-Verlag.

Rosvold, H.E., Mirsky, A.F., Sarason, I., Bransome, E.D., & Beck, L.H. (1956). A continuous performance test of brain damage. Journal of Consulting Psychology, 20, 343–350.

Rourke, B.P. & Adams, K.M. (1984). Qualitative approaches to the neuro-psychological assessment of children. in: R.E. Tarter & G. Goldstein (eds.). Advances in Clinical Neuropsychology, Vol.2. New York: Plenum.

Rourke, B.P., Bakker, D.J., Fisk, J.F. & J.D. Strang. (1983). Child Neuropsychology. New York: Guilford.

Semmes, J., Weinstein, J., Ghent, L. & Teuber, H-L. (1955). Spatial orientation in man after cerebral injury. Journal of Psychology, 39, 227–244.

Smith, K. & Griffiths, P. (1987). Defective lateralized attention for non-verbal sounds in developmental dyslexia. Neuropsychologia, 25, 259–268.

Spreen, O. & Gaddes, W.H. (1969). Developmental norms for 15 neuro-psychological tests age 6 to 15. Cortex, 5, 171–191.

Stoddart, C. & Knights, R.M. (1986). Neuropsychological assessment of children. in: J.E. Obrzut & G.W. Hynd (eds.). Neuropsychological Assessment and the School-Age Child. New York: Grune & Stratton.

Taylor, E. (1983). Hyperactivity: drug response and diagnostic validation. in: M. Rutter (ed.). Developmental Neuropsychiatry. New York: Guilford.

Taylor, H.G. & Fletcher, J.M. (1983). Biological foundations of specific developmental disorders: methods, findings and future directions. Journal of Clinical Child Psychology, 12, 46–65.

Teeter, P.A. (1986). Standard neuropsychological batteries for children, in: J.E. Obrzut & G.W. Hynd (eds.). Neuropsychological Assessment and the School-Age Child. New York: Grune & Stratton.

Walsh, K.W. (1978). Neuropsychology: A Clinical Approach. Edinburgh: Churchill Livingstone.

ATTENTION, CHILDREN AND HEAD INJURY

David A Johnson

INTRODUCTION

We are supposed to know what attention is, by the perpetual quoting
of William James, but it is clear from the literature and clinical
experience that we know very little of the nature and significance of
attentional disorder following head injury in children. Attention is
fundamental to the smooth, efficient, integrated and almost effortless
functioning of the healthy nervous system, and is highly dependent on the
integrity of the brain (Posner & Presti, 1987). The variety of attentional problems with which one is presented clinically suggests that the
reified construct of attention cannot be a single entity. If we examine
behaviour carefully we may infer that attention has distinct components,
which presumably reflect different aspects of brain state (Nissen, 1986).
Attempting an adequate definition of attention is, therefore, difficult.
It seems to represent an ability of the alert individual to process
information, direct and sustain selective mental effort for specific
periods of time to specific tasks. These key elements are often referred
to interchangably, so a brief description may be helpful:

Arousal-alertness. Phasic changes in arousal affect the speed with
which we become aware of and respond to stimuli. Without appropriate
arousal levels behaviour cannot be planned nor implemented. Lack of
control over arousal makes the normal registration of information impossible. The underaroused nervous system is unable to fully process information before it is lost or decays, so only partially coded information
may be stored. Conversely, increased arousal is generally accompanied by
increased performance up to an optimal point beyond which higher arousal
lessens performance. The system is overloaded and reacts with automatisms, or well-learned habits.

Information processing. Information received by the nervous system
is processed through a number of stages which transform and extract
details from the stimulus, up to the stage of response selection. It is
highly dependent upon arousal.

Selectivity. Selectivity allows the individual to effectively focus
or divide attentional resources, depending on the stimulus saliency and
situational demands. Selectivity is necessary to deal with the continuous
stream of information received through normal sensory input (Luria, 1973;
Moskovitch, 1979).

Effort. The coordinating element representing expenditure of mental
energy, necessary to maintain active processing of information.

Vigilance. Vigilance or sustained attention is phasic, and cannot be continuously maintained (James, 1899), because of limited capacity, or lack of control over other elements.

Capacity. Capacity is determined by the structural limits of the nervous system. Children may have generally smaller functional capacity (Chi & Gallagher, 1982), making it difficult to disentangle any structural deficits from an inability to deal with that limitation.

The broad dichotomy of involuntary (automatic), and voluntary (controlled) attention (James, 1899; Schneider & Schiffrin, 1977), may help elucidate the normal development of attentional processes and their traumatic disruption. Automatic attention operates involuntarily without conscious effort, and relies on stored experience and skills in long term memory. Attentional resources are required for fast and efficient multiple processing, with conservation and extension increasing with automaticity. Conversely, controlled attention operates when the amount, complexity or novelty of input exceeds available resources. It is voluntary, usually serial, slower, and demands more attentional resources, especially consciously controlled mental effort.

Attention essentially represents control over different levels of fundamental brain activity, which must combine to form a system of knowledge or long term memory. Knowledge allows greater efficiency in the acquisition of information. With practice behaviour becomes easier to pick up and more automatic, allowing more time to acquire new and potentially useful information. When a child first experiments with walking he must focus and sustain attention just to remain upright (Piontkowski & Calfee, 1979). The task is new, difficult and all demanding, so attentional processing is slow, deliberate and demands effort to be sustained. As with all new learning, few well learned automatisms exist and all controlled attentional resources are focused onto the present task. But the young child is naturally vulnerable to outside distractions or intrusions which interfere with attentional control and, therefore, performance.

Time pressure is crucial to efficient attention because it relates to the extent of automatisation and available resources (Kail & Bisanz, 1982; Van Zomeran, Brouwer & Deelman, 1984). Controlled attention may fail, for example, simply because of the pace of a task, when the resources become overloaded and attention disrupted. A divided attention deficit (Schneider & Shiffrin, 1977) may arise for several reasons: interference arising through lack of control, fatigue through inadequate resources, or when the processing rate is lower than the task demands. Developmental limitations of attention, as in the infant's walking example above, or in the case of the child's distractibility in early school, seem to parallel the breakdown of attention after head injury in both child and adult. It is clinically interesting to observe how significant head trauma can highlight the presence of such a dichotomous construct as automatic-controlled processing. Typically automaticity is lessened after cerebral injury, behaviour becomes voluntary, highly conscious, mentally and physically exhausting (c.f. Brodal, 1973).

From this highly simplified breakdown it is evident that the broad concept of attention must be carefully delineated not only if we are to explain post-traumatic functioning, but as a necessary prerequisite to the refinement and clinical implementation of attentional rehabilitation. It is no use whatsoever that we simply document that a child 'doesn't pay attention'. It may prove necessary to further analyse the components of attention (e.g. Chi & Gallagher, 1982) without necessarily reaching a stage of extreme reductionism. We may find that the underlying processes in attention develop at different rates, which would be of considerable practical importance in rehabilitation. For example, reaction time generally slows with age and is a sensitive indicator of cerebral dysfunction. On the basis of electromyographic and simple reaction time data, Chi and Gallagher (1982) suggest that response selection may be a primary source of developmental differences in reaction time. In rehabilitation such findings may suggest the need to focus on the speed at which information is presented, rather than speed of response.

NEUROLOGICAL CONTROL

Complex behaviours such as attention do not arise at birth but, as Vygotsky observed, are shaped by the adult who provides a clear external structure or framework to facilitate the infant's response. Throughout learning and development there are increasingly greater demands for concentration, selection of goals or targets, physical and mental effort. This follows a general sequence of external input leading, with practice, to internalisation and increasing automaticity. As behaviour changes so the underlying neurological organisation also changes (Luria, 1973, Das & Varnhagen, 1986). The child achieves the beginning of stable, controlled and socially-organised attention as he begins formal schooling. These '...social roots of the higher forms of voluntary attention...bridged the gap between the elementary forms of involuntary attention and the higher forms of voluntary attention...' (Luria, 1973 p.262-3).

Attentional control develops from the inherent plasticity of the nervous system (James, 1899), reflected by the development of self-awareness and self-regulation (Bromley, 1977; Gibson & Rader, 1979). The brain normally regulates its level of arousal as a function of the demands for attention (Kahneman, 1973). As the complexity of any task increases, so self-regulation becomes even more important in terms of effort and control of impulsive or incorrect responding. Simplified models of attention's neurological bases (Pribram & McGuinness, 1975; Mesulam, 1981) generally involve at least two reciprocal pathways between the brainstem, limbic and cortical regions, with complex interactions between structural and functional areas (Luria, 1973), and neurochemical substrates which may alter attention qualitatively (McGuinness & Pribram, 1980). The brainstem reticular activating system is the most fundamental of the brain's self-regulatory processes (Lindsley, 1960) and is generally regarded as the critical component in arousal and alertness. It receives large numbers of collaterals from many ascending and descending pathways, and provides major ascending cholinergic and monoaminergic pathways to interact with subcortical (thalamic and hippocampal), and highly developed cortical (frontal and parietal) systems. This neurological self-regulation may exist asymmetrically within the right cerebral hemisphere (Heilman & Van Den Abel, 1980; Mesulam, 1981; Tucker & Williamson, 1984) leading to differential responses on some tests of attention, such as reaction time.

PATHOLOGY

Many of the brain's structures and pathways associated with attention and memory are disrupted by head trauma. The actual pathology involved in any case will of course depend upon the mechanism and type of injury. In road traffic accidents, for example, the typically severe biomechanical forces involved in the rapid acceleration, rotation and deceleration of the soft brain within the rigid confines of the skull cause severe disruption of normal function throughout the brain, with focal areas of damage primarily in the anatomically prone orbito-frontal and antero-temporal regions. The resultant picture is likely to be a widespread combination of structural damage and metabolic disruption.

The peak incidence for children's head injury occurs at ages 2-3, 8-9 and 10-12 (Levin, Ewing-Cobbs & Benton, 1984; Johnson, 1985). Their pathophysiological response is characterised by low mortality but severe acute neurological damage differing from adults because of anatomical proportions, weight, and stage of myelination. Bruce et al., (1978) suggest that if the threshold for neurophysiological dysfunction is lower in children than for the same input force to the adult brain, then the recorded neurological picture will be worse in the child. Experimental and clinical studies have shown distinctive mechanisms of injury and patterns of recovery in young organisms, leading many authors to doubt that age confers any advantage in withstanding the effects of diffuse insult upon the immature brain (Shapiro, 1985). As early as 1942 Hebb suggested that the cognitive sequelae of brain injury are of greater severity and generality when damage occurs in early infancy than in later life, hindering the acquisition of new abilities while having less effect upon established skills. Age alone is an inadequate index of neurological and physiological maturation, however, as both are substantially influenced by genetic blueprints and the rearing environment (Jeffrey, 1980). Important variables in determining the type or severity of cognitive deficit include the functional maturation of involved tissue (especially the frontal lobes), age at injury, time since injury, experience and nutrition before and after trauma (St. James-Roberts, 1979). The consistent observation of a dose-response relationship strongly suggests, however, that neuropsychological disabilities following head-injury in children are caused directly by the cerebral insult (Chadwick et al., 1981).

Attention and memory seem to be particularly vulnerable to the effects of head-injury. The slowing of electrophysiological responses after concussion (Ommaya, 1979) may underlie the apparent slowing of cognition (Van Zomeran, 1981) and some aspects of memory deficit (Geschwind, 1982). A consistent relationship between speed of information processing and capacity of working memory has been reported (Chi & Gallagher, 1982), with the suggestion that the speed at which letters and words are processed, for example, may determine the remaining capacity in working memory for comprehension (Das & Varnhagen, 1986). This is clearly crucial to learning and memory and fundamental to the child's normal development, and may relate to the findings of Dickstein and Tallal (1987) discussed below. Deficits in attention and memory can easily lead to substantial learning difficulties and academic problems for the head-injured child, which arise only years after the original trauma. Although not yet adequately documented, the head injured child appears to have difficulty in focusing and sustaining attention over time, and in controlling distractibility. Poor performance on distraction tasks may be due to slowness, difficulties in focusing and sustaining attention, failure to inhibit strong response tendencies, or ignore irrelevant stimuli. This type of distraction through interference, or a difficulty in screening out irrelevant information, may particularly slow some components of attention (Ewing-Cobbs, Fletcher & Levin, 1985; Clark, Geffen & Geffen, 1986).

Despite its seemingly critical nature, attentional disorder after closed head-injury has been poorly demonstrated using achievement tasks that primarily tap structured cognitive resources (Stuss & Benson, 1986). Of the few studies which have attempted to evaluate memory and attention following head-injury in children most can be particularly criticised for their test selection. Although many authors affirm the importance of including suitable measures as a practical test of coping ability in the classroom (Chadwick et al., 1981), no seemingly adequate test is included in any of these studies (e.g. Leahy, Holland & Frattalli, 1987). Most have relied on the ubiquitous intelligence test, such as the Weschler Intelligence Scale for Children (WISC), or Halstead-Reitan battery (Fay & Janesheski, 1986), both of which have been criticised for their relative insensitivity and inaccuracy in individual diagnosis and prescription (Yule, 1978; Chadwick & Rutter, 1984). Authors frequently attempt to relate often spurious IQ estimates with the practical significance of specific difficulties on speeded tasks.   For example, Filley et al., (1987) attributed a WISC-R Verbal-Performance IQ discrepancy to Perform-ance Scale tests which '...put selective demands on attention and are likely to document gross deficits during a post-traumatic confusional state' (p.198). Academic problems in reading, spelling and arithmetic, dysphasia and memory impairment were all encountered in that study and were, presumably, equally attributable to selective demands on attention (sic). Poor arithmetical test performance alone may be due to problems in speed, tracking, sequencing, or spatial ability, so it is practically important to ascertain which aspects are impaired in the head-injured child. Similarly, deficits in speeded visuo-motor performance are con-sistently reported, primarily with the more severely injured child (Bawden, Knights & Winogren, 1985), but with little idea of its precise nature. Such reports highlight the absolute futility of using IQ figures in an attempt to explain neuropsychological function after head-injury. We should be guided by a recent report (Dickstein & Tallal, 1987) which suggests that some developmental dyslexic or dysphasic children do not suffer from specific language deficits, but a general capacity deficit. Such children may process information at a rate slow enough to lose temporally related information, or have limited capacity to rapidly process information simultaneously. There are clear parallels with the child who suffers post-traumatic difficulties in these areas, suggesting a common pathological substrate.

In discussing the educational implications of test performance deficits in the head-injured child, attention and memory receive scant consideration. Following an often dramatic early improvement from the unconscious to walking wounded stages, the head-injured child who has no obvious physical problems, such as a broken limb, will be pressured into resuming his pre-accident lifestyle as soon as possible. He faces an early return to school with its high stress on learning, complex reason-ing, problem solving, and adaptive behaviour, all areas in which it may be predicted that he will have problems. Educational placements are usually based on meaningless IQ and achievement test scores, which undoubtedly overestimate the head-injured child's ability. There is little doubt that many children who achieve normal intelligence test scores after head-injury do nonetheless have attentional and learning deficits and may be unable to function adequately in the normal classroom (Fay & Janesheski, 1986). In writing an essay, for example, speeded motor performance is only part of the classroom requirements. The information has initially to be adequately processed and fed back at many of atten-tion's neurophysiological and cognitive levels, before the final motor response is achieved. Consequently, the advocacy of using computer-assisted writing tools to improve classroom performance is to be dep-lored, given our imprecise and insufficient knowledge. Even the less severely head-injured child will be slow or distractible, and quite unable to function efficiently at optimal levels (Boll, 1983). Common problems after head-injury include difficulties in keeping up with what is said, shutting out both internal and external distractions, following lessons, instructions, or recalling information from memory on demand. In his attempts to concentrate harder and overcome these difficulties the child may exert greater effort but, with resources limited by the head-injury, the likely outcome is fatigue, controlled attention deficits and increasing failure. We should heed Teuber's insistence on the insensitivity of many traditional psychological tests, as our habits or skills which are overlearned and automatised may show little disruption, particularly after mild or moderate head-injury. It is primarily new learning that suffers, which is not of inconsequential importance for the child in education. A marked decline in educational achievement and transfer to special schools is not uncommon for the severely head-injured child, but it is far from clear what contributes to this change. The frequent and persistent deficits in WISC Performance IQ and manual dexterity share a common feature in that good performance depends upon the ability to respond quickly in visuo-spatial or motor skills. The underlying cause, or pathological substrate, may be structural, functional, cognitive, motor speed, or motivational. Which aspects of cognitive deficit are crucial to academic achievement after head-injury remains an unanswered question. It is practically most important, therefore, that psychologists and teachers understand how the head injured child processes information and arrives at a particular answer, rather than simply whether or not they can answer a question within a set time period, irrespective of their actual ability.

ASSESSMENT

The nature of these problems clearly show the need for accurate assessment which must '...systematically measure the adaptive abilities that reflect impairment of the various functional systems within the brain' (Fay & Janesheski, 1986 p.17). There is only a narrow range of standardised tests available for use with children, and concern about the downward extension of adult tests for children (Fletcher & Taylor, 1984). Because the organisation of abilities changes with age, it is essential to incorporate developmental principles into such test procedures (e.g. Chelune & Baer, 1986). Among the attentional tests reported, the Continuous Performance Test is widely used but there is a paucity of information on its psychometric properties (Chadwick & Rutter, 1984). Experimental tasks such as computerised mental rotation (Kail, 1986) or reaction time are not easily portable (Bakker & Vinke, 1985) and are restrictive in use. In their seminal studies, Chadwick et al., (1981) used a paced auditory serial addition task (PASAT) based on the attentional test for head-injured adults (Sampson, 1956). They found that head-injury had little effect upon performance, but only severely head-injured children were assessed, and only at 27 months follow-up. It may have been more applicable with the mild and moderate populations, or conducted earlier and serially. Performance on this type of test appears to require selective and sustained attention, stored memory components, mental transformations and has inherently strong control aspects, requiring the subject not to add his answer to the next number. In all, a need for sustained and controlled attention.

A revised paced auditory serial addition test for children (CHIPASAT) has subsequently been developed (Johnson, Roethig-Johnston & Middleton, 1988). The performance of normal school children showed that the number of correct responses declined significantly for all ages as presentation rate increased, without concomitant increases in errors. The speed of response increased exponentially with age, older children achieving more correct responses in every trial, concurring with the developmental change reported by Kail (1986). Younger children have a much slower speed of response and are more affected by increased presentation rate, perhaps because of less available automatic processing demanding more attentional resources in performing the task. Resources may increase gradually and continually with age, reflecting a general maturational change which alters the physiological limits on attention. The same pattern of development is reported for many speeded tasks, with response time decreasing steadily in middle childhood, and continuing at a slower decline subsequently, reflecting a functional maturity in early-mid adolescence. This suggests that neurological changes produced by head-injury could have considerable influence on attention and complex cognition relative to the child's development.

Increased speed of presentation demands an effective strategy for responding. In clinical use of the PASAT/CHIPASAT less effective strategies may be used overtly by the patient, as demonstrated by some of the normal younger children who used their fingers to add, obviously slowing responses considerably. As children develop they use increasingly sufficient and efficient procedures (Kail & Bisanz, 1982). Early procedures are partially correct, and elaborated during development in ways that increase proficiency. The same procedures may be used by individuals of different ages, but the components are performed more quickly with age. Repeated use or practice as a child develops may lead to their becoming generally more proficient in devising efficient strategies for task performance, which become increasingly automatic.

We are currently testing the hypothesis that head injured children show less efficient attention, performing at lower age levels on CHIPASAT, and that this reflects a pathological slowing of attention, with recovery following a developmental curve.

TREATMENT

The basis of structural damage and metabolic disruption following head-injury should focus our attempts at rational and effective treatment (Luria, 1963). Adequate assessment is, however, a necessary precursor for identifying what it is we should be treating. There seems little doubt that cognitive deficits persist after head-injury generally and, given the importance of cognitive demands placed upon the head-injured child, it is necessary to consider how much attentional deficit might contribute to this pervasive disability. Automaticity may never return to its previous level (Moskovitch, 1979) and the plasticity which marks learning (James, 1899) may be considerably more difficult to achieve, restricting cognitive development at stages which normally lay the foundation for adulthood. Accurate delineation of attentional deficits, whether speed or control, or combined with reading difficulties, for example, could be crucial to the child's development. As attention is fundamental to general brain function, attentional difficulties may represent one of a constellation of closely related deficits, all of which have far reaching effects upon the child's behaviour, academic achievement, and cognitive functioning. It is possible that even the more severely head-injured child may show some generalised improvement if we can effectively identify and treat underlying attentional problems (Whyte, 1986). We must be wary of how we measure the efficacy of retraining, however, as any benefits may be due to motivation rather than enhanced neural integration (Jeffrey, 1980). The vogue for computer-based attentional retraining (Tyerman, 1987) is a most pertinent example of this need.

Meaningful assessment and effective rehabilitation require an understanding of the relevant neurological processes. Knowledge of how the mediating structures develop will influence how we organise and control the treatment environment, our expectations of the child and his recovery. Reports of behavioural treatments for attentional disorder (Ylvisaker, 1985; Wood, 1986) are not encouraging, because of small and heterogenous populations and an apparent failure to incorporate the neurological basis of the disorder. This type of approach ignores the possibilities of direct intervention within the nervous system (Finger &

Stein, 1982) and a truly neurobehavioural approach (sic), as is typical of the traditional, narrow, and largely ineffective rehabilitation in this country.

A more direct approach to treatment is suggested by reports of Hemispheric Specific Stimulation (HSS) with dyslexic children (Spyer, de Jong & Bakker, 1987), which indicate that direct HSS resulted in eletrophysiological changes, notably in the parietal region, and improved reading performance. Given the theoretical importance of parietal function in attention, and the incidence of post-traumatic reading disorder (Chadwick et al., 1981) this clearly deserves investigation with head-injured children.

On the basis that differential aspects of attention are dependent upon brain state and the neurochemical substrates involved are those likely to have been disrupted by head injury, then the logical step is surely one which combines a pharmacological and cognitive approach. The vast majority of central monoaminergic (MA) systems originate in the brainstem (Clark, Geffen & Geffen, 1986), so it is not surprising to find substantial changes in MA activity following head trauma (Johnson, 1989a). Abnormalities within the catecholaminergic and cholinergic systems, for example, may be particularly important to early recovery, and may persist for varying periods after head injury. These same neurochemical systems have been implicated in a wide range of attention-related measures, so it is reasonable to suggest that such neurochemical abnormalities may form part of the substrate for persisting cognitive deficits. If we can modify neurophysiological processes pharmacologically, this could have important effects upon cognitive functions (Cope, 1986). Attentional processes could therefore be delineated and modified on a rational basis (Callaway, 1984). In spite of longstanding calls (Luria, 1963; Bach & Rita, 1980) there are few reports on neuropsychopharmacological intervention with the head injured population (Gualtieri, 1987) and even fewer with head injured children. Consequently we must glean information on the possibilities from other populations, notably Attention Deficit Disorder (ADD) and Hyperactive children. The use of stimulant drugs and cognitive training has proved an important role with ADD children. For both the ADD and the head-injured child, attentional difficulties may be due to problems in any or all of the subordinate processes of attention (Douglas, 1984).

There are two broad classes of relevant drug use which give brief examples of the possibilities in this area:

Stimulants. Methylphenidate is a commonly used stimulant in many populations. Clark, Geffen and Geffen (1986) found no significant effect on attentional performance or electrophysiological response latency in normal adults, other than a higher error rate in divided attention. The subjects complained of increased alertness and elation, wider field of attention, and increased distractibility, which implies less effort was required, but also a lack of internal control. In contrast, a 14 year old female with very severe head trauma, who could no longer learn, in part due to her almost total inability to attend and not be distracted, was given a trial of methylphenidate. This lead to dramatic improvement in attention span, responses to social rewards, and capacity for behavioural learning (Parmalee & O'Shanick, 1987). Use of another stimulant, Piracetam, has been reported to facilitate speed of reading in dyslexic children, especially when combined with HSS (Spyer, de Jong & Bakker, 1987). Increased vigilance may be one effect of this nootropic use (Cope, 1986), and so this class of drug needs further clinical application with head-injured children.

Anticholinergics. Luria (1969) suggested that the cholinergic system might be successfully manipulated to ameliorate some symptoms in early recovery. Given the postulated cholinergic roles in sleep, learning and memory, it is possible that persisting deficits in those areas (Johnson, 1989b) may be amenable to pharmacological modification. Cholinergics have an important role in the stimulus-evaluation stage of information processing, and a general priming function in behaviour (Panksepp, 1986). Scoploamine slows reaction time and P300 latency in a dose-response fashion, suggesting inhibition of the cholinergic based stimulus-evaluation (Callaway, 1984).

Neuropsychopharmacological approaches to rehabilitation must always be combined with other important variables, including small highly structured classrooms and teaching style, with slower presentation of smaller amounts of information to avoid overload and comprehension breakdowns. The caveat here is whether the side effects of drugs and the risk of undesirable behaviours (Glenn, 1986) outweigh the potential long-term benefits.

CONCLUSIONS

The goal of clinical neuroscience remains the understanding of cognition, behaviour and emotion (Kandel, 1982). To achieve this we must specify those neural systems which influence different aspects of cognition. By fractionating complex cognitive functions and delineating specific neural processes (Tucker & Williamson, 1984), we can apply this neurological knowledge to elucidate cognition, its disorders and treatment (Moskovitch, 1979). Attention has a crucial role in reaching that goal. The chief value of neuropsychological assessment is in the accurate delineation of cognitive and other deficits, quantifying not only the presence of dysfunction, but also the efficiency of functioning. Test results which give rise only to an undifferentiated diagnosis of something wrong with the brain, are of little practical or theoretical value. Paediatric neuropsychology is in a transitional stage, with interest in children's head-injury now beginning to emerge. We need to establish the value of existing tests, their use in pathological differentiation, and develop research tools for routine clinical use.

Attentional processes clearly involve more than one brain area and neurochemical system (Panksepp, 1986), but the suggestion that deficits in a conceptual fronto-limbic-reticular loop underlie pathological attention is insufficiently precise to be of any clinical guidance with head injured children. We need to be clear about which aspects of attention are implicated by the child's poor performance. We need to ascertain whether the child shows problems in arousal, attentional capacity, speed, selectivity, vigilance, or distractibility. The questions of poor control, disordered arousal (Brouwer, 1985; Klove, 1987) and persisting metabolic dysfunction after head injury (Alavi et al., 1986) should be used to elucidate the bases of impaired attention. Optimal performance can be disrupted by high or low arousal and may particularly reflect general impairment of frontal lobe control. Only then can we begin to design rational treatment. It is clinically important to be able to assess attention as a diagnostic aid and as a guide to recovery, and to establish the level of ability which, in the presence of other recovery, will allow the child to be appropriately placed in education.

Conclusions about good prognosis in children (Flach & Malmos, 1972) hardly seem warranted in the present state of inadequate assessment, the perpetual reliance on ubiquitous and meaningless IQ figures, and professional ignorance within education, psychology, and medicine. Teuber's dictum 'Absence of evidence is not evidence of absence' is most pertinent to the head-injured child with outwardly good physical recovery, but in whom the cognitive difficulties are hidden out of sight (Boll, 1983). If children do show a greater propensity for better physical recovery then we must be more alert to the hidden dangers of subtle but significant cognitive difficulties. Children who present with learning difficulties may have developed these as a result of the unnoticed and cumulative effects of earlier head-injury. It has been suggested that the incidence of subsequent head-injury is greater than expected for both age and sex in children, implying that initial post-traumatic deficits may increase the propensity for further trauma. It is easy to misread or misinterpret behaviours such as wandering attention or withdrawal, and not recognise cognitive deficits. Neuropsychological problems can be exaccerbated by failure of identification, potentially resulting in marked behavioural and academic disturbances, and yet further failure.

'The educational system does not teach 'attending' or 'remembering' ...(and) often assumes that these skills are automatic and intact' (Cohen, 1986 p.23). The perpetual classroom command 'PAY ATTENTION' at best acts to arouse the child for a few moments. Whereas the normal child will be able to drag his attention back to the task in hand, the head-injured child is unlikely to have sufficient control to do so. Good attention, say Gibson and Rader (1979) involves perceiving what has utility for what the child is doing, or intends to do, but motivation may also be a major problem for the head-injured child. In his most engaging discourse William James highlights the importance of interest and motivation in learning, giving many practical examples which would be invaluable aids in rehabilitation. '...the great thing in all education is to make our nervous system our ally instead of our enemy' (1899 p.66). It is with this in mind that we may begin to help the head-injured child.

ACKNOWLEDGEMENT

The test development reported here was financially supported by St. George's Hospital Special Trustees Research Fund.

REFERENCES

Alavi, A., Langfitt, T., Fazekas, F., Duhaime, T., Zimmerman, R. & Reivich, M. (1986). Correlative studies of head trauma (HT) with PET, MRI and XCT. Journal of Nuclear Medicine, 27, 918–919.

Bach, Y. & Rita, P. (1980). Recovery of Function: Theoretical Considerations for Brain-Injury Rehabilitation. Bern:Huber.

Bakker, D.J. & Vinke, J. (1985). Effects of hemispheric specific stimulation on brain activity and reading in dyslexics. Journal of Clinical and Experimental Neuropsychology, 7, 505–525.

Bawden, H.N., Knights, R.M. & Winogren, H.W. (1985). Speeded performance following head-injury in children. Journal of Clinical and Experimental Neuropsychology, 7, 39–54.

Boll, T.J. (1983). Minor head-injury in children: out of sight but not out of mind. Journal of Clinical Child Psychology, 12, 74–80.

Brodal, A. (1973). Self observations and neuroanatomical correlations after a stroke. Brain, 96, 675–694.

Bromley, D.B. (1977). Personality Description in Everyday Language. Chichester: Wiley.

Brouwer, W.H. (1985). Limitations of Attention After Closed Head-Injury. Netherlands: Rijksuniversitiet Groningen.

Bruce, D.A., Raphaely, R.C., Goldber, A.I., Zimmerman, R.A., Bilanuik, L.T., Schut, L. & Khul, D. (1978). Pathophysiology, treatment and outcome following severe head-injury in children. Child's Brain, 5, 174-191.

Callaway, E. (1984). Human information processing: some effects of methylphenidate, age and scopolamine. Biological Psychiatry, 19, 649-662.

Chadwick, O., Rutter, M., Schaffer, D. & Shrout, P. (1981). A prospective study of children with head injury: IV- specific cognitive deficits. Journal of Clinical and Experimental Neuropsychology, 3, 101-120.

Chadwick, O., Rutter, M., Thompson, J., Shaffer, D. (1981). Intellectual performance and reading skills after localised head-injury in children. Journal of Child Psychology & Psychiatry, 22, 117-139.

Chadwick, O. & Rutter, M. (1984). Neuropsychological assessment. in: M. Rutter (ed.) Developmental Neuropsychiatry. Edinburgh: Churchill-Livingstone.

Chelune, G.J. & Baer, R.A. (1986). Developmental norms for the Wisconsin Card Sorting Test. Journal of Clinical and Experimental Neuropsychology, 8, 219-228.

Chi, M.T.H. & Gallagher, J.D. (1982). Speed of processing: a developmental source of limitation. Topics in Learning & Learning disability, 2, 23-32.

Clark, C.R., Geffen, G.M. & Geffen, L.B. (1986). Role of monoamine pathways in attention and effort: effects of clonidine and methylphenidate in normal human adults. Psychopharmacology, 90, 35-39.

Cohen, S.B. (1986). Educational reintegration and programming for children with head-injury. Journal of Head Trauma Rehabilitation, 1, 22-29.

Cope, D.N. (1986). The pharmacology of attention and memory. Journal of Head Trauma Rehabilitation, 1, 34-42.

Das, J.P. & Varnhagen, C.K. (1986). Neuropsychological functioning and cognitive processing. in: J.E. Obzrut & G.W. Hynd (eds.) Child Neuropsychology Volume 1: Theory and Research. New York: Academic Press.

Dickstein, P.W. & Tallal, P. (1987). Attentional capabilities of reading-impaired children during dichotic presentation of phonetic and complex non-phonetic sounds. Cortex, 23, 237-249.

Douglas, V.I. (1984). Attentional and cognitive problems. in: M. Rutter (ed.) Developmental Neuropsychiatry. Edinburgh: Churchill-Livingstone.

Ewing-Cobbs, L., Fletcher, J.M. & Levin, H.S. (1985). Neuropsychological sequelae following paediatric head-injury. in: M. Ylvisaker (ed). Head-injury Rehabilitation: Children and Adolescents. London: Taylor & Francis.

Fay, G. & Janesheski, D. (1986). Neuropsychological assessment of head-injured children. Journal of Head Trauma Rehabilitation, 1, 16-21.

Filley, C.M., Cranberg, L.D., Alexander, M.P. & Hart, E.J. (1987). Neurobehavioural outcome after closed head-injury in childhood and adolescence. Archives of Neurology, 44, 194-201.

Finger, S. & Stein, D.G. (1982). Brain Damage and Recovery. New York: Academic Press.

Flach, J. & Malmos, R. (1972). Longterm follow-up of children with severe head-injury. Scandinavian Journal of Rehabilitation Medicine, 4, 9-15.

Fletcher, J.M. & Taylor, H.G. (1984). Neuropsychological approaches to children: towards a developmental neuropsychology. Journal of Clinical and Experimental Neuropsychology, 6, 34-56.

Geschwind, N. (1982). Disorders of attention: a frontier in neuropsychology. Philosophical Transcripts of the Royal Society of London, B298, 173-185.

Gibson, E. & Rader, N. (1979). Attention: perceiver as performer. in: G.A. Hale & M. Lewis (eds.). Attention and Cognitive Development. New York: Plenum Press.

Glenn, M.B. (1986). CNS stimulants: applications for traumatic brain-injury. Journal of Head Trauma Rehabilitation, 1, 74-76.

Gualtieri, C.T. (1987). Pharmacotherapy and the neurobehavioural sequelae of traumatic brain-injury. Unpublished manuscript.

Hebb, D.O. (1942). The effect of early and late brain injury upon test scores, and the nature of normal adult intelligence. Proceedings of the American Philosophical Society, 85, 275-292.

Heilman, K. & Van Den Abel, T. (1980). Right hemisphere dominance for attention. Neurology, 30, 327-330.

James, W. (1899). Talks to Teachers. London:Longman.

Jeffery, R. (1980). The developing brain and child development. in: M.C. Wittrock (ed). The Brain and Psychology. New York: Academic Press.

Johnson, D.A. (1985). Pediatric Head-injury in South West Thames. Unpublished data.

Johnson, D.A. (1989a). Indices of arousal in acute severe head trauma. In preparation.

Johnson, D.A. (1989b). Neurological indices of sleep and cognition after severe head trauma. In preparation.

Johnson, D.A., Roethig-Johnston, K. & Middleton, J. (1988). CHIPASAT: the development of an attentional test for head-injured children. I: information processing in a normal sample. Journal of Child Psychology and Psychiatry, 29, 199-208.

Kahnemann, D. (1973). Attention and Effort. New Jersey: Prentice Hall.

Kail, R. (1986). Sources of age differences in speed of processing. Child Development, 57, 969-987.

Kail, R. & Bisanz, J. (1982). Information processing and cognitive development. Advances in Child Development and Behaviour, 17, 45-81.

Kandel, E. (1982). The origins of modern neuroscience. Annual Review of Neuroscience, 5, 299-304.

Klove, H. (1987). Activation, arousal and neuropsychological rehabilitation. Journal of Clinical and Experimental Neuropsychology, 9, 297-309.

Leahy, L.F., Holland, A.C. & Frattalli, C.M. (1987). Persistent deficits following children's head-injury. Paper presented to International Neuropsychology Society, Washington, USA.

Levin, H.S., Ewing-Cobbs, L. & Benton, A.L. (1984). Age and recovery from brain damage. in: S.W. Scheff (ed.). Aging and Recovery of Function in the Central Nervous System. New York:Plenum Press.

Lindsley, D.B. (1960). Attention, consciousness, sleep and wakefulness. in: J. Field, W. Magoun & V.E. Hall (eds.). Handbook of Physiology 3: Neurophysiology. Washington:American Physiological Society.

Luria, A.R. (1963). Restoration of Function after Brain-injury. Oxford: Pergamon Press.

Luria, A.R., Naydin, V.L., Tsvetkora, L.S. & Vinarskaya, E.N. (1969). Restoration of higher cortical function following local brain damage. in: Vinken, P.J. & Bruyn, G.W. (Eds): Handbook of Clinical Neurology, Vol.3. North Holland, Amsterdam.

Luria, A.R. (1973). The Working Brain. Harmondsworth:Penguin.

McGuinness, D. & Pribram, K. (1980). The neuropsychology of attention: emotional and motivational controls. in: M.C. Wittrock (ed.). The Brain and Psychology. New York:Academic Press.

Mesulam, M.M. (1981). A cortical network for directed attention and unilateral neglect. Annals of Neurology, 10, 309-325..

Moskovitch, M. (1979). Information processing and the cerebral hemispheres. in: M.S. Gazzaniga (ed.). Handbook of Behavioural Neurology volume 2: Neuropsychology. New York:Plenum Press.

Nissen, M.J. (1986). Neuropsychology of attention and memory. Journal of Head Trauma Rehabilitation, 1, 13-21.

Ommaya, A.C. (1979). Indices of neural trauma. in: A.J. Popp (ed). Neural Trauma. New York:Raven Press.

Panksepp, J. (1986). The neurochemistry of behaviour. Annual Review of Psychology, 37, 77–107.

Parmalee, D.X. & O'Shanick, G.J. (1987). Neuropsychiatric intervention with head–injured children and adolescents. Brain Injury, 1, 41–48.

Piontkowski, D. & Calfee, R. (1979). Attention in the classroom. in: G.A. Hale & M. Lewis (eds.). Attention and Cognitive Development. New York: Academic Press.

Posner, M.I. & Presti, D.E. (1987). Selective attention and cognitive control. Trends in Neuroscience, 10, 13–16.

Pribram, K. & McGuinness, D. (1975). Arousal activation and effort in the control of attention. Psychological Review, 82, 116–149.

St. James-Roberts, I. (1979). Neurological plasticity, recovery from brain insult, and child development. in: H.W. Reese & L.P. Lipsitt (eds.). Advances in Child Behaviour and Development volume 14. New York:Academic Press.

Sampson, H. (1956). Pacing and performance in a serial addition task. Canadian Journal of Psychology, 10, 219–225.

Schneider, W. & Shiffrin, R.M. (1977). Controlled and automatic human information processing:1 – detection, search and attention. Psychological Review, 84, 1–66.

Shapiro, K. (1985). Head–injury in children. in: D.P. Becker & J.T. Povlishock (eds.). Central Nervous System Trauma: Status Report. Washington:National Institute of Health.

Spyer, G., de Jong, A. & Bakker, D.J. (1987). Piracetam and hemispheric specific stimulation. Paper presented to International Neuropsychology Society, Barcelona, Spain.

Stuss, D. & Benson, D.F. (1986). The Frontal Lobes. New York:Raven.

Tucker, D.M. & Williamson, P.A. (1984). Asymmetric neural control systems in human self-regulation. Psychological Review, 91, 185–215.

Tyerman, A.D. (1987). Personal communication.

Van Zomeran, A.H. (1981). Reaction Time and Attention after Head Injury. Lisse:Swets Zeitlinger.

Van Zomeran, A.H., Brouwer, W.H. & Deelman, B.G. (1984). Attentional deficits: the riddle of selectivity, speed and alertness. in: D.N. Brooks (ed.). Closed Head–injury. Oxford:Oxford University Press.

Whyte, J. (1986). Outcome evaluation in the remediation of attention and memory deficits. Journal of Head Trauma Rehabilitation, 1, 64–71.

Wood, R.L. (1986). Brain Injury Rehabilitation: a neurobehavioural approach. London:Croom Helm.

Ylvisaker, M. (1985). Head–injury Rehabilitation: children and adolescents. London:Taylor & Francis.

Yule, W. (1978). Diagnosis: developmental neuropsychological assessment. Advances in Biological Psychiatry, 1, 35–54.

TEMPORAL LOBECTOMY, COGNITION AND BEHAVIOUR: A BRIEF REVIEW WITH SPECIAL
REFERENCE TO THE REQUIREMENTS OF INFORMED CONSENT

Graham E Powell, Penny A Murphy and Tom McMillan

INTRODUCTION

Temporal lobe epilepsy has been perceived as a clinical entity since
the observations of Hughlings Jackson in 1888. It is characterised by a
specific type of seizure involving a brief period of dazedness with confused or semipurposive behaviour and by masticatory or sniffing movements, and is preceded by auras of physical experience such as epigastric
sensation or sensory hallucinations often of taste or smell (Falconer et
al., 1955). In more severe cases, an attack may develop into a grand-mal
seizure, but essentially temporal lobe seizures begin with epileptic
discharges from foci in one or both of the temporal lobes. According to
Falconer et al. (1955) a quarter to one third of all patients with
epilepsy demonstrate such EEG phenomena. The identification of this type
of seizure with temporal EEG foci paved the way for the operation of
temporal lobectomy for intractable conditions, an operation pioneered in
Canada by Wilder Penfield (e.g. Penfield & Steelman, 1947; Penfield &
Flanigin, 1950). Penfield's series began in 1939 and originally the
excisions of the temporal lobe spared the deeper parts, notably the
uncus, amygdala and hippocampus. In time, and with the development of
centres in other parts of the world, the operation came to be carried out
upon EEG evidence alone, whereas originally Penfield tended to operate
only upon those with an abnormality visible at operation, and the operation resolved into a standard en bloc resection that removed between 5.5
and 6.5 cm from the temporal pole and included the mesial structures of
amygdala, anterior hippocampus and uncus (Falconer, 1953; 1969). The
specimen is removed as one piece (in contrast to the original suction
technique) and is therefore available for pathological examination. Left
and right hemisphere resections are identical except for the fact that
the surgeon attempts to spare the posterior portion of the superior
temporal gyrus of the dominant lobe in order to minimise the effects of
the operation upon language.

The two major centres that have contributed to our understanding of
the efficacy and effects of the operation are the Montreal Neurological
Institute, continuing Penfield's series, and the Maudsley Hospital,
London. This latter series began in 1951 under Falconer and had reached
more than 300 patients by the mid-seventies (Falconer, 1974). Since then
a further hundred or so cases have been added in a new series under
Polkey (Powell, Polkey & McMillan, 1985), and it is the results from
these cases that will largely form the focus of this paper.

In a review of the world literature, Jensen (1975) showed a reasonable success rate and low morbidity and mortality. If those series in

which the lobectomy was complete (i.e. standard en bloc resection) are selected from the cases presented by Jensen, then worthwhile improvement of seizure frequency is seen in over 60% of patients (Polkey, 1982). Indeed, in certain patient subgroups, such as those with mesial temporal sclerosis, 60% of cases become seizure free, a high figure in any circumstances but especially so in view of the fact that these cases have all proved resistant to the effects of standard drug treatments.

However, all clinicians and researchers in the field are concerned to weigh carefully these obvious gains against the possible negative consequences of removing a substantial portion of brain tissue, such as intellectual deterioration, memory disturbance and language dysfunction.

COGNITIVE EFFECTS OF TEMPORAL LOBECTOMY

In order to review briefly the findings prior to the new Maudsley series, the cognitive effects of temporal lobectomy can be broken down under the following headings:

Short term effects on intelligence. Short term here means two weeks post-operatively for Montreal and four weeks post-operatively for the Maudsley. Intelligence declines by about 10-15 points after left lobectomy and by a smaller amount, perhaps 5 points, after right lobectomy (Meyer, 1959; Milner, 1975; Kimura, 1963). This decline tends to be on verbal scales after left lobectomy and non-verbal or performance scales after right lobectomy (Blakemore & Falconer, 1967).

Short term effects on memory. Left cases are poorer on tests of verbal memory such as paired associate learning, whereas right cases are poor on non-verbal memory tasks, such as maze learning and memory for faces. (Meyer, 1959; Jones, 1974; Jones-Gotman & Milner, 1978).

Short term effects on language. Falconer et al. (1955) reported that early in his series one third of dominant operations led to a degree of nominal dysphasia, but consequent upon this the operation was modified to spare more of the superior temporal gyrus. Even so, Serafetinides and Falconer (1963) still reported that 29 out of 56 left resections failed to name three or more of ten common objects. This finding is congruent with the disturbance of verbal IQ and verbal memory noted above.

Long term effects on intelligence. The intelligence of both left and right cases rises over time, sometimes to above baseline levels (Milner, 1975; Wilkins & Moscovitch, 1978). Sometimes this improvement is greater in right cases (Meyer, 1959) and long term differences between left and right cases on verbal and non-verbal IQ (in obvious directions) have been reported (Blakemore & Falconer, 1967).

Long term effects on memory. Persistent verbal memory deficits in left cases have been observed (Blakemore & Falconer, 1967; Rausch, 1977). Similar non-verbal deficits have been noted in right cases (Rausch, 1981; Jones-Gotman & Milner, 1978).

Long term effects on language. The Maudsley group have found the dysphasia after dominant lobectomy to be transient; only 5 of the first 100 cases had a mild but persisting nominal dysphasia (Falconer & Serafetinides, 1963; Serafetinides & Falconer, 1963).

The above studies are not without methodological inadequacies. There is a frequent failure to report pre-operative scores. Related to this there is a distinct tendency to attribute post-operative differences between left and right groups to the operation rather than to the possibility of pre-existing differences. Post operative testing is often at 2 weeks, and some would say this is too early and confounded by peripheral effects of neurosurgery. The distributions of scores on crucial variables is not described, for example Kimura (1963) and Blakemore and Falconer (1967) do not give standard deviations. Histograms of raw scores are not described or given, precluding the possibility of detecting subgroups within the data. Change scores across the operation are seldom given. Often significance tests are omitted. Long term and short term test results can be pooled in some studies making impossible the estimation of recovery curves. Left and right dominant cases can be combined in analyses, and finally the details of the resection are omitted and cases with rather different operations pooled for the purposes of analysis.

INVESTIGATIONS OF THE NEW MAUDSLEY SERIES

It is against this background that the results of the new Maudsley series were presented in detail (Powell, Polkey & McMillan, 1985; McMillan et al., 1987; Powell, Polkey & Canavan, 1987). In an attempt to remedy the above short-comings pre-operative and change scores were given; all post-operation testing was at four weeks; distributions were described and histograms of raw scores made available; testing for significance was exhaustive; right dominant cases were excluded from all major analysis; and only cases who underwent the standard operation were included.

The series selected according to these critera thus comprised 59 adults (34 male; 29 left lobectomy) of mean age about 25 years at the time of the operation. Five were left handed, their first seizure was on average reported between the ages of 8 and 10 and regular seizures began on the whole between 12 and 13. On average between 5 and 6 partial seizures were reported per week and the frequency of generalized seizures was typically very low. The average length of resection was 6 cm (see Powell et al., 1985 for details). Routine tests always included the assessment of verbal and non-verbal intelligence and verbal and non-verbal memory. Estimates were made of both immediate and delayed memory. Others tests were given as appropriate but not routinely, to investigate possible dysfunction outwith the temporal lobe, or to examine other aspects of temporal lobe functioning, (e.g. Powell, Sutherland & Aga, 1984; Bennett-Levy, Polkey & Powell, 1980). Investigation of children in the new Maudsley series, is currently underway and detailed results will not be presented here.

With regard to adults in the new series, scores on intelligence measures were within the normal range pre-operatively, and this is consistent with a policy of rejecting for the operation those candidates who were intellectually impaired or deteriorating in a manner suggestive of widespread, non-focal impairment. There were no significant differences on intelligence variables between left and right lobectomy cases, but there were some suggestive trends. For example only 33% of left cases had a higher verbal than non-verbal IQ as opposed to 57% of right cases (χ^2 = 2.29, n.s.).

Of major importance was the finding that the mean change scores across the operation were not significantly different from zero. This implies that over the course of time, experience and the results of previous studies have improved patient selection and screened out many of those liable to deteriorate intellectually. Change scores on intelligence were not significantly different for left and right groups, although some trends were evident. For example, in left cases verbal IQ fell by an average of −3.78 points while performance IQ rose by 3.83 points, whereas in right cases verbal IQ rose by 0.08 and performance IQ fell by 0.77 points. Overall, small and non-significant trends that existed pre-operatively were added to by way of small and non-significant trends across the operation, so that post-operatively the standard picture of left cases being lower than right cases on verbal IQ (91.38 vs 103.35, p<0.05) but higher on non-verbal IQ (105.50 vs 94.65, p<.05) was found. These findings suggest that in the past post-operative differences have in part been erroneously attributed to the operation exclusively, ignoring the contribution of pre-existing patterns.

The results on memory variables broadly parallel the above findings. Mean scores on memory tests pre-operatively were within the normal range, again reflecting that some candidates with poor memory functions were screened out on the grounds that this represented generalised dysfunction (see Powell et al. 1987 for the results of the intracarotid amytal test). Left and right cases did not differ significantly on any memory variable, although once again trends were found, with left cases scoring somewhat lower on both short and long term retention of prose passages, for example. As with intelligence, change scores on memory variables did not depart significantly from zero. This can be viewed as an improvement upon the results of the previous series. Again, there were non-significant trends in the change scores consistent with previous findings for laterality. For example, on immediate recall of prose passages, eight left cases improved and 15 deteriorated, while 12 right cases improved and eight deteriorated (χ^2 = 2.73, ns.). Once again, pre-operative trends added to change score trends resulting in at least one left-right difference post-operatively. As before left cases were significantly lower on immediate recall of prose passages from the Logical Memory Test of the Wechsler Memory Scale.

Taking a broader view of the data, the 17 cognitive variables described in Powell et al. (1985) were correlated with each other separately for left and right cases and for pre- and post-operative results. It was striking that more significant correlations for the right than the left group were found (76 vs. 35 pre- and 72 vs. 49 post-operatively). This is consistent with Semmes (1968) view that right functions are more diffusely represented and hence left lesions have specific effects that dissociate scores while right lesions have broad effects that maintain correlations between variables. Further, as the difference is evident pre-operatively one could propose a view that hemispheric differences in structure are present from early in life, given the high proportion of early onset cases in the series.

The next issue concerns the influence of individual variables. Considering histograms of change scores for verbal and non-verbal IQ, (figure 1) it is clear that some patients improve and some deteriorate. However, are these changes random and due to the errors of measurement of which all psychological tests are prone, or are they systematic and predictable on the basis of subject characteristics? Some of the main findings are set out below.

Pre-Operative Level of Functioning

Without doubt those patients scoring higher pre-operatively evidenced greater deterioration across the operation. For example, pre-operative delayed recall scores on Logical Memory correlated −0.72 (p<0.001) with change scores within the left group and −0.48 (p<0.05) within the right group.

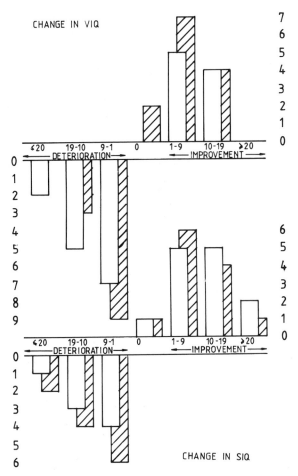

Figure 1. Histograms of change in verbal IQ (VIQ) and performance IQ (SIQ). Left hemisphere cases are depicted with open bars and right hemisphere cases with shaded bars.

Age of Onset of Regular Seizures

Pre-operatively, late onset cases were cognitively more able than early onset cases. For example, age of onset correlated with verbal IQ (0.45 in left cases, p<.05, and 0.63 right cases, p<.001). However, in terms of changes across the operation, late onset cases fared more poorly than early onset cases. Considering left cases, verbal IQ went down by −1.08 in the early onset group (seizures starting between the ages of 0 and 11 years) but by −7.30 in the late onset group. Similarly, for right cases, non-verbal IQ fell by 7.33 in the late onset group but increased by +6.33 in the early onset group (this result cannot be explained by regression to the mean or by the influence of the relationship between pre-operative level and change scores − see Powell et al., 1985 for details).

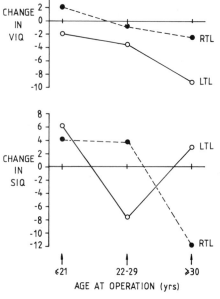

Figure 2. Mean changes in verbal IQ (VIQ) and performance IQ (SIQ) in left (LTL) and right (RTL) temporal lobectomy cases for three age groups.

Age at Operation

Older patients were cognitively more able pre-operatively on verbal tests but deteriorated most across the operation, as indicated in figure 2. Here is can be seen that the oldest left cases deteriorated more than younger groups on verbal IQ and that the oldest right cases deteriorated more than the younger groups on non-verbal IQ.

DISCUSSION

Taken together, (see Powell et al. 1985) these results suggest a model of the effects of temporal lobectomy. Early onset cases have organic damage present from a younger age than late onset cases. Early onset cases might therefore develop with only one 'effective' temporal lobe, with the damaged lobe contributing little to cognitive performance. This inhibits cognitive development in general because of great pressure upon lessened processing capacity. However, although early onset cases are disadvantaged in terms of development they are at an advantage with respect to the operation, which only removes tissue that contributed little to cognitive functioning. Conversely, in late onset cases the affected lobe which had been acquiring functions throughout its period of normal development, was removed at operation together with the epileptic focus. This model is supported by the results from neuro pathology data (McMillan et al., 1987). Those cases with hippocampal sclerosis (i.e. early onset caused by anoxia at birth) scored less well on IQ tests pre-operatively than did those with other pathologies (e.g. cysts and tumours that result in late onset), and across the operation IQ scores tended to

<u>increase</u> for the hippocampal group and <u>decrease</u> for the other pathology group.

Overall, it can be concluded, although temporal lobectomy has acceptable cognitive side-effects when viewed against the probability of a major reduction in seizures, there can be increased costs when offering the operation to those who are older, or intellectually more able, or who have late onset of seizures. One possible corrolary of these findings is that temporal lobectomy should be offered earlier rather than later to allow greater time for constructive compensation to take effect and to reduce the length of time that a young person has to develop within a context of disruption by the presence of damaged tissue and dysfunctional discharges. Accordingly, our current research centres upon the longer term cognitive and psychosocial effects of childhood lobectomy and these will be presented in due course.

Merely considering the matter of childhood lobectomy forces a more detailed examination of the ethical issues, partly because of complic-ations in obtaining informed consent, and also subjectively, because children seem more vulnerable. Some of the basic elements in informed consent are listed in Table 1. In a broad sense there are few obvious problems given conscientious medical management. In our experience, diagnostic tests are exhaustive, the rationale is acceptable, descrip-tions of the operation are forthright and accurate, the aim is obviously to reduce seizures, treatment options are pursued vigorously, positive and negative consequences are well understood and properly conveyed. If a problem exists it is that the aim of the operation is <u>not</u> always exclu-sively a reduction in seizures. It is true to say that all patients and their parents will hope for seizure reduction but it can sometimes appear that they hope for much more. Consider the following replies to the question 'Why did you agree to the operation?', which has recently been put to patients operated upon in childhood and their parents:

Patient A.B. 'How could I have a best friend when I was hardly ever at school?'

Patient C.D. 'I didn't like going anywhere before I had the operation in case I had a fit.'

Parent E.F. 'I was ashamed at the time when she had fits.'

Parent G.H. 'It was difficult to manhandle her as she got older.... I was worried all the time in case I was called home from work because she'd had a fit.'

These statements may reveal complex motives and aspirations. The patients and their parents clearly construed that a reduction in seizures would have personal, psychological and social consequences. Would A.B. in fact be more able to form close friendships? Would patient C.D. become less socially anxious? Is the personal difficulty that E.F. has in accep-ting her child's epilepsy sufficient grounds to give parental consent? Will parent G.H. worry less about her child?

In our current research we are examining more closely the changes in quality of life for children and their parents, and are carefully match-ing aspirations with outcome, defining psychological or behaviour outcome from a more individually centred and psychologically rigorous basis than evidenced by the relatively gross psychiatric and behavioural categories employed in other recent research (e.g. Vaernet, 1983; Meyer et al., 1986; Lindsay et al., 1984). In this manner the process of obtaining fully informed consent can be further improved and the results will bear

TABLE 1

Aspects of informed consent

1. An accurate diagnostic description

2. A convincing treatment rationale

3. A description of the operative procedure

4. Statement of the aims of the operation

5. Appraisal of treatment options

6. A statement of negative side effects

7. A statement of expected success in achieving
   the stated aims

upon the issue of whether the operation should indeed be offered earlier rather than later.

ACKNOWLEDGEMENT

Part of the work reported in this chapter was supported by Action Research for the Crippled Child and this assistance is gratefully acknowledged.

REFERENCES

Bennett-Levy, J., Polkey, C.E. & Powell, G.E. (1980). Self report of memory skills after temporal lobectomy — the effect of clinical variables. Cortex, 16, 543-557.

Blakemore, C.B. & Falconer, M.A. (1967). Long-term effects of anterior temporal lobectomy on certain cognitive functions. Journal of Neurology, Neurosurgery, and Psychiatry, 30, 364-367.

Falconer, M.A. (1953). Discussion of the surgery of temporal lobe epilepsy: the clinical study and selection of patients. Proceedings of the Royal Society of Medicine, 46, 971-974.

Falconer, M.A. (1969). The surgical treatment of temporal lobe epilepsy. in: R.N. Herrington, (ed.). Current Problems in Neuropsychiatry Ashford: Headley Brow.

Falconer, M.A. (1974). Mesial temporal (Ammon's Horn) sclerosis as a common cause of epilepsy: aetiology, treatment and prevention. The Lancet, ii, 767-770.

Falconer, M.A., Mill, D., Meyer, A., Mitchell, W. & Pond, D.A. (1955). Treatment of temporal lobe epilepsy by temporal lobectomy. A survey of findings and results. Lancet, i, 827-835.

Falconer, M.A. & Serafetinides, E.A. (1963). A follow up study of surgery in temporal lobe epilepsy. Journal of Neurology, Neurosurgery, and Psychiatry, 26, 254-165.

Jensen, I. (1975). Temporal lobe surgery around the world. Results, complications and mortality. Acta Neurologica Scandinavica, 52, 354-373.

Jones, M.K. (1974). Imagery as a mnemonic aid after left temporal lobectomy: contrast between material specific and generalized memory disorders. Neuropsychologia, 12, 21-30.

Jones-Gotman, M. & Milner, B. (1978). Right temporal lobe contribution to image mediated verbal learning. Neuropsychologia, 16, 61-71.

Kimura, D. (1963). Right temporal lobe damage: perception of unfamiliar stimuli after damage. Archives of Neurology, 8, 264-271.

Lindsay, J., Glaser, G., Richards, P. & Ounsted, C. (1984). Developmental aspects of focal epilepsies of childhood treated by neurosurgery. Developmental Medicine and Child Neurology, 26, 574-587.

McMillan, T.M., Powell, G.E., Janora, I. & Polkey, C.E. (1987). Relationships between neuropathology and cognitive functioning in temporal lobectomy patients. Journal of Neurology, Neurosurgery, and Psychiatry, 50, 167-176.

Meyer, F.B., Marsh, W.R., Laws, E.R. & Sharbrough, F.W. (1986). Temporal lobectomy in children with epilepsy. Journal of Neurosurgery, 64, 371-376.

Meyer, V. (1959). Cognitive changes following temporal lobectomy for relief of temporal lobe epilepsy. Archives of Neurology and Psychiatry, 81, 299-309.

Milner, B. (1975). Psychological aspects of focal epilepsy and its neurosurgical management. in: D.P. Purpura, J.K. Penry & R.D. Walter (eds.). Advances in Neurology No. 18. New York:Raven Press.

Penfield, W. & Flanigin, H. (1950). Surgical therapy of temporal lobe seizures. Archives of Neurology and Psychiatry, 64, 491-500.

Penfield, W. & Steelman, M. (1947). The treatment of focal epilepsy by cortical excision. Annals of Surgery, 126, 740-762.

Polkey, C.E. (1982). Neurosurgery. in: J. Laidlaw & A. Richens (eds.). A Textbook of Epilepsy. London:Churchill Livingstone.

Powell, G.E., Polkey, C.E. & Canavan, A.G.M. (1987). Lateralisation of memory functions in epileptic patients by use of the sodium amytal. Journal of Neurology, Neurosurgery, and Psychiatry, 50, 665-672.

Powell, G.E., Polkey, C.E. & McMillan, T. (1985). The new Maudsley series of temporal lobectomy 1: short term cognitive effects. British Journal of Clinical Psychology, 24, 109-124.

Powell, G.E., Sutherland, G. & Agu, G.A. (1984). Serial position, rehearsal and recall in temporal lobe epilepsy. British Journal of Clinical Psychology, 23, 153-154.

Rausch, R. (1977). Cognitive strategies – patients with unilateral temporal lobe excisions. Neuropsychologia, 15, 385-395.

Rausch, R. (1981). Lateralization of temporal lobe dysfunction and verbal encoding. Brain and Language, 12, 92-100.

Semmes, J. (1968). Hemispheric specialization: possible clues to mechanisms. Neuropsychologia, 6, 11-26.

Serafetinides, E.A., & Falconer, M.A. (1963). Speech disturbance in temporal lobe seizures: a study in 100 epileptic patients submitted to anterior temporal lobectomy. Brain 86, 333-346.

Vaernet, K. (1983). Temporal lobectomy in children and young adults. in: M. Parsonage (ed.). Advances in Epileptology: XIVth Epilepsy International Symposium. New York:Raven Press.

Wilkins, A., & Moscovitch, M. (1978). Selective impairment of semantic memory after temporal lobectomy. Neuropsychologia, 16, 73-79.

DYSPHASIA THERAPY: A RESPECTABLE OCCUPATION?

Rosalyn Shute and Krystyna Curtis

INTRODUCTION

The efficacy of dysphasia therapy has been a matter of considerable debate for some years. As noted by Benson (1979) there appears to be a long-standing belief among neurologists that such therapy is ineffective, and that any improvement which occurs is not produced by the treatment, but represents spontaneous recovery (e.g. Bay, 1973). After reviewing the evidence Miller (1984) also came to the conclusion that there is very little evidence in favour of the effectiveness of dysphasia therapy. Howard and Hatfield (1987) believe that the scientific community has come to see dysphasia therapy as intuitive and imprecise. It is, they suggest, a less respectable occupation than studying dysphasia for the purpose of testing theoretical models within the hard-nosed discipline of cognitive psychology. Newcombe (1985) also notes that, while the management of patients with neuropsychological impairments is very demanding, its yield for the citation index is small. Powell (1984), in a review of Miller's (1984) book, proposed that neuropsychological therapy 'should still be considered the province of the experimentalist, and not taught willy-nilly to other groups or professions who do not have the necessary scientific background'.

One of us (KC) has developed a project to help dyshasia sufferers in the Rhymney Valley, in South Wales (Curtis, 1986). Funded by Mid Glamorgan County Council's Adult Basic Education Service, it involves both professional educationalists and volunteer tutors. It is the only such scheme in existence in Wales, although several similar ones have been developed independently in England. Such schemes, assuming as they do that there is a role within dysphasia therapy for certain non-scientists, and even for some people who may not be professionals of any kind, might be seen as putting dysphasia rehabilitation well beyond the pale of respectability. It is the contention of the present authors that psychologists should give proper consideration to such schemes, for several reasons. Firstly, they should not be dismissed on the grounds that all attempts at dysphasia therapy are doomed to failure, since it is premature to conclude that dysphasia therapy is ineffective. Secondly, dysphasia sufferers and their families have immediate needs which such schemes can help to meet. Thirdly, educationalists and lay persons may have special contributions to make. Finally, it is proposed that the best chance of developing effective treatment programs will come from increased co-operation between all those interested in dysphasia, whatever their background; academic neuropsychology could also benefit in the long run since, as pointed out by Howard and Hatfield (1987), a theory is strengthened if it can predict how a deficit can be alleviated and the pattern of change that will result.

THE EFFICACY OF DYSPHASIA THERAPY

Considering first the question of the efficacy of therapy, while some reviewers, as already noted, can see little room for optimism, others reviewing the same evidence are convinced that dysphasia therapy does work (e.g. Shewan, 1986). A third viewpoint is that no conclusions can yet be drawn from the available evidence (Howard & Hatfield, 1987), because of drawbacks in experimental design (Newcombe, 1985) and inadequate assessment techniques (Code & Müller, 1983). One of the main problems is that most of the existing studies are group studies, using the Randomised Clinical Trial (RCT). In this dysphasics are randomly assigned to two groups, one receiving treatment and the other not: a greater improvement in the tested group would be taken as evidence in favour of the efficacy of treatment. Howard (1986) maintains that some basic assumptions of this design have not been met in studies of dysphasia therapy: the subjects should form a homogeneous group, treatment should be homogeneous, and differences between the treatments received by groups should be specifiable. In practice, these conditions are almost impossible to meet; for example, since the dysphasics in an RCT are almost certain to form a heterogeneous group, then a standardised treatment may be appropriate for some but not for others. The differentiation of the effects of treatment from other sources of variation presents a further problem: subjects may be recovering spontaneously at various unknown rates, and some who are supposed to be untreated will be receiving informal therapy from family and friends. The measurement of outcome is another source of difficulty, given the lack of appropriate and sensitive assessment procedures for the evaluation of individual patients (Code & Müller, 1983). Overall, then, the sum total of 'noise' in the experiment will mask any real benefits of treatment which may occur for some patients (Howard & Hatfield, 1987).

Shewan and Bandur (1986) suggest that group studies can be improved by using matched experimental and control subjects or by using statistical techniques such as analysis of covariance to reduce imbalances. They cite several studies of this type which have yielded positive results for therapy (e.g. Shewan & Kertesz, 1984).

However, there is a school of thought that really well-controlled group studies of therapeutic techniques generally are impossible in practice, and that the most fruitful way forward is through the use of single-case experimental designs (Holland, 1975; Barlow & Hersen, 1984; Howard & Hatfield, 1987). These avoid the difficult task of matching subjects by using each as his or her own control, and aim to demonstrate that improvement is treatment-specific and is not due to spontaneous recovery: they also avoid the ethical problem of withholding treatment from control-group subjects. Such single-case studies are beginning to apear in the literature; for example, Byng and Coltheart (1986) have demonstrated the effective re-learning of word pronunciation in a surface dyslexic patient by comparing practised and non-practised word sets which had not differed in terms of pre-test performance.

Evidence of this sort suggests that a pessimistic view of the future of dysphasia therapy is not warranted, particularly in view of the criticisms which can be levelled at most of the studies which have failed to produce positive results. Hopefully, well-designed studies will appear in increasing numbers but, in the meanwhile, is it reasonable to expect dysphasic people and their families to patiently await the results?

THE NEEDS OF DYSPHASIA SUFFERERS AND THEIR FAMILIES

In fact, it is already the case that many dysphasics receive little or no treatment, of even an experimental nature. Not all stroke victims are admitted to hospital, and those who are do not automatically have their language difficulties assessed. Some may receive speech therapy as in-patients, and some of these may receive further out-patient treatment for a few months, until they are discharged to make way for more pressing cases. However, many dysphasics and their families receive neither linguistic advice nor more general psychological support. As noted by Newcombe (1985): 'It is in the domain of long-term pastoral care that society fails the victims of disabling brain-damage, and neglects the heavy burden imposed indefinitely on their families'. At worst, dysphasic patients might find themselves to be explicitly written-off, as in the case of the woman who lay on her hospital bed after a massive stroke to hear the doctor telling her relatives that she would be a cabbage from then on; she understood perfectly, but was unable to produce a word in protest (Jordan & Law, 1986).

Far from accepting this prognosis the patient in question, Diana Law, founded ADA - Action for Dysphasic Adults - in 1980, so shocked was she by the condition and the ignorance that surrounds it, among professional groups as well as the general public. In the space of four years, ADA distributed 30,000 copies of its pamphlets advising those who care for dysphasic adults, and a single mention of ADA in a national newspaper brought in nearly 800 enquiries. This illustrates the size of the problem and the need which sufferers and their families feel for help and advice (ADA's correspondence has recently been analysed by Woodhouse and Müller in the first systematic attempt to identify the needs of the spouses of dysphasics). Howard and Hatfield (1987) have commented that dysphasia is a condition that demands a response; the activities of bodies such as ADA and The Chest, Heart and Stroke Association suggest that dysphasia sufferers and their families will remain vigorous in their pursuit of help when they perceive the existing services as inadequate, and that academic assertions about the unproven efficacy of therapy will not satisfy the potential consumers.

One argument that might be made is that, while dysphasics and their families clearly do need more information and support, this should be geared towards helping them to come to terms with their changed circumstances, rather than be aimed at linguistic improvement, and Newcombe (1985) has discussed the potential role of voluntary organisations in providing social support. Schemes like that in the Rhymney Valley have the potential for providing such support for dysphasics and their families while retaining a central emphasis on the development of communication skills. The underlying philosophy is one of providing a service to those who request it, on the understanding that positive results cannot be guaranteed. Such schemes can provide a safety net for those who find difficulty in obtaining help elsewhere; for example, if speech therapists followed the advice of Marshall (quoted by Edelman, 1986) they would concentrate their limited resources on their less severely affected clients, with the inevitable result that the most handicapped would receive little or no therapy. At the other end of the spectrum there are individuals whose impairment is considered too mild to warrant clinical treatment but who nevertheless desire help; for example, a pharmacist sought help from the Rhymney Valley scheme because a stroke had left him with spelling problems which, though slight, had robbed him of some professional confidence.

ADULT BASIC EDUCATION AND DYSPHASIA

When Adult Basic Education servies began in England and Wales, provision for special groups, such as dysphasics and the hearing impaired, was not envisaged. The Adult Literacy Campaign was launched in 1975 to cater for the needs of adults experiencing problems as a result of having left school with persisting basic difficulties in reading and writing. Today, most local education authorities provide Basic Skills tuition for adults. Being a form of remedial education, it necessitates one-to-one and small-group teaching situations. Since a high ratio of tutors to students is presupposed, and such schemes operate at the margin of local education authority budgets, trained volunteer tutors play a vital role.

The Rhymney Valley dysphasia project originated from an apparently normal Basic Skills referral, of a woman with severe reading and writing difficulties. In her case, however, it transpired that these difficulties were acquired as the result of brain damage sustained in a near-fatal car accident two years previously. The help of the community speech therapist was enlisted in assessing her difficulties and suggesting ways in which she might be helped. KC then spent two years researching and developing the dysphasia project, which was launched in 1984; referrals of some twenty-five dysphasic people have been made over the first three years.

Those who believe that dysphasia therapy should be the province of the experimental cognitive psychologist and the experimental clinician will have severe reservations about the development of such a scheme, perhaps arguing that education is not a proper discipline to be concerning itself with such matters, and that the background of educationalists and lay persons does not prepare them to deal with this complex clinical problem.

One view which can be taken is that dysphasia therapy is, essentially, re-education, a view prevalent in the United States after World War Two, when educationalists were much involved in the rehabilitation of head-injured veterans. This view has been challenged by Shewan and Bandur (1986), since they contend that it depends on a view of dysphasia as a language loss, which can be regained by repetition and rote learning. The present authors also regard it as inaccurate to regard dysphasia as a loss of language, but can see no good reason why this should therefore rule out the involvement of educationalists. Shewan and Bandur's criticism seems to be based on a rather narrow and outdated view of what education is about: that it is essentially didactic and based on repetition and rote learning of standardised materials. Shewan and Bandur believe that dysphasia therapy should aim to improve, re-organise or maximise the efficiency of the impaired language system. Again, the present authors concur with this view, but draw a different conclusion: whereas Shewan and Bandur hold that the nature of therapy rules out a role for re-education, the present view is that re-education must be about improving, re-organising or maximising the efficiency of the impaired language system. Hutchinson, of the National Institute for Adult Education, has given a definition of adult education which seems very far removed from the narrow view discussed above: '...all responsibly organised opportunities which enable men and women to enlarge and interpret their own living experience' (Hutchinson, 1963). On this basis, then, the provision of dysphasia therapy within an educational context is valid, and the argument then shifts to its responsible organisation. Consideration must next be given, therefore, to the repercussions of organising such schemes under the umbrella of Adult Basic Education services.

For reasons outlined earlier, Adult Basic Education services in England and Wales are only viable because of the involvement of volunteer tutors. This raises a political problem, since some of those wishing to see the development of better professional services of various kinds may fear that the involvement of volunteers gives policy-makers an excuse for failing to provide greater financial resoures (for example, for increasing speech therapy services). In fact, educationalists involved in dysphasia therapy through Adult Basic Education are vigorous in their promotion of speech therapy services, which their schemes are designed not to supplant, but to augment, and liaison with speech therapists is actively sought.

Apart from the political question about the role of lay volunteers, there is the further question of whether they can be capable of contributing usefully to dysphasia rehabilitation programmes. A study of the use of volunteers was carried out at University College Hospital, and the results published in 1979 (Meikle et al., 1979). Patients either received therapy from speech therapists or from lay volunteers with speech therapists' backing. Unfortunately, the study suffered from the weaknesses inherent in group studies discussed earlier, and there was no untreated control group. Meikle and Wechsler (1983) reported that, although no firm conclusions could be drawn from the study, the scheme was felt, qualitatively, to be so worthwhile that funding was sought to continue it after the trial ended. Another study, by David et al. (1982) suffered from similar methodological drawbacks: patients improved equally on the Functional Communication Profile whether they had received therapy from speech therapists or volunteers. However, the data suggested that these improvements were due to therapy over and above spontaneous recovery, since there was no evidence of greater improvement in the most recently diagnosed patients, in whom the most rapid rate of spontaneous recovery would be expected. So far, then, the statistical evidence on the effectiveness of volunteer tutors is very thin, but the qualitative evidence is positive. Newcombe (1985) has suggested that such studies could include another group – those treated by volunteers who do not feel constrained to mimic professional therapists, but who are free to evolve social programmes tailored to the needs of individual patients. Although the value of such a system remains to be tested experimentally, this is precisely what happens in the Rhymney Valley project. Such a system has the potential for providing services for dysphasic adults not currently available elsewhere, and is based on a view of dysphasia as more than a mere linguistic problem.

As pointed out by Code and Müller (1983), it is an unchallenged fact that dysphasia causes, for both patients and their families, massive psychosocial problems which remain largely unassessed and untreated. They also suggest that a patient's degree of recovery in communicative abilities may be closely related to the level of psychosocial adjustment, and a number of writers on dysphasia (e.g. Eisenson, 1973) have suggested that issues of psychosocial adjustment should be an integral part of speech therapy. Code and Müller (1983) have suggested that group treatment might be valuable in this respect, since it constitutes a semi-naturalistic situation, and is a step nearer to real life. Russian workers (e.g. Luria's pupil, Tsvetkova, 1980) have also noted the value of group work in promoting self-confidence, a positive self-image and an improved desire to communicate. Adult Basic Education schemes go one step further than group treatment in a clinical setting, since they provide the opportunity for dysphasic people to come together to develop their communication skills within their own community, and provide a potential medium for the provision of other kinds of support for dysphasics and their families.

One great advantage of a local voluntary scheme is its flexibility. Dysphasic patients often miss speech therapy appointments because of transport difficulties or illness, and informal arrangements with volunteers can be adjusted to such problems much more readily. Flexibility is also available in terms of the type of environment which can be provided. The importance of providing the best milieu for rehabilitation was noted by Goldstein (1942). Apart from the obvious desirability of providing a milieu in which the student feels good, an atmosphere which is conducive to relaxation can result in improved linguistic performance (Marshall & Watts, 1976). In the UCH study it became apparent that some patients' linguistic performance was better in their own homes, which may have been because they felt more relaxed there; others, however, performed optimally under test conditions at the clinic. Adult Basic Education schemes are able to provide whatever medium suits the individual: a person may begin by receiving home visits, then progress to classes, but still working on a one-to-one basis; finally, group work may be incorporated when the individual is ready for it. Thus a variety of social environments becomes available to the individual, within the community, but nevertheless understanding and accepting of his or her difficulties. Providing conditions which optimise performance is likely, in turn, to have a positive effect on motivation.

This theme of treating dysphasic people as individuals is central to the ABE philosophy. Frequently, someone who suffers from unexpected and severe disability is plunged into depression, lethargy and helplessness (Sarno, 1981), and all too easily becomes a passive patient whose condition is managed by professionals (Howard & Hatfield, 1987). Progress towards becoming a well-functioning member of society again is perhaps further exacerbated by the 'does-he-take-sugar syndrome'. In the Rhymney Valley scheme, those who come for help are not regarded as patients but as students, who play an active part in deciding what suits them best: whether to work individually or in groups, at home or in class, which volunteers they prefer to work with and which particular activities and subject matter they prefer. Indeed, whether to become, or remain, involved in the scheme at all.

This great individualisation of treatment programs is another reason for the involvement of trained volunteer tutors, as an enormous amount of preparation time is necessary. Each student's particular linguistic and numeracy problems are analysed: a speech therapist's report may be available, and is used in conjunction with other tests (including a screening test developed by KC for use by volunteers) and interviews with relatives. The particular problems and interests of the student then determine which activities and materials are used; these frequently have to be prepared specially, and the volunteers provide a diverse pool of interests and expertise, which maximises the chances of matching up a student with a volunteer with shared interests. A further likely advantage lies in the fact that the volunteers provide a variety of speech models.

It would be possible for schemes of a similar nature to be set up through local hospitals, as happened at UCH. However, there are certain advantages in organising them through Adult Basic Education. Firstly, there is an existing nationwide network of services, with a parent body (the Adult Literacy and Basic Skills Unit) through which information and expertise can be disseminated. Secondly, although Adult Basic Education was originally set up to remediate literacy skills, it has since developed to meet the needs of other groups, such as those with numeracy problems, the hearing-impaired and the mentally handicapped; thus expertise has been built up in training professional and volunteer tutors to deal with a variety of special needs, and in setting up and maintaining appropriate education programs (n.b. Adult Basic Education is probably the only existing service with experience in the remediation of numeracy skills in adults). Thirdly, some dysphasics may regard it as nearer to 'normality' and less of a stigma to attend sessions at a local college rather than a hospital. It should also be recognised that educationalists without scientific training will nevertheless be well-placed to understand issues of rehabilitation when their own background is in remedial education.

It has been argued thus far that Adult Basic Education schemes may have an important part to play in providing services for dysphasic people, but there still remains an important problem. Given that dysphasia specialists cannot agree on the nature of dysphasia and its remediation, what methods should Adult Basic Education adopt? Howard and Hatfield (1987) have delineated eight different schools of therapy, including didactic, behaviour modification, stimulation, re-organisation of function, pragmatic, neo-classical, neurolinguistic and cognitive neuropsychology. They believe that a magpie-like approach, picking bits and pieces from different methods, is becoming increasingly untenable. Adult Basic Education schemes are in their infancy, and their practitioners do not pretend, at this stage, to be anything other than magpies. Dysphasia therapy is an ongoing, developing discipline, and an open-minded approach is necessary. In her project, KC uses whatever methods seem appropriate for a particular student at a particular time for a particular purpose, but finds the writings of cognitive neuropsychologists particularly helpful in motivating remedial techniques.

Before concluding, the following anecdotal examples are included to give the flavour of the Rhymney Valley project, and to illustrate the kind of ways (other than the strictly linguistic) in which a voluntary scheme of this nature can help individuals.

H., aged 75, and a stalwart of his local choir, was becoming depressed because his stroke had turned him into a letter-by-letter reader, which meant that he could not learn the words of new songs. His progress through rehabilitation was clearly too slow to solve his immediate problem, so the musician husband of one of the volunteers put the words and piano accompaniments on tape, which enabled H. to learn the songs aurally and remain in his choir.

A., rendered an expressive dysphasic and hemiplegic by a stroke in her mid-forties, learned to drive an adapted car. The neurologist who had to certify her intellectual competence would not permit her to write down answers to his questions, and she feared that she would no longer be permitted to drive, which she likened to being 'put in prison'. KC wrote to the neurologist, explaining that A. had difficulty in initiating verbalisations and used written letters as a cueing device. A. was granted a licence and has since driven all over the country. Last year, following weeks of preparation in classes, she was word perfect at her wedding ceremony.

L. became dysphasic in his late twenties, unable to write or speak, and displayed great emotional distress when he first attended classes. A former engineer, he is now re-developing his mathematical abilities, displays his sense of humour and is the class expert on Makaton sign language, learned from his speech therapist.

Humour, incidentally, is considered an important ingredient in rehabilitation in the Rhymney Valley project. Its probable value and underuse in clinical settings has been noted by Foot (1986), and it has been demonstrated that exposure to laughter can improve the linguistic performance of dysphasics (Potter & Goodman, 1983).

CONCLUSIONS

The present writers believe that the unproven efficacy of dysphasia therapy shuld not be permitted to lead to neglect of the urgent needs of dysphasia sufferers and their families. The evidence is suggestive that dysphasia therapy can work under the right circumstances, and that Adult Basic Education has a particular role to play in catering flexibly for individual needs within the community, taking account of the whole person, not just the linguistic deficit. It would be a mistake for psychologists to dismiss such efforts as well-meaning but ill-advised. The responsible organisation of such schemes necessitates the breaking down of interdisciplinary barriers. The educationalists and medical profession are already beginning to work together, having recently formed HIRE (Head Injury Re-Education) in association with HEADWAY. This organisation aims to form a national body for educational therapists which would then lobby for educational provision for all age groups of head-injured people while in hospital and during rehabilitation, to provide a continuing educational input following hospital treatment and/or rehabilitation, and to provide training and resources for both professional and volunteer staff. Such a system would clearly benefit from co-operation with psychologists in referral, assessment, advice, evaluation and research. Perhaps, by developing interdisciplinary co-operation and understanding, dysphasia therapy will once more become a respectable occupation.

REFERENCES

Barlow, D.H. & Hersen, M. (1984). Single Case Experimental Designs: Strategies for Studying Behavior Change (2nd Edit.). New York: Pergamon.

Bay, E. (1973). Der gegenvärtige Stand der Aphasieforschung. Nervenartzt, 44, 57-64.

Benson, D.F. (1979). Aphasia rehabilitation. Archives of Neurology, 36, 187-189.

Byng, S. & Coltheart, M. (1986). Aphasia therapy research: methodological requirements and illustrative results. in: E. Hjelmquist & L.B. Nilsson (eds.). Communication and Handicap. Amsterdam: Elsevier.

Code, C. & Müller, D.J. (1983). Perspectives in aphasia theray: an overview. in: C. Code & D.J. Müller (eds.). Aphasia Therapy. London: Edward Arnold.

Curtis, K.J. (1986). ABE and the re-education of brain-injured people. Adult Education, 59, 44-47.

David, R.M., Enderby, P. & Bainton, D. (1982). Treatment of acquired aphasia: speech therapists and volunteers compared. Journal of Neurology, Neurosurgery and Psychiatry, 45, 957-961.

Edelman, G. (1986). Aphasia – a complex phenomenon. Therapy Weekly. 28 August, p.4.

Eisenson, J. (1973). Adult Aphasia: Assessment and Treatment. New Jersey: Prentice Hall.

Foot, H. (1986). Humour and laughter. in: O. Hargie (ed.). A Handbook of Communication Skills. London: Croom Helm.

Goldstein, K. (1942). After Effects of Brain Injuries in War. London: Heinemann.

Holland, A.L. (1975). The effectiveness of treatment in aphasia. in: R.H. Brookshire (ed.). Clinical Aphasiology Conference Proceedings. Minneapolis: BRK Publishers.

Howard, D. (1986). Beyond randomised controlled trials: the case for effective case studies of the effects of treatment in aphasia. British Journal of Disorders of Communication, 21, 89-102.

Howard, D. & Hatfield, F.M. (1987). Aphasia Therapy: Historical and Contemporary Issues. Hove: Lawrence Erlbaum Associates.

Hutchinson, E.M. (1963). Introduction to Adult Education. National Institute for Adult Education.

Jordan, L. & Law, D. (1986). Left speechless. Community Care, 20 March, 25-27.

Marshall, R.C. & Watts, M. (1976). Relaxation training: effects on the communicative ability of aphasic adults. Archives of Physical Medicine and Rehabilitation, 57, 464-467.

Meikle, M.S. & Wechsler, E. (1983). The use of volunteers in the treatment of dysphasia following cerebrovascular accident. in: C. Code & D.J. Müller (eds.). Aphasia Therapy. London: Edward Arnold.

Meikle, M., Wechsler, E., Tupper, A., Benenson, M., Butler, J., Mulhall, D. & Stern, G. (1979). Comparative trial of volunteer and professional treatments of dysphasia after stroke. British Medical Journal, 2, 87-89.

Miller, E. (1984). Recovery and Management of Neuropsychological Impairments. Chichester: Wiley.

Newcombe, F. (1985). Rehabilitation in clinical neurology: neuropsychological aspects. in: J.A.M. Frederiks (ed.). Handbook of Clinical Neurology, Vol.2(46): Neurobehavioural Disorders. Amsterdam: Elsevier.

Potter, R.E. & Goodman, N.J. (1983). The implementation of laughter as a therapy facilitator with adult aphasics. Journal of Communication Disorders, 16, 41-48.

Powell, G. (1984). Review of Miller (1984). Bulletin of the BPS, 37, 417-418.

Sarno, M.T. (1981). Recovery and rehabilitation in aphasia. in: M.T. Sarno (ed.). Acquired Aphasia. New York: Academic Press.

Shewan, C.M. (1986). The history and efficacy of aphasia treatment. in: R. Chapey (ed.). Language Intervention Strategies in Adult Aphasia. (2nd Edit.). Baltimore: Williams and Wilkins.

Shewan, C.M. and Bandur, D.L. (1986). Treatment of Aphasia: a Language-Oriented Approach. London: Taylor and Francis.

Shewan, C.M. & Kertesz, A. (1984). Effects of speech and language treatment on recovery from aphasia. Brain and Language, 23, 272-299.

Tsvetkova, L.S. (1980). Some ways of optimisation of aphasics' rehabilitation. International Journal of Rehabilitation Research, 3, 183-190.

Woodhouse, L. & Müller, D.J. Caring for the carers: current levels of support for famlies of dysphasic adults. Journal of the Royal Society of Health, in press.

FAMILY BASED MEMORY REHABILITATION AFTER TRAUMATIC BRAIN INJURY

W M McKinlay and A Hickox

INTRODUCTION

In this chapter it will be argued that it is important to provide
memory rehabilitation aimed at 'real life' memory problems following
severe head injury. The rationale and methods of our present study will
be described together with some preliminary findings.

Serious head injury is one of the most common causes of disability
in young adults throughout the westernised world (e.g. Rimel & Jane,
1983). It is estimated that in the UK there are 150 people wih major
disability resulting from head injury per 100,000 population (Field,
1976). Given that 15 to 35 years of age is the time of peak incidence of
injury (e.g. Medical Research Council Coordinating Group, 1982) and that
life expectation is not known to be reduced, this means that very many
years of 'disabled surviving' result from severe head injury.

What are the most important disabilities which result from brain
injury? Perhaps surprisingly, even after very severe injury, physical
disability is not usually of major importance. Thus, in McKinlay et al.'s
study (1981) of very severely injured patients, 50 out of 55 patients
were independently mobile by 6 months after injury and a further 3 managed with a stick or crutch leaving only 2 out of 55 who were confined to
a wheelchair. However, whereas serious physical disability is uncommon,
cognitive, behavioural and personality changes are much more common, are
associated with stress in close relatives (McKinlay et al., 1981), and
persisted at 5 years post-injury in Brooks et al.'s follow-up (1986).
Moreover, these are also the problems which militate against return to
work. In a further study, Brooks et al. (1987) followed up 98 patients
between 2 and 7 years after injury: 86% were employed before but only 20%
after injury. The factors associated with a failure to return to work
were cognitive, behavioural and personality changes.

This chapter is concerned with rehabilitation of memory and so the
behavioural and personality changes will not be discussed in any detail.
However, as regards the cognitive changes, memory problems are the most
common and persistent according to the accounts of relatives. For
example, in two studies (Mckinlay et al., 1981; Brooks et al., 1986) concerning the outcome in patients with 'very severe' injuries (median post-
traumatic amnesia - PTA 21 days), memory difficulties were reported in
73% of cases at 3 months, 69% at 12 months, and 67% at 5 years post-
injury. Thomsen reported on a very long term follow-up of patients with
very severe injuries indeed (Thomsen, 1987): there were memory problems
in 80% of her cases at 2 1/2 years post-injury and in 75% at 10 to 15
years post-injury. Oddy et al. (1985) reported on a further group of very
severely injured patients. According to relatives, 79% had memory prob-

lems at 6 years post-injury although only 53% of patients themselves admitted this problem. McKinlay and Brooks (1984) had also reported the phenomenon of lack of agreement between patients and relatives. This lack of agreement and the obvious lack of insight of some patients have led researchers to obtain the accounts of relatives separately from those of patients. In the study of return to work already mentioned (Brooks et al., 1987), memory deficit was one of the key barriers to resumption of employment, with immediate recall of Logical Memory (Wechsler, 1945) emerging as the best cognitive predictor in a multiple regression analysis.

Memory deficits following severe head injury may usefully be divide into 'early' and 'late' deficits. In the early stages after injury a period of PTA is characteristic and indeed duration of PTA has been described as 'the best yardstick' for assessing severity of head injury. This applies to nearly all civilian injuries, which are 'blunt', that is, they are not caused by gunshot or other missiles: missile wounds have different characteristics and PTA does not have the same value in such cases. The concept of PTA has recently been reviewed by Teasdale and Brooks (1985). PTA is the time after injury which cannot subsequently be recalled by the patient. 'Islands' of memory do not count as signalling the end of PTA: it is the recovery of continuous memory which marks the end of PTA. The significance of PTA may be illustrated by Jennett and Teasdale's findings. Reporting on 486 patients 6 months post-injury they noted that 83% of those with less than 14 days of PTA made a 'good re-covery' while only 27% of those with over 28 days of PTA did so (Jennett & Teasdale, 1981, p.326, Table 6). However, it must be noted that their definition of 'good recovery' is a broad one (see Jennett & Teasdale, 1981, Ch.13) and need by no means imply freedom from neuropsychological and personality changes of some significance.

The nature of the 'late' memory deficit (i.e. following the acute period of PTA) has been reviewed in a number of papers and chapters. The review of the quantitative research by Schacter and Crovitz (1977) and Brooks's chapter (1984) should receive particular mention. On psycho-metric tests in general clinical use, forwards digit span is generally normal or near normal but few other memory tasks are performed normally. Recall of stories, learning of paired associates, and recall of visuo-spatial material all tend to be impaired. The pattern of deficits is generally held to reflect impaired long-term memory (LTM) and indeed experimental as well as clinical studies support this contention (e.g. Brooks, 1975). Whether this deficit is due to impaired registration, storage, or recall, or to combinations of these is harder to say. Levin et al. (1979) studied a group of patients with 'severe' or 'very severe' head injuries, using the Buschke Selective Reminding Task (Buschke, 1973). They found evidence of defective storage in some cases and of defective retrieval in some too, and concluded that there was marked heterogeneity in the nature of memory impairment. It has also been sug-gested (see Newcombe, 1982) that impaired attentional processes may lead to failure to attend to to-be-remembered material.

In addition to these memory difficulties there may also be other cognitive deficits, particularly deficits in attention (Van Zomeren, Brouwer & Deelman, 1984), although general intelligence is usually not grossly impaired (e.g. Newcombe, 1982). The nature of the attentional deficit is addressed in the excellent review by Van Zomeren et al. (1984). Briefly, the facet of attention for which there is clear evidence of impairment after head injury is 'divided attention'. The authors explain that:

The term 'divided' in this context refers to the fact that the available processing capacity must be divided over several cognitive operations required for task performance (Van Zomeren, Brouwer & Deelman, 1984, p.85).

Such impairment is also referred to as reduced speed of information processing (IP). When speed of IP is reduced it becomes impossible to deal with as much available information as usual and more information will be inclined to go unnoticed.

What emerges is a picture of patients who seem absent-minded and whose memory of recent events and their sequence may be patchy. Studies of 'real life' memory failures add a further source of information. Sunderland and his colleagues (Sunderland, Harris & Baddeley, 1983; Sunderland, Harris & Gleave, 1984) have found that the most common complaints include absent-mindedness, failure to pass on messages, and failure to remember the sequence and details of recent events (see Table 1). A further important finding by Sunderland and his colleagues concerns the measurement of 'real-life' or 'everyday' memory (Sunderland, Harris & Baddeley, 1983). They found that the relationship between formal testing and measures of everyday memory was weak for patients recently discharged from hospital (mean 11 weeks) after head injury. As regards patients seen between 2 and 8 years after injury, whose memory deficits were stable, there was a stronger relationship between test scores and reported everyday reported everyday memory. However, the relationship with everyday memory was only reasonably consistent on 2 of the formal tests, namely story recall and verbal associate learning. Even here, the degree of association ranged from Spearman's Rho=0.72 ($p<0.01$, 1 tail) down to some very modest and non-significant correlations depending on the precise comparisons made. It is quite clear from these findings that everyday

TABLE 1

Memory Failures in Everyday Life Following Severe Head Injury
(adapted from Sunderland et al., 1984)

Items discriminating severe head injuries from controls (minor head injuries) included:

Losing things around the house

Not remembering a change in your daily routine

Forgetting that you were told something yesterday or a few days ago

Letting yourself ramble on in conversation

Forgetting important details of what you did or what happened the day before

Forgetting to pass on a message

Forgetting what you have just said

Having difficulty picking up a new skill

Unable to follow the thread of a newspaper story

Asking the same question twice

Having to go back and check whether you have done something

memory is not necessarily reflected by formal test scores. This is not to discredit formal tests which can provide a detailed description of the nature and extent of memory failure. However, it is likely that reported everyday memory failures will reflect other factors beside memory ability per se, perhaps including the interests and occupation of the individual and the demands these place on memory.

The same paper (Sunderland, Harris & Baddeley, 1983) also provides evidence which bears on the issue of the validity of questionnaire and checklist measures of everyday life memory. The validity of the patients' questionnaire was suspect: it was out of step with the other 3 everyday memory measures used. Morever, there wout of were strong a priori grounds for believing that memory failure should be more frequent among the head injured group than amongst orthopaedic controls, who were also included in the study, and the patients' questionnaire alone of the measures did not show this expected difference. The authors note that this is perhaps not surprising since such a questionnaire is in itself a memory task, requiring the patient to think back and survey recent events. The patients' checklist (a record of memory failure made at the time), and both the checklist and questionnaire completed by relatives showed reasonable consistency each with the other as well as the expected difference between head injuries and controls.

Reports on memory remediation have been appearing in the neuropsychological literature for some time, including both attempts at reinstating memory processes and teaching compensation strategies for defective memory. Methods have included computer-administered practice of memory laden tasks (e.g. Gianutsos & Gianutsos, 1979), the use of visual imagery (e.g. Patten, 1972; Wilson, 1982) and the use of peg methods (Moffat, 1984). Generally, the material learned by subjects in such studies has been a list of fixed information - e.g. the names of staff and other patients. However, those are not the kinds of task with which patients mostly seem to have difficulty in everyday life. This limited relevance may help explain why, despite some gains on formal testing, results have often been disappointing in terms of real-life gains. In addition, some of these strategies themselves make heavy demands on the processing capacities of the individual and sometimes patients simply forget to use them (see Gloag, 1985). One interesting study which deserves to be considered in this context is by Harris (1980). He canvassed a panel of students, whose need for memory aids and mnemonics and whose intellectual capacity to understand and use them might be supposed to be above average. Many of the students were aware of 'internal' mnemonic strategies but very few had used them in the last week; while, in contrast, simple memory aids were widely used (Table 2). Methods which healthy students presumably find unwieldy seem unlikely to find favour with cognitively impaired post head injury patients.

Following on from these considerations, the present study has four elements which are seen as being of key importance.

(1) The memory strategies used should be simple and should not themselves impose any more burden than necessary on the patients' limited information processing capacity (see Van Zomeran, Brouwer & Deelman, 1984). This should make possible greater acceptance of the methods by patients.

(2) In view of the problems of patients forgetting to use mnemonics and aids (see Gloag, 1985) the help of relatives, acting as co-therapists, will be used to try to achieve over-learning.

(3) Clear documentation and homework assignments will be available to back up training sessions and remind patients and relatives of what they are to do.

TABLE 2

Memory Aids Students Use (adapted from Harris, 1980)

INTERNAL	Ever	More than once in last week	EXTERNAL	Ever	More than once in last week
Mental retracing	97	23	Memos to self	97	43
A-Z searching	80	3	Special place	100	40
First letter			Diary	93	43
mnemonics	73	3	Ask someone to		
Rhymes	57	0	remind	97	37
Loci method	13	7	Shopping list	93	13
Story method	23	0	Write on hand	53	20
Face-name assoc.	13	3	Cooking alarm	53	7
Peg method	7	0	Ring on calendar	40	10

(4) In view of the lack of real-life prediction available from tests and the evidence that patients' retrospective questionnaires are not valid (Sunderland, Harris & Baddeley, 1983), the main outcome measures will be <u>checklists</u> of 'real-life' memory failures completed at the time by both patients and relatives.

THE STUDY

A multiple baseline across subjects design was used. Subjects were recruited to the project and assessed. There then followed a baseline period: subjects were randomly assigned a baseline period of 4, 5, 6, 7, or 8 weeks. During baseline the frequency of memory difficulties was recorded using a checklist completed by relatives as well as patients. The length of the baseline period was the independent variable. Any changes which are attributable to training should only occur after the baseline has ended and training has begun (see Figure 1).

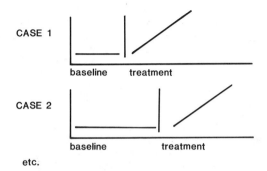

Figure 1. Multiple baseline across subjects' design: in the present study cases were randomly assigned baselines of 4, 5, 6, 7 or 8 weeks.

Adults (16–60 years) with severe head injury (PTA of 2 days or more) and without previous CNS damage or a history of drug/alcohol dependence or severe communication difficulties were accepted. Clinical psychometric assessments of IQ, memory, and concentration were included, but the key dependent measures were frequency counts of memory failures. These were recorded jointly at the time of the failure by patients and relatives. In addition, relatives and patients completed questionnaires about the patients' memory failures (Sunderland, Harris & Gleave, 1984; Broadbent et al., 1982).

Four memory aids/mnemonics were devised or adapted from the literature on cognitive remediation.

(1) The first problem to be tackled was the failure of patients to remember the sequence and details of recent events. The DAILY ACTIVITY SCHEDULE (DAS) is a simplified diary which allows a whole week to be scanned at a time, and by using pictograms and simple wording is readily understood even by patients with limited concentration or other cognitive impairments.

The DAS takes the form of a grid, like a timetable, with a square for each hour of the day for 7 days. The patient was instructed to make one or two word entries and draw 'pictograms' to provide an easily scanned record of his/her activities. Future commitments were entered in red ahead of time: these might include regular events such as remembering to take a pill or perhaps a social engagement. The DAS is illustrated in Figure 2.

The purpose of the DAS is to cue recall of recent events, provide a summary record of what the patient has been doing, and to provide an aid to structuring the days.

(2) A DAILY DIARY was then introduced for those patients who had more detailed tasks to remember. This was simply a list of things to be done in the coming day, and the times at which to do them. Patients were required to tick off items as they completed them. These included minor tasks which were to be completed in the course of the day like shopping for certain items or posting a letter.

(3) The PQRST method (Robinson, 1970) was originally a study method and has been described in various texts aimed at students. It has also been used in neuro-rehabilitation (Glasgow et al., 1977). A simplified version of this was prepared. The aim was to help patients remember what they read – newspapers, books, their own diary, job instructions, etc. It provided a structured approach to reading any piece of material. The purpose of including this method was that a more structured approach would be expected to facilitate encoding, and indeed Wilson (1987) has recently provided evidence of enhanced recall of material read using this method. The stages of PQRST are summarised in Table 3. Study forms were provided to help patients work through these stages until they became thoroughly familiar with them and they also made a self-rating of how good they considered their recall to be.

(4) A PINBOARD was put in a place the patient passed regularly, and on this were put messages, memos, articles being studied using PQRST, etc. While this was a very obvious suggestion to make, we again gave very definite guidelines on how to use this. It was to be located in whichever room was most used. Articles being studied with PQRST and sections for each family member's incoming messages were displayed. Indeed, other family members were positively encouraged to use it to

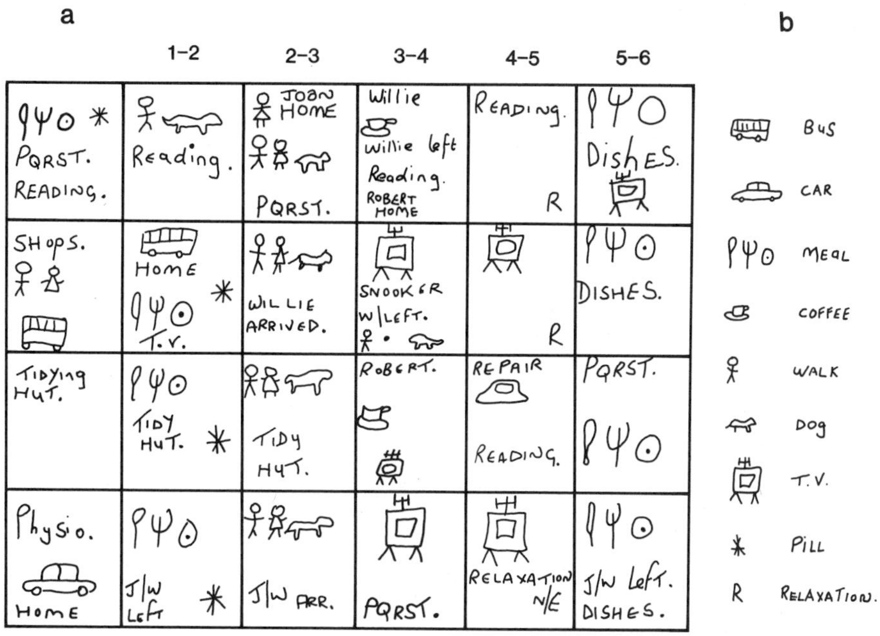

Figure 2. Daily activity schedule (DAS): (a) section of a completed DAS; (b) example of 'pictograms'.

pass messages to each other to make the patient feel less like the odd one out.

In all this the relative's help was seen as crucial. A relative who would help with training was identified at the outset. This relative was present and took part in every session (although opportunities were also provided for patient and relative to air concerns separately). The relative was involved in two main ways. Firstly, he/she helped by recording memory failures - as they occurred - on a checklist: this record formed a key outcome measure. Secondly, he/she was to prompt the patient in the use of the techniques listed above. For example, the DAS was to be carried by the patient at all times, in the same place, and the relative provided whatever prompts were necessary to ensure that this became habitual. For example, a physical and verbal prompt might be necessary at the outset which would be faded down to the level of an occasional verbal reminder, which would be faded out altogether in time.

Data from three of the first carefully documented cases are given in Table 4 and Figures 3 and 4. It can be seen from Table 4 that all three cases had extensive PTA and all were classified as 'extremely' severe blunt head injuries on this basis. They were at least 18 months post-injury and so would be unlikely to be showing significant spontaneous recovery of memory functions (see e.g. Brooks, 1984). All were in full-time occupations at the time of injury but had been unable to resume these. The main presenting problem in each case was poor memory. Standard psychometric tests of memory, Logical Memory, Paired Associate Learning, Rey-Osterrieth Complex Figure - see e.g. Lezak (1983) produced scores well below what would be expected given their premorbid level of ability (assessed using the NART - Nelson, 1982; and see chapter by Crawford, this volume).

TABLE 3

Simplified Summary of the PQRST Method
(adapted from Robinson, 1970)

PREVIEW	Briefly skim to learn the general content. Look for.... headings, main subjects.
QUESTION	Ask and write down key questions. These might be...who? what? when? where? OR ... what are the 3 or 4 main points?
READ	Read actively, with the goal of answering the questions. Read slowly and carefully - intend to remember.
STATE	Go over the outline of what you've read...Then lay it aside and recap. If you need to, read again to fill in the gaps.
TEST	Test yourself by answering the questions you posed earlier.

TABLE 4

Description of Cases

AGE	48	23	21
PTA	2 months	3 months	6 months
TIME SINCE INJURY	4 years	18 months	18 months
OCCUPATION			
- BEFORE	Boilermaker	Business trainee	University student
- NOW	Unemployed	Unemployed	Unemployed
MAIN PROBLEM	Poor memory	Poor memory	Poor memory
RELATIVE HELPING	Wife	Parents	Mother
COGNITIVE STATUS			
- PREMORBID IQ	113	115	118
- MEMORY TESTS	2-3 sds below mean	1 sd above to 2 sds below mean	1 sd above to 2 sds below mean

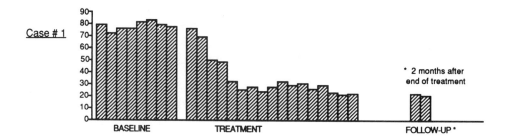

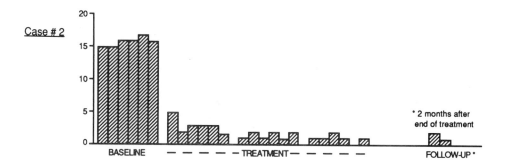

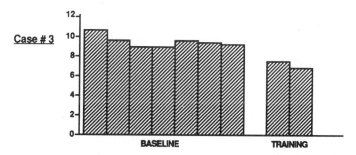

Figure 3. Total number of reported memory failures per week as recorded jointly by relatives and patients using checklists.

DISCUSSION

The dependent measure used in this study was a record of the frequency of memory failures. The record was made at the time by relatives and patients jointly using checklists. It is encouraging that stable baselines have been obtained with these measures. This confirms that these patients have plateaued in terms of memory recovery and suggests that use of the checklists will enable training effects to be identified. Taking the three cases presented together, there is a trend in the expected direction. Improvements in these cases ALWAYS and ONLY occur after the onset of training. In cases 1 and 2 the gains were maintained at a 2 month follow-up. The initial level of memory failures with which the patients presented varied considerably, from over 70 per week to around 15 per week. Decline, during the training procedure, was very gradual in case 1: several weeks elapsed, during which the four techniques were introduced in turn, before the frequency of memory falures reached its final level.

Case 3 must be regarded as a failure at this time as he dropped out

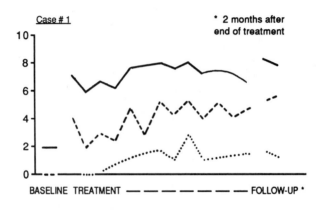

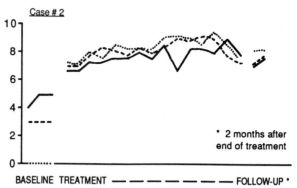

Figure 4. Patients' self-ratings of how well they remembered material studied using the 'PQRST' method. Ratings were made at various times after studying the method, a scale where IO = good and O = poor was used. Continuous line = after 1/2 hour, broken line = after 1 hour, dotted line = after 24 hours.

of the trial. Our initial impression is that unrealistically high expectations made him unwilling to work hard towards limited goals. In analysing data from the whole group (which is intended to number about 30 to 40 in the completed study) attention will be paid to the role of expectations in influencing compliance with training. It may be that additional training procedures aimed at having the patient acknowledge his/her deficits (as suggested by Johnson, 1987) would be a useful adjunct.

Some comment should be made on the self-ratings of how well PQRST helped cases 1 and 2 to remember material which they had studied. We do not contend that such self-ratings provide any objective evidence for the efficacy of PQRST. However, they do reflect the extent to which the patients themselves considered the method to be helpful; and attention to patients' own perceptions is important if methods of this sort are to be used regularly by patients. A much wider range of measures has been used than is contained in this preliminary report. For example, other measures of memory, and measures of mood and of burden on family members have been included. A longer follow-up is also planned (1 year). Analysis of these data will provide a more complete picture and certainly collection of further cases is necessary before firm conclusions can be reached. For example, all the cases reported here are of above average estimated premorbid IQ. Over the course of the study, a wider range of premorbid IQs will be included as this may influence willingness and ability to use the methods employed in the study.

The use of adequate documentation and the involvement of relatives as co-therapists were conceived as key elements of the study. Relatives have generally been keen to help, but a range of relationship problems has emerged in some cases. Our initial impression is that generally these can be ameliorated by counselling, but they add a further dimension to developing training procedures of this sort.

ACKNOWLEDGEMENTS

This research was supported by Grant Number K/OPR/2/2/C751 from the Chief Scientist Office of the Scottish Home and Health Department. We wish to thank John Gray and Miren Ortega for their helpful comments on the draft of this chapter.

REFERENCES

Broadbent, D.E., Cooper, P.F., FitzGerald, F. & Parkes, K.R. (1982). The cognitive failures questionnaire (CFQ) and its correlates. British Journal of Clinical Psychology, 21, 1-16.
Brooks, D.N. (1975). Long and short term memory in head injured patients. Cortex, 11, 329-340.
Brooks, N. (1984). Cognitive deficits after head injury. in: N. Brooks (ed.). Closed Head Injury. Oxford: Oxford University Press.
Brooks, N., Campsie, L., Symington, C., Beattie, A. & McKinlay, W. (1986). The five year outcome of severe blunt head injury: a relative's view. Journal of Neurology, Neurosurgery and Psychiatry, 49, 764-770.
Brooks, N., McKinlay, W., Symington, C., Beattie, A. & Campsie, L. (1987). Return to work within the first seven years of severe head injury. Brain Injury, 1, 5-19.
Buschke, H. (1973). Selective reminding for analysis of memory and learning. Journal of Verbal Learning and Verbal Behaviour, 12, 543-550.
Field, J.H. (1976). Epidemiology of Head Injuries in England and Wales. London: HMSO.
Gianutsos, R. & Gianutsos, J. (1979). Rehabilitating the verbal recall of brain-injured patients by mnemonic training: an experimental demonstration using single-case methodology. Journal of Clinical Neuropsychology, 1, 117-135.
Glasgow, R.E., Zeiss, R.A., Barrera, M. & Lewisohn, P.M. (1977). Case studies on remediating memory deficits in brain damaged individuals. Journal of Clinical Psychology, 33, 1049-1054.
Gloag, D. (1985). Rehabilitation after head injury: 1 - cognitive problems. British Medical Journal, 290, 834-837.
Harris, J.E. (1980). Memory aids people use: two interview studies. Memory and Cognition, 8, 31-38.
Jennett, B. & G. Teasdale (1981). Management of Head Injuries. Philadelphia: F.A. Davis Company.
Johnson, R.P. (1987). Modifying the denial of symptoms following severe head injuries. Clinical Rehabilitation, 1, 319-323.
Levin, H.S., Grossman, R.G., Rose, J.E. & G. Teasdale (1979). Long-term neuropsychological outcome of closed head injury. Journal of Neurosurgery, 50, 412-422.
Lezak, M.D. (1983). Neuropsychological Assessment (2nd Edit.). New York: Oxford University Press.
Medical Research Council Co-ordinating Group (1982). Research aspects of rehabilitation after acute brain damage in adults. Lancet, ii, 1034-1036.

Moffat, N. (1984). Strategies of memory therapy. in: B.A. Wilson & N. Moffat (eds.). Clinical Management of Memory Problems. London: Croom Helm.

McKinlay, W.W., Brooks, D.N., Bond, M.R., Martinaga, D.P. & Marshall, M.M. (1981). The short term outcome of severe head injury as reported by relatives of the injured persons. Journal of Neurology, Neurosurgery and Psychiatry, 44, 527-533.

McKinlay, W.W. & Brooks, N. (1984). Methodological problems in assessing psychosocial recovery following severe head injury. Journal of Clinical Neuropsychology, 6, 87-99.

Nelson, H.E. (1982). National Adult Reading Test (NART). Windsor: NFER-Nelson.

Newcombe, F. (1982). The psychological consequences of closed head injury: assessment and rehabilitation. Injury, 14, 111-136.

Oddy, M., Coughlan, T., Tyerman, A. & Jenkins, D. (1985). Social adjustment after closed head injury: a further follow-up seven years after injury. Journal of Neurology, Neurosurgery and Psychiatry, 48, 564-568.

Patten, B.M. (1972). The ancient art of memory: usefulness in treatment. Archives of Neurology, 26, 25-31.

Rimel, R.W. & Jane, J.A. (1983). Characteristics of the head injured patient. in: M. Rosenthal, E.R. Griffith, M.R. Bond & J.D. Miller (eds.). Rehabilitation of the Head Injured Adult. Philadelphia: F.A. Davis Company.

Robinson, F.P. (1970). Effective Study. New York: Harper.

Schacter, D.L. & H.F. Crovitz (1977). Memory function after closed head injury: a review of the quantitative research. Cortex, 13, 150-176.

Sunderland, A., Harris, J.E. & Baddeley, A.D. (1983). Assessing everyday memory after severe head injury. in: J.E. Harris & D.E. Morris (eds.). Everyday Memory, Actions and Absentmindedness. London: Academic Press.

Sunderland, A., Harris, J.E. & Baddeley, A.D. (1983). Do laboratory tests predict everyday memory? a neuropsychological study. Journal of Verbal Learning and Verbal Behaviour, 22, 341-357.

Sunderland, A., Harris, J.E. & Gleave, J. (1984). Memory failures in everyday life following severe head injury. Journal of Clinical Neuropsychology, 6, 127-142.

Teasdale, G. & Brooks, N. (1985). Traumatic Amnesia. in: P.J. Vinken, G.W. Bruyn & H.L. Klawans. (eds.) Handbook of Clinical Neurology. Vol.45.

Thomsen, I.V. (1987). Late psychosocial outcome in severe blunt head trauma: a review. Brain Injury, 1, 5-19.

Van Zomeren, A.H., Brouwer, W.H. & Deelman, B.G. (1984). Attentional deficits: the riddles of selectivity, speed and alertness. in: N. Brooks (ed.). Closed Head Injury. Oxford: Oxford University Press.

Wechsler, D. (1945). A standardised memory scale for clinical use. Journal of Psychology, 19, 87-95.

Wilson, B. (1982). Success and failure in memory training following a cerebral vascular accident. Cortex, 18, 581-594.

NEUROPSYCHOLOGICAL CAUSES FOR AGORAPHOBIA?

David J Weeks and Kate Ward

INTRODUCTION

Benedikt (1870), the first clinician to describe what is now termed agoraphobia, concluded that dizziness was the central problem and suggested that this dizziness was caused by a disorder of the ocular muscles. Westphal (1871) rejected this notion; he gave the name agoraphobia to a syndrome experienced by patients walking in public places and open spaces. This consisted of severe panic attacks, dizziness, fear of losing balance, nausea, anxiety, palpitations and trembling, and a host of other symptoms usually attributed to an overaroused autonomic nervous system. Westphal singled out anxiety as the cardinal symptom.

Since 1871, psychiatrists generally have accepted that agoraphobia is a functional disorder, and that the symptoms of agoraphobia are overt signs of underlying emotional conflicts. Marital problems have recurred as explanatory concepts (Fry, 1962; Liotti & Guidano, 1976; Milton & Hafner, 1979). Cognitive explanations have also been mooted (Cordes, 1871; Frances & Dunn, 1975; Beck, 1976; Guidano & Liotti, 1983).

Westphal's infuential paper would seem to have diverted aetiological considerations away from hypotheses that considered an organic basis for at least a proportion of agoraphobic cases. This is surprising: his original paper was based on observations of only three male patients. The usual approximate estimate given since is that two thirds of patients have been women (Marks, 1969). In the clinics that the senior author works in, this proportion exceeds ninety per cent. Some authors have had serious doubts whether agoraphobia should be viewed as a unitary diagnostic entity. Snaith (1981) has written that it is 'a misleading diagnostic label for a group of conditions which are not homogeneous and have in common only a certain type of feared situation'. Other clinical scientists have expressed similar reservations (Shafer, 1975; Hallam, 1978; Marks, 1981; Gelder, 1982). It is possible that the diagnosis of agoraphobia may actually conceal several distinct but overlapping syndromes. The distinctions made appear to be significant in that they may have implications for treatment, and perhaps also for prognosis. Agoraphobia has always been a rather anomalous disorder, sometimes stubbornly refractory to treatments which are otherwise effective for similar patients, e.g. systematic desensitisation, flooding, etc. Agoraphobia also has internally contradictory aspects, encompassing features which at first seem incompatible, e.g. fears of open spaces and crowded spaces; different emotions appearing in rapid succession in the same individual: anticipatory anxiety, fear, panic, impatience, anger, unhappiness, and so on.

Marks (1981) has drawn attention to one such condition which has been, and can be, easily mistaken for agoraphobia. He names this new

305

disorder 'space phobia' or 'pseudoagoraphobia'. In Marks' series of patients, who were on average thirty years older than 'typical' agoraphobics, those who feared falling responded less favourably to a trial of standard behaviour treatment, and eighty per cent of them had evidence suggestive of various organic diseases. These included tinnitus, cervical spondylosis, pyramidal and cerebellar signs, nystagmus, hypertension and carotid bruit. Marks argued that these diverse abnormalities reflect a common disorder, most probably a derangement of oculo-vestibular mechanisms.

The hypothesis that organic neuropsychological deficits of this nature are involved is specific to agoraphobia, and falsifiable. It also helps to explain why elderly agoraphobics may fall over initially, and why they have subsequent attacks that seem to be independent of other stressful life-events and preceding psychological anxiety. As other researchers (Wolfson et al., 1981) have pointed out, 'Patients are often emotionally upset after an episode of vertigo (in Wolfson et al. terminology, vertigo is 'an hallucination of motion'), and particularly when it develops without warning, they may become extremely frightened'. Hood (1975) also found a high prevalence of anxiety neurosis (41%) in patients referred with vestibular disorders who were found to have an abnormal response to caloric stimulation. There is also the recent pilot study conducted by Jacob et al. (1985). They found that a high frequency of panic disorder patients who complained of dizziness and unsteadiness showed abnormal vestibular function in the absence of a specific neurological disorder: 67% of the patients showed positional or spontaneous nystagmus, 56% had abnormal responses to caloric stimulation, 35% to rotational tests and 32% to posturography. Pure tone audiograms were abnormal in 26% and accoustic reflexes in 44% of the patients.

Despite this, because agoraphobia has in the past been classified under the more general rubric of a neurotic disorder, much of what patients have said about their experiences have been dismissed or invalidated as one more part of their neurotic pathology. For instance, after adducing a little evidence and much conjecture for an interpersonal-stress hypothesis, Guidano and Liotti (1983) then observe (disbelievingly): 'It is almost a rule that patients deny that this contextual condition can explain the origin of their disturbances, that they consider it only a general source of tension, or that they think it somehow important, but attribute their main complaints to a mysterious and independent somatic illness'. And later they assert, without any evidence produced whatever, '... every state of autonomic arousal that does not seem subject to self-control through "willpower" is not considered to be of an emotional nature (by an agoraphobic) but rather a symptom of a physical or psychic illness ... agoraphobics see themselves as somehow weak ... and physically inferior because of an illness ... As long as they are able to maintain control over their own "weakness", and over the dangers of the unfamiliar environment, they are safe'. A more properly scientific attitude would call for a more balanced stance of healthy scepticism, awaiting properly conducted controlled trials.

To further complicate the issue, however, even proponents of the possibility of underlying physical causes for agoraphobia and/or 'space phobia', only regard it as a comparatively rare clinical picture (Gelder, 1982). Therefore, fairly large numbers of agoraphobics, representative of all age groups, from late adolescence to old age, would need to be tested. As the rare organic dysfunction hyothesis is specific to agoraphobic-like syndromes, one appropriate control group would be sufferers of all other phobic syndromes exclusive of agoraphobia. Therefore, the first priority in research in this area should be to corroborate the existence of these neuropsychological abnormalities, to see how prevalent they are in unselected representative phobia patients referred from general practice or general adult psychiatry.

METHOD

Subjects

Three different groups of patients were utilised in this study. These consisted of consecutive referrals for treatment to two outpatient clinics at the Royal Edinburgh Hospital, the Andrew Duncan Clinic or the Jardine Clinic, from October, 1985 to October, 1987. Patients were requested to participate voluntarily in this research project if they suffered from a phobia or any other neurotic disorder. There were four refusals at this initial stage. Two of these patients were subsequently diagnosed as agoraphobic; one other patient had an acute anxiety disorder, and the fourth patient had a hypochondriacal neurosis. The non-patient control subjects were drawn randomly from a larger community volunteer control subject panel.

Only physically healthy patients and subjects were included in the study. No subjects were included in the study if they were found to be suffering from an organic cerebral impairment, schizophrenia, mania, other psychoses, or endogenous depressive illness. Three potential subjects were excluded from the study on these criteria. One was diagnosed as suffering from motor-neuron disease and a second from suspected myalgic encephalomyelitis. A third patient was excluded on the grounds that he had been diagnosed by a consultant psychiatrist two years previously as suffering from schizophrenia. See Table 1 for a description of the four samples used in the study.

TESTS

The neuropsychological tests were derived from the Manual for the Seven-Year Paediatric-Neurologic Examination according to the thoroughly described National Collaborative Perinatal Project protocol (PED-76) (Shaffer et al., 1985). These were augmented by tests derived from the Quick Neurological Screening Test (QNST) (Mutti, Sterling & Spalding, 1978). Both researchers received special training and much preparatory practice in the use of these tests prior to the commencement of the research. In addition, each subject received the Embedded Figures Test (Witkin et al., 1971), was tested with an electronic three-choice reaction timer (Byrne, 1976) and given tests of olfactory threshold and discrimination. Clinical diagnosis was accomplished independently and blindly to the results of the neuropsychological tests, by extended clinical interview based on the Present State Examination (PSE) (Wing, Cooper & Sartorius, 1975). This was augmented by data from the Fear Questionnaire (Marks & Mathews, 1979) and the Wakefield Depression Self-Rating Scale (Snaith et al., 1971).

PROCEDURE

Each patient referred was assigned by secretarial staff to the psychological tester, who remained blind to the referring doctor's diagnosis. Prior to the tests, each subject was given a brief description of what the tests involved, and requested not to divulge the specific nature of their behavioural or emotional difficulties to the tester. The neuropsychological tests were then administered in the following order, under the following broad classifications: visual reactions, balance in

TABLE 1

Description of Patient Groups and Normal Control Group

	AGORAPHOBICS (n=53)	OTHER PHOBICS (n=43)	ANXIETY PATIENTS (n=38)	NORMAL CONTROLS (n=41)
Age	45.4 (14.5) (range 18-77)	43.4 (16.6) (range 20-79)	46.7 (17.8) (range 22-78)	45.5 (17.7) (range 16-84)
Sex Distribution % Female	91%	86%	77%	71%
Social Class	3.3 (1.5)	3.1 (1.3)	2.9 (1.2)	2.6 (1.2)
Education (Yrs)	10.9 (1.8)	12.8 (3)	12.7 (2.8)	13.7 (3.1)
Duration of Symptoms (Yrs)	13.6 (12.4)	14.1 (10.8)	6.9 (8.4)	--
Total Fear Self-Rating (Fear Questionnaire)	66.5 (24.1)	43.4 (16.5)	34.9 (22.6)	15.9 (10)

* Figures in parentheses refer to standard deviations.
(There were no significant group differences in
lateralisation of functions).

walking tasks, coordination of bodily movements, laterality, muscle tone
and power, tests for abnormal bodily movement, Embedded Figures Test,
choice reaction tests, and olfactory tests.

On a subsequent occasion, each subject was administered a full and
independent diagnostic interview consisting of the measures outlined
above. To be assigned to either of the three patient groups, which were
agoraphobic disorder, other phobic disorder, or anxiety-related disorder,
only patients who conformed to the stringent diagnostic criteria of DSM-
III (American Psychiatric Association, 1980) were accepted into the trial
and included in the following descriptive data analyses.

RESULTS

Three of the tests of eye reactions and movements showed the phobic
groups to have more abnormalities than the control groups. As can be seen
in Table 2, the agoraphobics were found to specifically have the greatest
difficulties in tracking a moving object in all directions with one eye
covered. Both eyes were approximately equally affected.

There were no differences between the four groups in respect to
divergent or convergent squints, unequal pupil sizes under equal standardised lighting conditions, pupil size reactions to direct bright light,

TABLE 2

Eye Reactions and Movements (% abnormal)

	AGORAPHOBICS (n=53)	OTHER PHOBICS (n=43)	ANXIETY PATIENTS (n=38)	NORMAL CONTROLS (n=41)
Consensual Pupil Size, Reaction to Light	20.4%	22.1%	15.0%	12.5%
Accommodation	29.2%	22.8%	15.0%	12.5%
Tracking Objects in Motion	22.1%	3.3%	8.3%	3.7%

TABLE 3

Balance Tests (% abnormal)

	AGORAPHOBICS (n=53)	OTHER PHOBICS (n=43)	ANXIETY PATIENTS (n=38)	NORMAL CONTROLS (n=41)
Heel-to-toe walking, (forwards), smoothness	9.1%	11.3%	5.8%	4.3%
Heel-to-toe walking (backwards), smoothness	19.6%	17.0%	12.2%	8.1%
Heel walking, abnormal movements of upper body	50.0%	32.8%	33.0%	23.0%
Walking on sides of feet, abnormal movements of upper body	53.0%	45.4%	33.3%	32.0%
Toe walking, abnormal movements of upper body	16.0%	9.2%	13.3%	0.0%
Romberg position	18.4%	10.9%	13.3%	7.4%
Hopping: Rhythmic irregularities	29.0%	19.4%	15.0%	7.5%
Tiptoe standing	78.7%	68.7%	60.0%	54.1%

conjugate gaze to follow in either the horizontal or the vertical, conjugate gaze to command in either the horizontal or the vertical, or the presence of nystagmus.

Eight of the tests of balance (see Table 3) showed all three of the clinical groups to have more abnormalities in this area than the normal control group. Most notable were adventitious movements of the upper body while the subjects walked on their heels or toes. These abnormal dyskinesic movements included fasciculations, tremor, and choreo-atheto-dystonic movements. However, the majority appeared to be the effects of excessive muscle tension in these test situations (Table 5). There were no differences between the four groups in respect to their normally walking fluent gait; pelvic drop was only exhibited by two agoraphobics and one normal control subject.

Finger-to-nose pointing (Table 4) with eyes closed, a test of co-ordination, showed both phobic groups committing more errors of accuracy. In addition, these two groups also exhibited more direction changes or halts in doing this, without intention tremor. Two agoraphobics and one normal control subject also exhibited this kind of difficulty with an additional intention tremor. The agoraphobic group showed specifically more mirror movements of the opposite foot during rapid rhythmical tapping of each foot than did any of the other groups. Only marked abnormalities were scored.

The agoraphobic group found the Embedded Figures Test more difficult than the other groups; their total time to solve all the problems was 23.7 minutes, as compared to 19 minutes for the other phobic group, 18.6 minutes for the anxiety patient group, and 12.1 minutes for the normal group. The choice reaction times for all the groups are presented in Table 6; these are broken down into Decision Time, or the speed of internal information processing, and Movement Time, or the speed of peripheral motor movement (Byrne, 1976).

There were no group differences on any of the tests of olfaction; these included tests of threshold, same-different discrimination or supra-threshold simple recognition. There was however a substantial age effect for all groups above age 61. There were also no demonstrable speech deficits, other than one elderly social phobic and one anxious patient, both of whom showed only slighty halting speech.

TABLE 4

Bodily Co-ordination (% abnormal)

	AGORAPHOBICS (n=53)	OTHER PHOBICS (n=43)	ANXIETY PATIENTS (n=38)	NORMAL CONTROLS (n=41)
Finger-to-nose pointing, accuracy	32.3%	21.0%	6.7%	17.3%
Finger-to-nose pointing, smoothness	14.3%	14.4%	0.0%	3.7%
Toe taps, mirror movements	25.0%	9.4%	16.7%	2.3%

TABLE 5

Bodily Coordination (% abnormal)

	AGORAPHOBICS (n=53)	OTHER PHOBICS (n=43)	ANXIETY PATIENTS (n=38)	NORMAL CONTROLS (n=41)
Muscle tone (% rigid)	24.8%	21.0%	20.0%	7.5%
Muscle power (% weakness)	6.2%	9.6%	3.3%	2.5%
Arm-leg extension, unusual finger or hand position	3.1%	8.0%	3.3%`	0.0%

TABLE 6

Choice Reaction Time Speeds (milliseconds)

	AGORAPHOBICS (n=53)	OTHER PHOBICS (n-=43)	ANXIETY PATIENTS (n=38)	NORMAL CONTROLS (n=41)
Decision time	384 (138)	410 (144)	417 (145)	345 (128)
Movement time	331 (118)	404 (170)	378 (158)	300 (110)

* (Standard deviations in parenthesis)

DISCUSSION

This is the first large-scale research project to show that agoraphobics do have specific neurological and neuropsychological dysfunctions that in number and severity are greater than comparable control groups. Because of these, agoraphobics may seem at times overwhelmed by irrelevant visual stimuli within a test configuration or their immediate evironment. Because of their balance deficits, this disability might be compounded when they are in movement. These findings need corroboration by neurological research. All that this research has found are the above-noted group differences, not the aberrant physiological mechanisms which may underlie them. The present researchers are currently examining a range of other psychological, environmental, and dietary variables, and their relationship to the visual, balance and coordination deficits shown above. The purposes of this more comprehensive approach are to exclude those factors that are not involved, and to attempt to formulate an integrated model as suggested recently by Jurgen Margraf and his colleagues (Margraf, Ehlers & Roth, 1986).

There may indeed be something of practical value in the notion that some agoraphobia patients do have valid neuropsychological abnormalities. Were this to be true, this approach could have implications for problem analysis and treatment. It seems imprudent to believe that all the symptoms and responses reproduced by agoraphobic patients can be attributed to their elevated and generalised fear levels alone. Further, their fear, and its related sequelae, i.e. anticipatory anxiety, hyperventilation, autonomic nervous system hyper-arousal, could conceivably be effects or intervening variables rather than causes.

If the organic deficit hypothesis were correct, potential new treatment modalities could be constructed. These could involve retraining in coordination and graceful balancing of the walking body, postural control, visual exercises, or bio-feedback treatment for these patients' proprioceptive, visual-perceptual, or hand-eye coordination abnormalities. Such treatment might also involve over-learning peripheral, seemingly unrelated components of the walking process. Such interventions might consist of deliberate combinations of both straightforward behavioural systematic desensitisation and physical therapy, as shown to good effect by Feldman and Di Scipio (1972).

ACKNOWLEDGEMENTS

The researchers are delighted to express our gratitude to the Phobic Research Campaign, 10 Silverknowes Bank, Edinburgh EH4 5PB, who made this research possible by a generous grant. We would also like to thank Dr David Shaffer, MB, MRCP, FRCPsych, DPM, of the Columbia University College of Physicians and Surgeons, New York, for his help.

REFERENCES

American Psychiatric Association (1980). DSM-III Diagnostic and Statistical Manual of Mental Disorder (3rd Edit.). Washington, D.C.: APA.

Beck, A.T (1976). Cognitive Therapy and the Emotional Disorders. New York: International Universities Press.

Benedikt, V. (1870). Uber Platzschwindel. Allgemeine Wiener Medizinische Zeitung, 15, 488.

Byrne, D.G. (1976). Choice reaction times in depressive states. British Journal of Social and Clinical psychology, 15, 149-156.

Cordes, E. (1871). Die Platzangst (Agoraphobie): symptom einer Erschopfungsparese. Archiv fur psychistrie und Nervenkrankheiten, 3, 521.

Feldman, M.G. & Di Scipio,W.J. (1972). Integrating physical therapy with behaviour therapy. Physical Therapy, 52, 1283-1285.

Frances, A. & Dunn, P. (1975). The attachment-autonomy conflict in agoraphobia. International Journal of Psychoanalysis, 56, 435-439.

Fry, W.F. (1962). The marital context of the anxiety syndrome. Family Process, 1, 245-252.

Gelder, M.G. (1982). Agoraphobia and space phobia. British Medical Journal, 284, 72.

Guidano, V.F. & Liotti, G. (1983). Cognitive Processes and Emotional Disorders. New York: The Guilford Press.

Hallam, R.S. (1978). Agoraphobia: a critical review of the concept. British Journal of Psychiatry, 133, 314-319.

Hood, D.J. (1975). The definition of vestibular habituation. in: R.F. Nauton (ed.). The Vestibular System. New York: Academic Press.

Jacob, R.G., Moller, M.B., Turner, S.M. & Wall, C. (1985). Otoneurological examination in panic disorder and agoraphobia with panic attacks: a pilot study. American Journal of Psychiatry, 142, 715-720.

Liotti, G. & Guidano, V.F. (1976). Behavioural analysis of marital interaction in agoraphobic male patients. Behaviour Research and Therapy, 14, 161–162.

Margraf, J., Ehlers, A. & Roth, W.T. (1986). Biological models of panic disorder and agoraphobia – a review. Behaviour Research and Therapy, 24, 553–567.

Marks, I.M. (1969). Fears and Phobias. London: William Heinemann Medical.

Marks, I.M. (1981). Space phobia: a pseudo-agoraphobic syndrome. Journal of Neurology, Neurosurgery and Psychiatry, 44, 387–391.

Marks, I. & Mathews, A.M. (1979). Brief standard self-rating for phobic patients. Behaviour Research and Therapy, 17, 263–267.

Milton, F. & Hafner, J.R. (1979). The outcome of behaviour therapy for agoraphobia in relation to marital adjustment. Archives of General Psychiatry, 36, 807–811.

Muti, M., Sterling, H.M. & Spalding, N.V. (1978). QNST: Quick Neurological Screening Test. Novato, California: Academy Therapy Publications.

Shafer, S. (1975). Agoraphobia. British Medical Journal, i, 40.

Shaffer, D., Schonfeld, I., O'Connor, P.A., Stokman, C., Trautman, P., Shafer, S. & Ng, S. (1985). Neurological soft signs. Archives of General Psychiatry, 42, 342–351.

Snaith, P. (1981). Clinical Neurosis. Oxford: Oxford University Press.

Snaith, R.P., Ahmed, S.N., Mehta, S. & Hamilton, M. (1971). Assessment of the severity of primary depressive illness – Wakefield self-assessment depression inventory'. Psychological Medicine, 1, 143–149.

Westphal, C. (1871). Die Agoraphobie: eine neuropathische Erscheinung. Archiv fur Psychiatrie und Neruenkrankheiten, 3, 138.

Wing, J.K., Cooper, J.E. & Sartorius, N. (1975). The Measurement and Classification of Psychiatric Symptoms. Cambridge: Cambridge: University Press.

Witkin, H.A., Oltman, P.K., Raskin, E. & Karp, S.A. (1971). Manual for the Embedded Figures Test, Palo Alto, California: Consulting Psychologists Press.

Wolfson, R.J., Silverstein, M., Marlowe, F.I. & Keels, E.W. (1981). Clinical Symposia – Vertigo. Summit, New Jersey: Ciba.

NEUROPSYCHOLOGICAL EVIDENCE FOR LOCALISATION OF VISUAL SENSORY FUNCTIONS

J T L Wilson, G N Dutton and K D Wiedmann

INTRODUCTION

Over recent years there has been a considerable advance in our understanding of the organisation of the cerebral cortex. It is now widely accepted that the visual cortex is subdivided into a number of areas each of which selectively analyses a particular stimulus attribute (Van Essen, 1979; Zeki, 1978). The evidence for this view derives almost entirely from neurophysiological and neuroanatomical studies. In contrast, neuropsychological evidence for localisation of sensory functions remains sparse: there have only been isolated reports of patients with specific visual sensory deficits. Yet such evidence is of particular significance since it serves to provide information not only about cortical functions, but also about the specific manner in which the human cortex is organised. Neuropsychological studies may therefore serve as a bridge between neurophysiological or neuroanatomical conceptions of functional organisation and our understanding of human visual functions. The purpose of this chapter is to consider selectively the neuropsychological evidence and examine its implications for current views of cortical organisation. In addition we will also describe and discuss a patient who shows a perceptual impairment in the ability to perceive vertical contour.

ORGANISATION OF THE VISUAL CORTEX

Neurophysiological evidence demonstrates that the visual cortex contains 12 or more maps of the visual field (Van Essen, 1979; Kaas, 1987; Zeki, 1978). Neurons within these maps are characterised by their discrimination for particular attributes of the stimulus. For example, neurons in area MT show selectivity for stimulus speed and direction of movement (Maunsell & Van Essen, 1983; Zeki, 1974), while cells in V4 respond selectively to stimuli of different colours (Zeki, 1977). Some information about other aspects of the stimulus such as contour orientation is maintained in these areas. However, the emphasis is on information concerning movement and colour, respectively, suggesting that each of these maps is responsible for analysing this particular stimulus dimension. The visual areas are also interconnected in a manner which implies a hierarchical organisation; a specific scheme has been proposed by Van Essen and Maunsell (1983). Within this scheme each level of the hierarchy contains a number of different areas, and it is possible to trace pathways linking a number of areas within the hierarchy. It has been proposed that there are two multistaged systems: an occipito-parietal route which is responsible for the representation of space, and in infero-temporal pathway responsible for perception of objects (Ungerleider & Mishkin, 1982; Mishkin, Ungerleider & Macko, 1983). The scheme outlined by Van Essen and Maunsell (1983) leaves open the possibility that there are further specialised pathways in visual cortex. The overall picture of cortical organisation given by this work is of multiple, specialised visual areas in primate visual cortex, the precise organisation of which will vary from species to species (Kaas, 1987); these areas are both hierarchically connected, and form diverging and converging pathways.

NEUROPSYCHOLOGICAL EVIDENCE FOR SPECIFIC SENSORY DISORDERS

It is generally accepted that current neurophysiology implies a high degree of localisation of function in visual cortex (Phillips et al., 1984). If this is indeed the case then one would expect to find patients who had disorders in processing specific stimulus attributes as a result of posterior brain lesions. However, such cases are reported only rarely in the literature. At present it is not clear why such cases are so uncommon. It is usually assumed that sensory functions are bilaterally represented, and therefore that a unilateral lesion should produce a deficit restricted to the contralateral half-field of vision. Bilateral, symmetrical lesions of the occipital lobes are relatively uncommon and therefore an absolute loss of a particular sensory function must consequently be rare. It is also possible that even when such deficits occur they have been thought to be hysterical in origin and have not been fully investigated, or they may occur in the context of additional cognitive disorders which are of greater functional significance for the patient (Walsh, 1985). Moreover, such cognitive dysfunction may preclude awareness of any deficit on the part of the patient. Apart from studies dealing with patients with lesions of striate cortex, psychophysical investigation of patients with occipital lobe damage is uncommon (Warrington, 1985).

When single cases do occur there are two stumbling blocks in the interpretation of the evidence they provide. First, a double dissociation is required to demonstrate that two functions are distinct (Teuber, 1955). In order to demonstrate that functions A and B are separate one must demonstrate not only that A can be impaired and B spared, but that the converse also occurs, that B can be impaired and A spared. Therefore, a single case can never be sufficient to establish that two functions are separate. Second, specialisation of function and localisation of function are not equivalent. Localisation of cortical function on the basis of lesions is problematic. It is often difficult to establish the true extent of lesions using current neuroimaging techniques. Cases in which lesions are verified by post-mortem anatomy are the exception (Newcombe et al., 1987). Furthermore, lesions are probably never confined to cortex only, but almost always involve subcortical tissue. It is usually impossible to determine to what extent the subcortical lesion is critical to the disruption of function.

What then can neuropsychology contribute? It is noteworthy that views concerning cortical organisation such as that advocated by Ungerleider and Mishkin (1982) imply particular patterns of dissociation: functions of different pathways should doubly dissociate, while functions of the same pathway should show only single dissociations. In other words a hierarchy of functions implies that only single dissociations should occur between the relevant functions, while parallel systems should show double dissociation of functions. Current neurophysiology also makes specific predictions about the anatomical locations in which the lesions which are associated with a particular functional disorder should be found. It is unlikely that neuropsychological studies can provide the main source of information concerning functional localisation. For

316

example, imaging of lesions, at its most accurate, provides localisation in terms of the gyri affected, but gyri are very variable and do not correspond to cytoarchitectonic borders (Bailey & von Bonin, 1951). The information which is available is nonetheless relevant and provides an important source of information concerning human cortical organisation.

Movement

Riddoch (1917) described nine cases of penetrating head injury in whom perception of movement was dissociated from perception of stationary stimuli. In all patients visual fields for movement were more extensive than visual fields for stationary stimuli. In four patients he was able to chart some recovery of vision for objects and movement. In these cases perception of moving stimuli recovered earlier than perception of stationary stimuli, and recovery was more complete for movement perception. Teuber et al. (1960) confirmed these observations in their series of patients with penetrating head injuries. However, they claimed that the reverse never occurred, that is, greater impairment of the perception of movement than the perception of form. They therefore argued that these observations imply that 'there is an order of fragility for visual functions, rather than a separate localisation' (Teuber et al., 1960, p97).

Evidence that, although rare, selective impairment of movement perception does occur has subsequently been presented by Zihl et al. (1983). Their patient was a 43 year old woman who had suffered bilateral posterior brain damage due to an infarct. This damage was extensive and included areas in occipital, parietal and temporal lobes of both hemispheres. In contrast the visual disorder found by Zihl et al. (1983) on testing was seemingly quite specific. The patient was unable to perceive movement faster than about 10 deg/s, but could perceive slowly moving stimuli in the centre of her visual field. She was unable to perceive long-range apparent movement. Unfortunately, she was not tested under optimal conditions for the perception of short-range apparent movement (Braddick, 1974). However, since she could perceive slow real movement, it seems probable that under appropriate conditions she would have been able to perceive short-range apparent movement. She had normal visual acuity, and visual fields; she also had normal foveal colour discrimination, and binocular depth perception. She was able to recognise tachistoscopically presented pictures and words, and she had normal critical flicker fusion thresholds; however, when she was tested on a task requiring discrimination of double and single brief stimuli she was unable to perform the discrimination (Wilson & Singer, 1981). Interestingly, she reported a difficulty in decoding facial expressions; however, this aspect of visual functioning and other, cognitive, visual functions were not formally assessed in this patient. Ungerleider and Mishkin (1982) propose that the movement areas in visual cortex are part of a spatial pathway, and it is thus of interest to establish whether movement processing dissociates from spatial localisation or not. Zihl et al. (1983) report that their patient had accurate saccadic localisation for stationary targets, but it would also have been valuable to establish whether she could reach accurately for targets.

The patient described by Zihl et al. (1983) thus appears to demonstrate a rather pure disorder. This was not a global impairment of movement perception but rather a loss of the ability to see fast movement. The occurrence of such a disorder contradicts the claim made by Teuber et al. (1960) and is consistent with the idea that movement perception is accomplished by a system which is functionally and anatomically distinct. Zihl et al. (1983) argue that their findings are consistent with the results of single unit recording from area MT (Maunsell & Van Essen, 1983; Zeki, 1974).

317

Meadows (1974) reviews early reports of disorders of colour perception which are due to cerebral lesions. He distinguishes between disorders of colour perception, and disorders in which colour perception is not impaired but the patient shows a deficit in naming colours. The former have been called cerebral achromatopsias or cerebral 'colour blindness' and the latter colour anomias or colour agnosias. In addition to describing the features of cerebral achromatopsia Meadows (1974) also reports a single case, and the same case has subsequently been studied in detail by Pearlman et al. (1979). Patients with cerebral achromatopsia typically complain that colours are less bright or that everything appears grey. The patient reported by Meadows (1974) complained that 'everything looked black or grey'. The patient was unable to discriminate different kinds of food on the basis of colour, but when asked to name the normal colours of common objects he was able to do so correctly. This patient also showed normal stereopsis, and made only two minor errors on the Ishihara pseudoisochromatic plate test for congenital colour deficiencies. Mollon et al. (1980) described a case of cerebral achromatopsia and demonstrated that the retinal mechanisms for processing colour were still intact in their patient by measuring increment thresholds for coloured stimuli against coloured backgrounds. On neuropsychological testing achromatopsia is often associated with prosopagnosia and impaired topographical memory (Meadows, 1974). However, the three disorders may be dissociated suggesting that they are functionally distinct.

Achromatopsia is associated with damage to the anterior inferior part of the occipital lobes, and most patients with complete achromatopsia have demonstrable bilateral lesions (Meadow, 1974). Pearlman et al. (1979) argue that achromatopsia results from damage to an area homologous to the V4 complex in rhesus monkey described by Zeki (1977). The idea that patients with cerebral achromatopsia have a lesion in such an area is quite compelling; however, some caution should be expressed concerning whether the same functional systems and anatomical locations are being identified in both species. It has been shown that in rhesus monkeys V4 is involved in colour constancy, but is not required for wavelength discrimination (Wild et al., 1985), but patients with achromatopsia have a more profound defect of colour perception than simply a loss of colour constancy. Furthermore, Mollon et al. (1980) point out that, since achromatopsia may follow encephalitis, the deficit need not arise from a lesion at a circumscribed anatomical location but is also consistent with the idea that patients have selectively lost one class of nerve fibre.

Location

The extensive and confusing literature on neuropsychological disorders of space perception is reviewed by De Renzi (1982). Many aspects of disordered space perception reflect high-level deficits, but two which may have a sensory basis will be briefly considered here. The first concerns localisation of position in space, and the second concerns depth perception and is dealt with in the following section.

Holmes (1918) described a syndrome of visual disorientation one feature of which was an inability to locate the position of a stimulus by vision alone. This form of defective localisation cannot be explained purely as a motor disorder, and is not simply due to field defects. An indication of the prevalence of deficits of localisation comes from a study of 49 patients with penetrating head injuries carried out by Ratcliff and Davies-Jones (1972). Subjects were required to indicate the position of a target presented at a selected point on a perimeter by making a smooth reaching movement and touching it with an index finger. None of the patients with anterior lesions were impaired on this task, but 36 out of 40 patients with posterior lesions had defective localisation. In these, unselected, cases the impairment was confined to stimuli presented in the peripheral visual field, and severe disorders of localisation were restricted to the half field contralateral to the site of the lesion. They conclude that some degree of defective localisation is a common consequence of posterior brain damage, and is particularly associated with lesions to the parietal lobe. Ratcliff and Davies-Jones (1972) did not assess other visual functions in their patients, however, Warrington (1985) reports that impaired performance on a perimetric localisation task is dissociable from deficits of acuity, shape discrimination and colour perception.

Clear evidence that localisation can be spared and other visual functions disrupted comes from studies of the effects of damage to striate cortex (Poeppel et al., 1973; Weiskrantz et al., 1974). Weiskrantz et al. (1974) showed that their patient, D.B., could reach accurately to targets presented in his blind hemifield despite having no conscious awareness that a target had been presented. Eye movements to targets are less accurate than reaching in these patients. However, Zihl (1980) has shown that accuracy of saccadic localisation increases with practice. Weiskrantz (1987) has demonstrated that D.B. does not have residual form discrimination in his blind hemifield, and furthermore that his detection of targets is not an artefact of scattered light. The ability shown by patients with 'blindsight' implies that localisation is a specialised visual function and, indeed, one which does not require an intact striate cortex.

A distinction between pattern recognition and spatial vision was proposed by Newcombe and Russell (1969) on the basis of a double dissociation found in their series of patients with penetrating head injuries. This double dissociation is exemplified by two single cases described by Newcombe et al. (1987). Both patients had preserved intellectual abilities as assessed by the Mill Hill Synonyms Test and Raven's Progressive Matrices. However, one patient was impaired on a maze learning task but not on a face recognition task, while the other was impaired on face recognition but showed normal maze learning performance. The patient with the maze learning deficit had a parietal lesion, and the patient with the face recognition problem had a temporal lesion.

The occurrence of double dissociations between deficits of localisation and impaired acuity and object perception supports the idea that localisation is accomplished in a separate pathway (Ungerleider & Mishkin, 1982). The neuropsychological evidence also confirms that the parietal lobe is particularly associated with space perception.

Depth

Riddoch (1917) reported the comments of a patient who was unable to appreciate depth or thickness in objects: 'Everything seems to be really the same distance away. For example, you appear to be as near to me as my hand' (he was holding his hand 1 1/2 inches from his face and I was sitting about 5 feet away from him)' (Riddoch, 1917, p.47).

A loss of all sense of depth is a rare consequence of brain damage. However, a specific loss of stereopsis is not uncommon (Danta et al., 1978). Stereopsis may be permanently lost even though visual acuity and binocular integration are theoretically sufficient for depth perception (Poeppel et al., 1978). Hamsher (1978) demonstrated that impaired global stereopsis, as assessed using random-letter stereograms, is associated with lesions of the right hemisphere. It is thus well established that a selective loss of stereopsis can occur as a result of brain damage. It is perhaps surprising, however, that stereopsis can be disrupted by unilateral lesions well outside the occipital regions, and Danta et al. (1978) were led to conclude that stereopsis is not a localised function but rather involves widespread areas of the brain.

Form

Form perception is a broad and ill-defined area which includes perception of contour, shape and objects. Although there are clearly a number of aspects to form perception it is unclear what precise distinctions should be made. Neuropsychological evidence may have an important contribution to make to the subdivision of this domain.

Warrington (1985) described dissociations between shape discrimination, visual acuity, colour perception and visual localisation in a group of 5 patients. All patients were considered to have had an acute episode of cortical blindness from which they had made a partial recovery, and they all had bilateral occipital infarctions verified by CT scanning. Patients were given a task which required discrimination between a square and a rectangle (Efron, 1968), and a task which involved detection of a fragmented stimulus against a random pattern background (Warrington & Taylor, 1973). In addition, patients were tested on their ability to locate stimuli by pointing to targets presented using a perimeter, on their visual acuity, and on their colour discrimination using the Farnsworth-Munsell 100 Hue Test or the Holmgren wool test. Warrington (1985) reports that four of the five patients had impaired shape discrimination, and that this occurred, in individual cases, with preserved acuity, colour perception and visual localisation. She also describes a patient with very impaired acuity and colour perception who performed perfectly normally on the shape discrimination tasks. Warrington's findings show that perception of form, perception of colour and localisation are dissociable. Interestingly, her results also provide evidence of a further dissociation within the form perception domain: 'There would appear to be at least partial independence in the mechanisms subserving discrimination of an edge (as measured by minimal separable acuity) and discrimination of an edge as an integral part of a shape' (Warrington, 1985, p.259). A double dissociation between pattern recognition and visual acuity has been described by Sprague et al. (1981) in ablation studies with cats. It appears therefore that not only is form perception distinct from other functions such as colour vision but also that patients may show a selective loss of particular aspects of form perception.

We have recently had the opportunity to test a patient who shows a deficit in the ability to perceive an elementary aspect of form, and her case history will therefore be summarised here. SL is a 38 year old woman. Two years prior to neuropsychological testing she had pneumonia while she was pregnant and was admitted comatose to intensive care. During the time she was in intensive care she had repeated periods of hypotension. When she recovered she complained of a visual problem, and specifically a difficulty in reading. Over the past two years she has had repeated conventional ophthalmological testing. The results from these examinations are consistent, and are briefly as follows. There is no history of strabismus or other visual disorder, and no current astigmatism or refractive error. There is no disorder of eye movements. She initially had moderately depressed visual acuity (distance acuity: right eye 6/24, left eye 6/36, binocular 6/18); but on most recent testing this has resolved. She has a small homonymous paracentral scotoma immediately to the left of fixation. The results of the ophthalmological examinations are consistent with the presence of a visual deficit of neurological

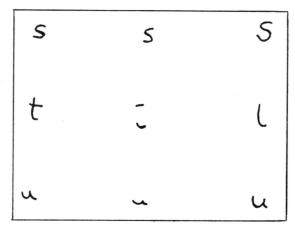

Figure 1. Left, examples of target letters that SL was asked to copy. Centre, her copies when the target letters were oriented vertically. Right, her copies when the target letters were rotated through 90 degrees.

origin, but do not explain the magnitude of her difficulty in reading.

An intriguing feature of her reading problem was that she reported greater difficulty reading print than cursive handwriting. Investigation of her reading indicated that her difficulty lay in recognising individual letters, which she reported as seeing only partially. We asked her to copy letters of the alphabet as she saw them. She employed free viewing but was instructed not to turn her head. In performing this task she consistently omitted the vertical portion of the letters (Fig.1). This occurred both with letters oriented normally, and copying letters rotated through 90 degrees. She had been unaware that it was consistently the vertical components of the letters which she did not see until it was pointed out to her. In order to document the disorder we measured SL's contrast sensitivity to gratings at various orientations using a computerised procedure. Contrast sensitivity was depressed at all spatial frequencies for vertically as compared to horizontally oriented gratings. Contrast sensitivity functions were obtained for low (.5 cycles/deg) and intermediate (6 cycles/deg) frequency gratings at four orientations (0, 45, 90 and 135 degrees to the horizontal). She exhibited a marked loss of sensitivity to gratings oriented at 90 degrees, and she showed intermediate sensitivity to gratings oriented at 45 and 135 degrees. The effect of orientation was present at both intermediate and low spatial frequencies, but was rather less pronounced in the latter case.

SL has little or no difficulty in recognising or naming objects. Her short-term visual memory span and her ability to learn novel patterns are within normal limits. Her Verbal IQ (Wechsler Adult Intelligence Scale) is 118. Her Performance IQ is distinctly lower, 92. However, the errors she made on the performance tests tended to be consistent with her perceptual problems. Her poorest scores were on Digit Symbol (scaled score 5) and Picture Completion (scaled score 7). For example, on the Picture Completion subtest she took 17 seconds to identify a line drawing of a door, but took only a further 8 seconds to correctly report that the door handle was missing. Her ability on the other Performance measures was within normal limits (Block Design: 9; Picture Arrangement: 9; Object Assembly: 10).

Both CT and MRI scans were performed. The results of the scans were consistent. However, the MRI scans allowed the lesion to be visualised more readily in three dimensions. The scans showed a well-defined lesion in the inferior portion of the right occipital lobe. The history of the patient suggests that additional diffuse damage may have been present, and was not demonstrated by neuroimaging.

The deficit shown by this patient supports the claim that there are functionally separate mechanisms in the visual system selectively processing different orientations (Blakemore & Campbell, 1969). The case described only demonstrates a single dissociation: it is conceivable that perception of vertical contour is particularly susceptible to brain damage. However, Regan and Maxner (1987) report that patients with Parkinson's disease show a selective loss of sensitivity to horizontal gratings. It appears therefore that sensitivity to vertical and horizontal are capable of double dissociation. It is surprising that a selective loss of sensitivity to vertical should occur as a result of an infarct since it suggests that, at some level, there is a separate anatomical location for processing information concerning this orientation. There is little direct neurophysiological support for such an idea. However, Barlow (1981) speculates that stimulus attributes such as orientation may show nontopographic mapping in the visual cortex, and the deficit shown by the patient is consistent with this idea.

CONCLUSIONS

We have selectively reviewed cases of impaired visual sensory functions arising from cortical lesions, and some common themes emerge. Sensory deficits arising from cortical lesions are rarely absolute. For example, the patient described by Zihl et al. (1983) retained some ability to perceive movement, although it is worth noting that references to this study often imply that the patient had a global impairment of movement perception. Most, if not all, sensory deficits which affect the whole visual field arise from bilateral lesions. A unilateral lesion generally gives rise to a defect in the contralateral half-field. Apparent exceptions to this rule may stem from a non-sensory contribution to visual functions. Detection of sensory deficits often requires specific testing. Although patients may be aware of a visual problem, they are often unaware of the precise nature of their disorder. When testing of a particular aspect of vision is carried out on a group of neuropsychological patients, sensory deficits are often found to be quite common (Danta et al., 1978; Ratcliff & Davies-Jones, 1972). It is also worth stressing that the dissociations described are between performance on different tests, rather than between different functions. It is therefore preferable that functions be assessed by a variety of measures rather than a single test. There is clearly a need for further systematic study of the consequences of posterior lesions.

In addition to supporting the proposed distinction between form perception and localisation in space, the neuropsychological evidence suggests that there are separate pathways or areas for movement perception, colour vision, and depth perception. Further fractionation may be possible within each domain. The case described by Zihl et al. (1983) suggests that perception of fast and slow movement may be at least partly independent, and may parallel the distinction made between long-range and short-range apparent movement (Anstis, 1978). In the domain of form perception Warrington (1985) reports a dissociation between edge discrimination in an acuity task, and discrimination of an edge as part of a shape. Furthermore we describe a single case suggesting that perception of vertical contour may be functionally distinct from perception of other orientations. It is conceivable that there are a large number of nontopographic maps subserving specific visual functions. The cases reviewed provide evidence for specialisation of function in the visual system. Specialisation of function does not imply localisation of function in distinct anatomical areas, and the evidence for precise localisation is often lacking. Noneteheless, separate localisation remains the most plausible reason for selective disruption of function by discrete brain lesions.

ACKNOWLEDGEMENTS

The Carnegie Trust provided help to JTLW during testing of patient SL. KDW was supported by an MRC project grant.

REFERENCES

Anstis, S.M. (1978). Apparent motion. in: R. Held, H.W. Leibowitz & H.L. Teuber (eds.). Handbook of Sensory Physiology (Vol.7) Perception. Berlin: Springer.

Bailey, P. & von Bonin, G. (1951). The Isocortex of Man. Urbana: University of Illinois Press.

Barlow, H.B. (1981). Critical limiting factors in the design of the eye and visual cortex. Proceedings of the Royal Society of London, B212, 1-34.

Blakemore, C. & Campbell, F.W. (1969). On the existence of neurons in the human visual system selectively sensitive to the orientation and size of retinal images. Journal of Physiology, London, 203, 237-260.

Braddick, O. (1974). A short-range process in apparent motion. Vision Research, 14, 519-527.

Danta, G., Hilton, R.C. & O'Boyle, D.J. (1978). Hemisphere function and binocular depth perception. Brain, 101, 569-589.

De Renzi, E. (1982). Disorders of Space Exploration and Cognition, Chichester: Wiley.

Efron, R. (1968). What is perception? Boston Studies in the Philosophy of Science. New York: Humanities Press Inc.

Holmes, G. (1918). Disturbances of visual orientation. British Journal of Ophthalmology, 2, 449-468; 506-516.

Kaas, J.H. (1987). The organisation of neocortex in mammals: implications for theories of brain function. Annual Review of Psychology, 38, 129-151.

Maunsell, J.H.R. & Van Essen, D.C. (1983). Functional properties of neurons in middle temporal visual area of the macaque monkey. I. Selectivity for stimulus direction, speed, and orientation. Journal of Neurophysiology, 5, 1127-1147.

Meadows, J.C. (1974). Disturbed perception of colours associated with localised cerebral lesions. Brain, 97, 615-632.

Mishkin, M., Ungerleider, L.G. & Macko, K.A. (1983). Object vision and spatial vision: two cortical pathways. Trends in Neurosciences, 6, 414-417.

Mollon, J.D., Newcombe, F., Polden, P.G. & Ratcliff, G. (1980). On the presence of three cone mechanisms in a case of total achromatopsia. in: G. Verriest (ed.). Colour Vision Deficiencies. Bristol: Hilger.

Newcombe, F., Ratcliff, G. & Damasio, H. (1987). Dissociable visual and spatial impairments following right posterior cerebral lesions: clinical, neuropsychological and anatomical evidence. Neuropsychologia, 25, 149-161.

Newcombe, F. & Russell, W.R. (1969). Dissociated visual perceptual and spatial deficits in focal lesions of the right hemisphere. Journal of Neurology, Neurosurgery and Psychiatry, 32, 73-81.

Pearlman, A.L., Birch, J. & Meadows, J.C. (1979). Cerebral colour blindness: an acquired defect of hue discrimination. Annals of Neurology, 5, 253-261.

Phillips, C.G. Zeki, S.M. & Barlow, H.B. (1984). Localisation of function in the cerebral cortex: past, present and future. Brain, 107, 327-361.

Poeppel, E., Brinkman, R., von Cramon, D. & Singer, W. (1978). Association and dissociation of visual functions in a case of occipital lobe infarction. Archiv fuer Psychiatrie und Nervenkrankenheiten, 225, 1-21.

Poeppel, E., Held, R. & Frost, D. (1973). Residual visual function after brain wounds involving the central visual pathways in man. Nature, London, 243, 295-296.

Ratcliff, G. & Davies-Jones, G.A.B. (1972). Defective visual localisation in focal brain wounds. Brain, 95, 49-60.

Regan, D. & Maxner, C. (1987). Orientation selective visual loss in patients with Parkinson's disease. Brain, 110, 415-432.

Riddoch, G. (1917). Dissociation of visual perceptions due to occipital injuries with especial reference to appreciation of movement. Brain, 40, 15-57.

Sprague, J.M., Hughes, H.C. & Berlucchi, G. (1981). Cortical mechanisms in pattern and form perception. in: O. Pompeiano & C. Ajmone Marsan (eds.). Brain Mechanisms and Perceptual Awareness. New York: Raven Press.

Ungerleider, L. & Mishkin, M. (1982). Two cortical visual systems. in: D.J. Ingle, R.J.W. Mansfield & M.S. Goodale (eds.). The Analysis of Visual Behaviour. Cambridge, Mass.: MIT Press.

Van Essen, D.C. (1979). Visual areas of the mammalian cerebral cortex. Annual Review of Newuroscience, 2, 227-263.

Van Essen, D.C. & Maunsell, J.H.R. (1983). Hierarchical organisation and functional streams in the visual cortex. Trends in Neurosciences, 6, 370-375.

Walsh, K.W. (1985). Understanding Brain Damage. Edinburgh: Churchill Livingstone.

Warrington, E.K. (1985). Visual deficits associated with occipital lobe lesions in man. in: C. Chagas, R. Gatass & C. Gross (eds.). Pattern Recognition Mechanisms. Berlin: Springer.

Warrington, E.K. & Taylor, A.M. (1973). Contribution of right parietal lobe to object recognition. Cortex, 9, 152-164.

Weiskrantz, L. (1987). Residual vision in a scotoma. Brain, 110, 77-92.

Weiskrantz, L., Warrington, E.K., Sanders, M.D. & Marshall, J. (1974). Visual capacity in the hemianopic field following a restricted occipital ablation. Brain, 97, 709-728.

Wild, H.M., Butler, S.R., Carden, D. & Kulikowski, J.J. (1985). Primate cortical area V4 important for colour constancy but not wavelength discrimination. Nature, London, 313, 133-135.

Wilson, J.T.L. & Singer, W. (1981). Simultaneous visual events show a long-range interaction. Perception and Psychophysics, 30, 107-113.

Zeki, S.M. (1974). Functional organisation of a visual area in the posterior bank of the superior temporal sulcus of the rhesus monkey. Journal of Physiology, London, 236, 549-573.

Zeki, S.M. (1977). Colour coding in the superior temporal sulcus of the rhesus monkey visual cortex. Proceedings of the Royal Society of London, B197, 195-223.

Zeki, S.M. (1978). Uniformity and diversity of structure and function in rhesus monkey prestriate cortex. Journal of Physiology, London, 277, 273-290.

Zihl, J. (1980). 'Blindsight': improvement of visually guided eye movements by systematic practice in patients with cerebral blindness. Neuropsychologia, 18, 71-77.

Zihl, J., Von Cramon, D. & Mai, N. (1983). Selective disturbance of movement vision after bilateral brain damage. Brain, 106, 313-340.

INSPECTION TIME: EXPERIMENTAL ADVANCES AND CLINICAL PROSPECTS

Ian J Deary

INTRODUCTION

Unlike many of the papers in this volume this chapter deals with
neither a clinical syndrome nor an established set of neuropsychological
tests. However, the relatively new technique of Inspection Time (IT) has
features that indicate its potential clinical usefulness. Substantial
reviews of the work on visual inspection time have been compiled by Brand
and Deary (1982) and Nettelbeck (1987) and it is not my intention to
replicate these efforts here. Instead, a brief resume of the theoretical
basis for the measure and a summary of the main experimental findings
will be offered by way of an introduction. The main body of the chapter
is devoted to the development of an auditory inspection time test. The
chapter ends with some suggestions for further development work on and
some clinical applications for IT Tests.

The IT measure was devised to test a theory of perception developed
by Vickers and his colleagues (Vickers, Nettelbeck & Willson, 1972;
Vickers & Smith, 1986). Vickers' theory states that the perception of a
target stimulus in a two choice decision task takes place by the accumul-
ation of evidence for each of the alternatives in quantal units called
'inspections'. During stimulus presentation the perceptual system sets up
two counters and a decision is made when the accumulated evidence in
favour of one of the alternatives has passed a certain threshold. The
theory also states that if a discrimination is very easy then only a
single inspection is required to make a correct choice. The theory offers
the possibility of measuring a fundamental aspect of perception: the time
required by an organism to make a single inspection of a stimulus.

A visual task was devised to measure subjects' visual IT (Vickers,
Nettelbeck & Willson, 1972). Stimuli consisted of two vertical black
lines on a white background and were presented tachistoscopically. The
line lengths were markedly different (e.g. 5cm versus 7cm) and the two
lines were placed 2cm apart. The subjects' task was to indicate which of
the lines (left or right) was longer. No estimate of response time was
necessary and, unusually for a decision task, subjects were requested to
respond at their leisure. The effective stimulus presentation time (i.e.
the stimulus onset asynchrony) was varied using a psychophysical method
and a normal ogive fitted to the data when stimulus duration is plotted
versus percentage of correct responses. All stimulus lines are backward
masked to prevent further information being extracted from the stimulus
when the presentation is finished. Typically, subjects achieve nearly
100% correct responses at longer stimulus durations and performance falls
off to chance levels as stimulus presentation time shortens. The inspection time for any one subject is defined as the stimulus duration (in ms)
at which the subject achieves a predetermined level of accuracy (this is

taken arbitrarily and is often 85%, 90% or 97.5% making comparison of absolute IT levels impossible across different studies).

INSPECTION TIME AND INTELLIGENCE

A report by Nettelbeck and Lally (1976) ensured that IT would not remain an obscure psychophysical index. They correlated ten subjects' IT durations with their Wechsler Adult Intelligence Scale (WAIS) scores (the ten subjects covered a wide range, from IQ 47 to 119, giving a high standard deviation which is likely to inflate the correlation). The correlations between WAIS scores and IT (which was tested on two occasions) were -0.89 and -0.92. The finding of a large negative correlation between IQ and IT (brighter subjects require less stimulus presentation time in order to make a correct decision) was replicated by Lally and Nettelbeck (1977) and Brand and his students (Brand, 1981). By 1982 Brand and Deary had reviewed nine experiments where IT was correlated with psychometric intelligence scores and, by including only those studies which had used culture fair tests on samples with a mean IQ of about 100, reported a median correlation of -0.80. These early results led to speculation that IT might provide a fairer way to test intelligence and provoked some controversy (Mackintosh, 1981; Brand & Deary, 1982; Nettelbeck, 1982).

Many studies, using larger subject samples, were conducted between 1982 and 1987 and these have provided a more modest estimate of the IT-IQ correlation while demonstrating the robust nature of the relationship. Nettelbeck's (1987) recent review provides an exhaustive account of the IT and intelligence literature. He collected 24 studies which examined the relationship between general intelligence and IT and the mean correlation was -0.34 (range 0.10 to -0.61) with 16 of the 24 reporting a significant negative correlation. Verbal IQ and IT were correlated in 12 studies with a mean correlation of -0.27, seven studies reported a significant negative correlation. Performance IQ and IT were studied in 9 experiments with an average correlation in retarded subject samples of -0.45. Non-retarded subject samples had a mean correlation of -0.33. Seven of the 9 studies reported significant negative correlations.

Two factors make these correlations under-estimates of the 'true' value. First, the test-retest reliability for the IQ tests and the IT tests is not perfect. Nettelbeck (1987) calculated an average test-retest reliability of 0.74 for IT (measured in 16 studies). Second, although the early studies of IT occasionally included mentally retarded subjects and large IQ ranges (see Mackintosh, 1986 and Vernon, 1986 for a discussion of this and Deary, 1988a for a reply), the more recent studies have tended to do the opposite, by often studying undergraduates. This restriction of ability range in samples also deflates correlations and an estimate of the true IQ-IT correlation when corrected for these effects is in the region of -0.50. Recent studies by Young (1987) and Deary (1987a) have corroborated this estimate. In summary, there is a large body of evidence which supports the finding that perceptual intake speed, as indexed by IT, has a moderately high correlation with psychometric IQ scores.

The finding is robust. It has been replicated in undergraduates (Longstreth et al., 1986; Mackenzie & Bingham, 1985; Mackenzie & Cumming, 1986; Deary, 1987a), in children (Anderson, 1986;1987; Hosie, reported in Brand & Deary, 1982; Young, 1987; Deary, 1987b) and in mentally retarded groups (see Nettelbeck, 1987). IT correlates wih IQ under different experimental conditions: stimuli consisting of two, three and four lines, two lights, animal names and stimuli pictures, coloured lines, horizontal lines, alphanumeric characters and tones of different pitch have proved successful (Brand & Deary, 1982; Nettelbeck, 1987) and different psycho-physical procedures such as adaptive staircases, e.g. PEST (Taylor & Creelman, 1967), and methods of constant stimuli yield correlations in the expected direction. IT stimuli have been presented via tachisto-scopes, light emitting diodes and computer monitor screens in different experiments and all have been effective.

AUDITORY INSPECTION TIME

What is the explanation of the IQ-IT correlation? Brand and Deary (1982) suggested that IT measures peceptual intake speed and that this speed may be a fundamental individual difference with an ontogenic relat-ionship to intelligence (Brand, 1984). Habituation studies in infants, where visual processing speed is inferred from an infant's looking times at successive presentations of a simple stimulus and correlated with later IQ (e.g. Bornstein, 1985), provide support for this notion. How-ever, some have contended that the IQ-IT correlation exists because high IQ subjects adopt more effective task strategies, or discover tricks (such as the apparent motion effect in visual IT as studied by Mackenzie & Bingham, 1985 and Mackenzie & Cumming, 1986), when performing the IT task. This view denies that IT is a basic measure: rather, IT is viewed as a higher cognitive skill with a difficulty that is akin to IQ test items (see Egan, 1986 and Deary, 1988a for a discussion of these ideas). It is no surprise, then, given that all higher mental tests show a pos-itive correlation, that these two indices of higher mental function cor-relate.

If the IT-IQ correlation is due to high IQ subjects finding specific strategies or tricks that lead to fast inspection times then it is reas-onable to hypothesise that different IT tests will require different strategies to solve them. Therefore, if IT is tested in two different modalities strategy theorists should predict a near-zero correlation between the IT estimates. On the other hand, if IT is a fundamental limitation of perceptual processes related to nervous structure or func-tioning then cross-modal IT estimates should show positive correlations. A small group of studies tend to favour the latter view.

Deary (1980, and summarised in Brand & Deary, 1982) devised an auditory IT (AIT) test as follows. Designed to be analogous to the visual IT test, subjects were required to discriminate the temporal order of two tones of markedly different pitch (i.e. they had to report whether a 770 and 880 Hz tone pair had been presented in the order 'high-low' or 'low-high'). Subjects heard a cue, tone 1, a 500ms gap and tone 2. The tones were forward and backward masked by white noise. The duration of both tones was identical and could be varied from several seconds to a few milliseconds. Subjects gave their responses verbally with no time pres-sure. AIT duration estimates correlated at -0.66 (p<.02) with Mill Hill Vocabulary scores and -0.70 (p<.01) with Raven's Progressive Matrices scores. The sample size was small (n=13) and included two mentally re-tarded subjects. In the same experiment visual IT estimates correlated at 0.99 with AIT durations but the result was dependent upon the inclusion of mentally retarded subjects.

Nettelbeck, Edwards and Vreugdenhil (1986) reported a correlation of 0.39 between auditory and visual IT estimates in an undergraduate sample. This study made improvements to the AIT task and in a sample with a restricted range of ability, obtained a correlation of -.38 between AIT and Raven's Advanced Progressive Matrices scores. Using an AIT task more like that of Deary (1980), Irwin (1984) tested fifty 12 year old children on auditory and visual IT and found that they correlated at 0.17 (Kendall's tau; Pearson's r=0.05).

From these three preliminary studies certain issues became clear. First, retarded subjects should not be included in IT investigations of normal subjects as they provide outliers in the data sets. Second, as Irwin (1984) noted, the AIT task, when it is masked with white noise, allows some subjects to achieve AIT scores as low as 6ms. At these durations the frequency spectra of the 770 and 880 Hz tones overlap to a considerable degree and may be testing a subject's pitch discrimination rather than their ability to resolve the temporal order of the tones. Therefore, a more effective backward mask was needed that elevated the AIT estimates. Third, Deary (1980) and Nettelbeck (1987) noted that some subjects find the AIT test difficult, even at very long tone durations. More detailed study of these subjects is required but for the present it appears reasonable to exclude these subjects from the data analyses for the same reasons that one would not include subjects with poor vision in the visual IT analyses. Irwin (1984) makes no mention of this and the possible inclusion of those subjects who were not able to perform the discrimination at any duration may have artificially lowered his correlations.

NEW EXPERIMENTS WITH AUDITORY INSPECTION TIME

A recent study by Deary (Deary, 1987; Deary et al., 1989) attempted to resolve some of the difficulties mentioned above. An improved IT task was devised. After a cue tone, subjects heard tone 1 followed by tone 2 with no gap between them. The backward mask immediately followed the second tone and was a warble consisting of alternate 10 ms bursts of the two stimulus tones. Undergraduates were given the AIT test using the method of constant stimuli and underwent three forms of the visual IT test using the PEST adaptive procedure. The three visual IT tests were the standard vertical lines test, a horizontal lines test and a test using geometric shapes (Longstreth et al., 1986). Subjects were also tested on the Alice Heim 5 test - an IQ test which discriminates among high ability subjects.

As expected, about one third of our sample could not make the pitch discrimination reliably. The correlation between AIT and IQ was -0.31 (n=40, p<0.05) while the visual IT tests correlated with IQ at -0.33 for the vertical lines test (n=51, p=0.02), -0.29 for the Longstreth test (n=32, p=0.10) and -0.32 for the horizontal lines test (n=20, n.s.). When these correlations are corrected for restriction of ability range in our sample the levels come close to the expected true value estimated by Nettelbeck (1987), i.e. -0.57, -0.60, -0.54 and -0.59 respectively. The new AIT task results in an average AIT of 75.8ms for our sample which is outside the range of levels where frequency spectra problems exist. The n-weighted mean of the intra-visual IT test correlations is 0.44. The mean of the three visual IT-AIT correlations was 0.30. In a population of restricted ability range and with tests which have reliabilities below 0.75 these correlations are underestimates but they corroborate the notion that some general variance is shared by performance estimates on visual and auditory IT tasks.

Our next experiment attempted to test an hypothesis put forward by Irwin (1984) who suggested that AIT was testing pitch perception rather than speed of auditory processing. There is some evidence that pitch perception ability is related to psychometric intelligence (Deary, 1988b; Raz, Willerman & Yama, 1987) and with the original AIT test such confounding of pitch perception and discrimination ability was a possibility. Deary and Egan (see Deary, 1987b) tested 120 schoolchildren (60 boys, 60 girls) of mean age 11.5 years on the Mill Hill Vocabulary Test and on Raven's Progressive Matrices. Subjects were given the same AIT test as that described above in our work with undergraduates. Subjects also undertook the Bentley Tests of Musical Ability which includes a 20-item pitch discrimination test. About 50% of schoolchildren, compared to 67% of undergraduates, were able to perform the AIT task. In boys the AIT task correlated at -0.35 (n=29, p<0.05) with both IQ tests. In girls the AIT test correlated at -0.40 (n=24, p<0.05) with the Mill Hill Vocabulary Test and at -0.09 (n=24, n.s.) with Raven's Progressive Matrices.

The pitch perception subtest of the Bentley Scales was administered twice, on separate days, and the test-retest reliabiity was 0.54 (n=120, p<0.001). For boys the correlations between Raven's Matrices and pitch peception (n=60) on the two occasions were 0.21 (p=0.05) and 0.09 (n.s.). The correlations between pitch perception and Mill Hill Vocabulary (n=57) were 0.32 (p=0.007) and 0.21 (p=0.06). For girls the correlations between Raven's Matrices and pitch perception (n=59) on the two occasions were -0.04 (n.s.) and 0.09 (n.s.). The correlations between pitch perception and Mill Hill Vocabulary were (n=59) 0.21 (p=0.05) and 0.22 (p=0.04).

Therefore, we replicated the AIT-IQ correlation and the results indicated that in boys AIT related to general intelligence while in girls AIT was related only to verbal intelligence. The pitch perception results were similar. Pitch perception is related only to verbal IQ in girls while in boys it appears to be related to general intelligence. In boys (n=29) AIT correlated with pitch perception at -0.16 (n.s.) and at 0.14 (n.s.). In girls (n=24) the correlations were -0.33 (p=.06) and -0.40 (p=0.03). When the pitch perception scores were partialled out the AIT-IQ correlations remained significant and almost unchanged from those reported above. Therefore, the AIT-IQ correlation is not dependent upon pitch perception ability.

CONCLUSIONS AND FUTURE DEVELOPMENTS

Our recent work on AIT confirms: that this psychophysical index correlates at moderate levels with psychometric intelligence; that there is some shared variance between estimates of IT tested in different modalities; and that performance differences on AIT are not due to individual differences in pitch perception ability. In conclusion, inspection time: has a large empirical literature which confirms its relationship to higher order abilities; has some claim to be considered as a fundamental property of perceptual systems; and derives from a well-developed theory of perception. These factors make it a potentially useful and interesting experimental and clinical neuropsychology test and our ongoing work is using IT in these areas.

We have shown that if evoked potentials are collected and averaged while subjects are performing the visual IT task then a P200 index (defined as the time to develop the P200 peak, which is calculated by measuring the time it takes to reach the P200 peak from the average epoch potential baseline) correlates at 0.44 (p<0.05) with IT performance (-Zhang, Caryl & Deary, 1988a). When age is controlled IT performance correlates at 0.55 (p<0.01) with P200 latency (Zhang, Caryl & Deary, 1988b). These experiments support the view that IT indexes the rate of transfer of information from a sensory register to short term memory.

Our clinical work is beginning to examine IT performance in the early stages of Alzheimer's disease, in Korsakoff's psychosis and in AIDS-related dementia. Also, IT is being used by us to examine the effects of various central nervous system depressants and stimulants on information processing rates. In these areas IT provides a quick, reliable and, given a short period of practice, practice-resistant index of perceptual intake speed. IT has the advantages of simplicity and discrimination: it is easy enough to be performed by young children but it may be applied to many subject populations (children, old people, mentally retarded people, undergraduates, Alzheimer's disease patients) with few problems relating to ceiling and floor effects.

IT is now becoming well-established as an important index of perceptual functioning that has a modest correlation with psychometric intelligence. Future work should be directed toward examining the development of IT, its physiological basis and its sensitivity and specificity as a clinical and neuropsychological tool.

REFERENCES

Anderson, M. (1986). Inspection Time and IQ in young children. _Personality and Individual Differences_, 7, 677–686.

Anderson, M. (1988). Inspection time, information processing and the development of intelligence. _British Journal of Developmental Psychology_, 6, 43–58.

Bornstein, M. (1985). How infant and mother jointly contribute to developing cognitive competence in the child. _Proceedings of the National Academy of Sciences of the U.S.A._, 82, 7470–7473.

Brand, C. (1981). General intelligence and mental speed: Their relationship and development. _in_: M.P. Friedman, J.P. Das & N. O'Connor (eds.). _Intelligence and Learning_. New York: Plenum.

Brand, C.R. (1984). Intelligence and inspection time: an ontogenic relationship? _in_: C.J. Turner & H.B. Miles (ed.). _The Biology of Human Intelligence: Proceedings of the twentieth annual symposium of the Eugenics Society, London, 1983_. Nafferton, U.K.: Nafferton Books.

Brand, C.R. & Deary, I.J. (1982). Intelligence and 'inspection time'. _in_: H.J. Eysenck (ed.). _A Model for Intelligence_. Berlin and New York: Springer.

Deary, I.J. (1980). How general is the mental speed factor in general intelligence? Unpublished thesis for the Honours Degree (B.Sc. Med. Sci.) in Psychology, University of Edinburgh.

Deary, I.J. (1987a). Visual and auditory inspection time: Their interrelationship and correlation with IQ in high ability subjects. Paper presented at the third biennial meeting of the International Society for the Study of Individual Differences, Toronto, June 1987.

Deary, I.J. (1987b). Intelligence, auditory inspection time and musical ability in schoolchildren. Paper presented to the British Psychological Society, Scottish Branch, Developments in Clinical and Experimental Neuropsychology, Rothesay, September 1987.

Deary, I.J. (1988). Basic processes in human intelligence. _in_: H.J. Jerison & I. Jerison (eds.). _Intelligence and Evolutionary Biology_. Berlin and New York: Springer.

Deary, I.J. (1988). The nature of intelligence: simplicity to complexity and back again. _in_: D. Forshaw & M. Shepherd (eds.). _Maudsley Essay Series in the History of Psychiatry and Psychology_. London: Vade Mecum, in press.

Deary, I.J., Caryl, P.G., Egan, V. & Wight, D. (1989). Auditory and visual inspection time: Their interrelationship and correlation with intelligence in high ability subjects. Manuscript submitted for publication.

Egan, V. (1986). Intelligence and inspection time: do high IQ subjects use cognitive strategies? _Personality and Individual Differences_, 7, 695–700.

Irwin, R.J. (1984). Inspection time and its relation to intelligence. _Intelligence_, 8, 47–65.

Lally, M. & Nettelbeck, T. (1977). Intelligence, inspection time and response strategy. American Journal of Mental Deficiency, 84, 553-560.

Longstreth, L.E., Walsh, D.A., Alcorn, M.B., Szeszulski, P.A. & Manis, F.R. (1986). Backward masking, IQ, SAT and reaction time: inter-relationships and theory. Personality and Individual Differences, 7, 643-652.

Mackenzie, B. & Bingham, E. (1985). IQ, inspection time and response strategies in a university population. Australian Journal of Psychology, 37, 257-268.

Mackenzie, B. & Cumming, S. (1986). How fragile is the relationship between inspection time and intelligence: the effects of apparent motion cues and previous experience. Personality and Individual Differences, 7, 721-729.

Mackintosh, N.J. (1981). A new measure of intelligence? Nature, 289, 529-530.

Mackintosh, N.J. (1986). The biology of intelligence? British Journal of Psychology, 77, 1-18.

Nettelbeck, T. (1982). Inspection time: An index for intelligence? Quarterly Journal of Experimental Psychology, 34A, 299-312.

Nettelbeck, T. (1987). Inspection time and intelligence. in: P.A. Vernon (ed.). Speed of Information Processing and Intelligence. Norwood, N.J.: Ablex.

Nettelbeck, T., Edwards, C. & Vreugdenhil, A. (1986). Inspection time and IQ: evidence for a mental speed-ability association. Personality and Individual Differences, 7, 633-641.

Nettelbeck, T. & Lally, M. (1976). Inspection time and measured intelligence. British Journal of Psychology, 67, 17-22.

Raz, N., Willerman, L. & Yama, M. (1987). On sense and senses: intelligence and auditory information processing. Personality and Individual Differences, 8, 201-10.

Taylor, M.M. & Creelman, C.D. (1967). PEST: efficient estimate on probability functions. Journal of the Accoustical Society of America, 4, 782-787.

Vernon, P.A. (1986). Inspection time: does it measure intelligence? Personality and Individual Differences, 7, 715-720.

Vickers, D., Nettelbeck, T. & Willson, R.J. (1972). Perceptual indices of performance: the measurement of 'inspection time' and 'noise' in the visual system. Perception, 1, 263-295.

Vickers, D. & Smith, P.L. (1986). The rationale for the inspection time index. Personality and Individual Differences, 7, 609-624.

Young, R. (1987). Intelligence and inspection time in 6 year-old children. Unpublished thesis for the Honours Degree (B.A.) in Psychology, University of Adelaide.

Zhang, Y., Caryl, P.G. & Deary, I.J. (1989a). Evoked potential correlates of inspection time. Personality and Individual Differences, in press.

Zhang, Y., Caryl, P.G. & Deary, I.J. (1989b). Inspection time and P200: The relationship between two perceptual intake indices. Manuscript submitted for publication.

ADDRESSES OF PRINCIPAL AUTHORS

John A.O. Besson
Dept. of Mental Health
University of Aberdeen
Aberdeen, UK.   AB9 2ZD

Janet Cockburn
Rivermead Rehabilitation Centre
Abingdon Road
Oxford, UK.   OX1 4XD

John R. Crawford
Dept. of Psychology
University of Aberdeen
Aberdeen, UK.   AB9 2UB

Ian J. Deary
Dept. of Psychology
University of Edinburgh
Edinburgh, UK.   EH8 9JZ

Anthony S. David
Institute of Psychiatry
De Crespigny Park
Denmark Hill
London, UK.   SE5 8AF

Arthur A. Dunk
Gastroenterology Research Unit
Aberdeen Royal Infirmary
Aberdeen, UK.   AB9 2ZB

Klaus P. Ebmeier
Dept. of Mental Health
University of Aberdeen
Aberdeen, UK.   AB9 2ZD

Hadyn D. Ellis
Dept. of Applied Psychology
U.W.I.S.T.
Cardiff, UK.   CF3 7UX

Peter Griffiths
Dept. of Psychology
University of Stirling
Stirling, UK.   FK9 4LA

David A. Johnson
Dept. of Neuropsychology
Atkinson Morley Hospital
Wimbledon, London, UK.   SW20 0NE

Robert H. Logie
Dept. of Psychology
University of Aberdeen
Aberdeen, UK.   AB9 2UB

Louis E.F. MacDonell
Highland Psychiatric Research Group
Craig Dunain Hospital
Inverness, UK.   IV3 6JU

Andrew R. Mayes
Dept. of Psychology
University of Manchester
Manchester, UK.   M13 9PL

William M. McKinlay
Dept. of Surgical Neurology
Western General Hospital
Edinburgh, UK.   EH4 2XU

Ziyah Mehta
Neuropsychology Unit
The Radcliffe Infirmary
Oxford, UK.   OX2 6HE

Ed Miller
Dept. of Clinical Psychology
Addenbrooke's Hospital
Cambridge, UK.   CB2 2QQ

A. David Milner
Dept. of Psychology
University of St. Andrews
St. Andrews, UK.   KY16 9JU

Daniela Montaldi
Wellcome Neuroscience Group
University of Glasgow
Great Western Road
Glasgow, UK.   G12 0AA

Denis M. Parker
Dept. of Psychology
University of Aberdeen
Aberdeen, UK.   AB9 2UB

Alison Peaker
Dept. of Clinical Psychology
Elmhill House
Royal Cornhill Hospital
Aberdeen, UK.   AB9 2ZY

Catherine Y. Peng
Dept. of Psychology
University of Oxford
Oxford, UK. OX1 3UD

Douglas D. Potter
Psychological Laboratory
University of St. Andrews
St. Andrews, UK.   KY16 9JU

Graham E. Powell
Dept. of Psychology
University of Surrey
Guildford, UK.   GU2 5XH

Rosalyn H. Shute
Dept. of Applied Psychology
U.W.I.S.T.
Cardiff, UK.   CF3 7UX

David J. Weeks
Jardine Clinic
Royal Edinburgh Hospital
Edinburgh, UK.   EH10 5HF

Klaus D. Wiedmann
Dept. of Psychology
University of Stirling
Stirling, UK.   FK9 4LA

J.T. Lindsay Wilson
Dept. of Psychology
University of Stirling
Stirling, UK.   FK9 4LA

INDEX